Current Topics in Heart Failure

Supplement to
Basic Research in Cardiology, Vol. 86, Suppl. 3 (1991)

Editors:
G. Elzinga (Amsterdam), R. Jacob (Tübingen), Th. Kenner (Graz)

Rainer W. Gülch,
Gerolf Kissling (eds.)

Current Topics in Heart Failure

Experimental and Clinical Aspects

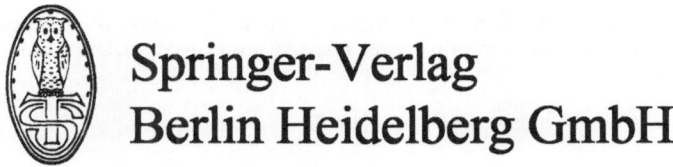

Springer-Verlag
Berlin Heidelberg GmbH

The editors:
Prof. Dr. Rainer W. Gülch
Prof. Dr. Gerolf Kissling
Physiologisches Institut II
der Universität Tübingen
Gmelinstraße 5
7400 Tübingen

ISBN 978-3-7985-0894-1   ISBN 978-3-662-30769-4 (eBook)
DOI 10.1007/978-3-662-30769-4

Basic Res. Cardiol, ISSN 0300-8428
Indexed in Current Contents.

Copyright © 1991 by Springer-Verlag Berlin Heidelberg
Originally published by Dr. Dietrich Steinkopff Verlag GmbH & Co. KG, Darmstadt in 1991

Medical editor: Sabine Müller – English editor: James C. Willis – Production: Heinz J. Schäfer

Preface

The clinical aspect of heart failure is characterized by a mismatch between the pumping capability of the heart and either the venous supply or the requirements of the systemic circulation. Since this disease has always played a dominant role in the field of clinical cardiology, the clinicians have been forced to become intensively involved in problems of its etiology, diagnosis, and therapy. The increasing realization of the complexity of this illness has, however, made it necessary to integrate basic medical sciences more deeply into cardiological scientific discussions. This has helped to clarify quite a number of pathophysiological aspects, resulting in a greater understanding of cardiac insufficiency. The danger, however, of involvement of such diverging disciplines in this particular research is that each field tends to become too insular, thus leaving the clinicians in the awkward situation of having to weave the individual facts together as a synopsis to form a composite picture of heart failure.

It was, thus, our endeavor to deepen the dialogue between clinical disciplines and basic research at the Sixth Erwin Riesch Symposium in Freudenstadt, 11–14 October, 1990, the proceedings of which represent a collection of all the contributions presented. The multiplicity of the problems of heart failure is reflected in the variety of the contributions, which deal with: chronic reactions of the heart; biochemical, molecular-biological, and immunological aspects; neuroendocrine mechanisms, as well as with therapeutical and cardioprotective principles of heart failure. We are strongly convinced that precisely this inevitable heterogeneity in the themes of the various contributions provides useful impulses for further discussions and understanding of this subject.

With this volume, we also wish to honor Prof. Dr. med. Ruthard Jacob, Director of the Institute of Physiology, University of Tübingen, on the occasion of his 65th birthday. Professor Jacob, who has been editor of Basic Research in Cardiology since 1973, has given major impetus to establishing the internationally high reputation which this periodical has earned in the field of cardiology. On this occasion, we would also like to acknowledge that pathophysiology of the heart has always played a central role in Prof. Jacob's scientific work, and that he is particularly open to clinical questions.

A scientific venture with such an international participation can, of course, only be realized with solid financial support. We are thus gratefully indebted to the generous support given by the Erwin Riesch foundation and the following pharmaceutical companies: Bayropharm GmbH; Boehringer Mannheim GmbH; Braun Melsungen AG; Bristol Arzneimittel; Byk Gulden Pharmazeutika; Cassella AG, Ciba-Geigy GmbH; Giulini Pharma GmbH; Gödecke AG; Hoffmann-La Roche AG; Intersan GmbH; Knoll AG; Madaus AG; Merck; Minden Pharma GmbH; Pfizer GmbH; Pohl-Boskamp GmbH & Co; Sandoz AG; Schwarz-Pharma AG; Squibb-von Heyden GmbH; Winthrop GmbH.

In addition, we would like to express our special thanks to Dr. Dietrich Steinkopff Verlag, Darmstadt, which has made it possible to publish all oral contributions in the form of this supplement to "Basic Research in Cardiology".

Tübingen, July 1991

Prof. Dr. R. W. Gülch
Prof. Dr. G. Kissling

Contents

Foreword V

Part I: Chronic Reactions of the Heart to Overload: Hypertrophy and Dilatation

The functional ambivalence of adaptive processes – Considerations based on the example of the hemodynamically overloaded heart
Jacob, R. 3

Experimental congestive heart failure due to myocardial infarction: Sarcolemmal receptors and cation transporters
Dhalla, N.S., I.M.C. Dixon, H. Rupp, J. Barwinsky 13

Myocardial fibrosis: role of ventricular systolic pressure, arterial hypertension, and circulating hormones
Weber, K.T., C.G. Brilla, J.S. Janicki, H.K. Reddy, S.E. Campbell 25

Effects of nifedipine and moxonidine on cardiac structure in spontaneously hypertensive rats (SHR) – Stereological studies on myocytes, capillaries, arteries, and cardiac interstitium
Mall, G., D. Greber, H. Gharehbaghi, G. Wiest, K. Amann, T. Mattfeldt 33

Principal considerations on the stroke volume-heart size relationship based on different heart models
Gülch, R.W., B. Dierberger, M. Brändle 45

Part II: Biochemical, Molecular-biological and Immunological Aspects of Heart Failure

The role of adrenergic system in regulation of cardiac myosin heavy chain gene expression
Gupta, M.P., M. Gupta, R. Zak 57

The metabolic syndrome and signal transduction of gene expression
Rupp, H. 65

A new concept for the mechanism of Ca^{++}-regulation of muscle contraction.
Implications for physiological and pharmacological approaches to modulate
contractile function of myocardium
Brenner, B.   83

Large and rapid changes of myofibrillar total calcium during the cardiac cycle.
Electron probe microanalysis of voltage-clamped guinea-pig ventricular myocytes
Wendt-Gallitelli, M.F., G. Isenberg, T. Voigt, C. Ross   93

Are antisarcolemmal (ASAs) and antimyolemmal antibodies (AMLAs)
"natural" antibodies?
Maisch, B., L. Drude, C. Hengstenberg, M. Herzum, G. Hufnagel,
K. Kochsiek, A. Schmaltz, U. Schönian, M.D. Schwab 101

Chemiluminescence as a marker of myocardial ischemia
Török, B. 115

Part III: Significance of Neuroendocrine Mechanisms for the Development of Heart Failure

Role of neuroendocrine mechanisms in the pathogenesis of heart failure
Riegger, A.J.G. 125

Modulation of baroreflex and baroreceptor function in experimental heart failure
Zucker, I.H., W. Wang 133

Does converting enzyme inhibition change the neuronal and extraneuronal
uptake of catecholamines?
Dominiak, P., A. Blöchl 149

Part IV: Therapeutical Principles from a Pathophysiological Point of View

Compensatory mechanisms for cardiac dysfunction in myocardial infarction
Ertl, G., P. Gaudron, C. Eilles, W. Schorb, K. Kochsiek 159

The effect of decreased left-ventricular afterload on cardiac performance
in the normal and hypertrophied rat heart
Kissling, G., M. Brändle 167

Function and structure of the failing left-ventricular myocardium in aortic
valve disease before and after valve replacement
Krayenbuehl, H.P., O.M. Hess, E.S. Monrad, J. Schneider, G. Mall, M. Turina . . 175

Protective effect of ACE- and kininase-inhibitor on the onset of cardiomyopathy
Nagano, M., M. Kato, M. Nagai, J. Yang 187

Contents

Effects of long-term medication for essential hypertension on cardiac hypertrophy and function
Takeda, N., I. Nakamura, T. Hatanaka, T. Iwai, A. Tanamura, Y. Obara,
M. Nagano 197

Part V: Cardioprotection: Dietetic and Pharmacological Treatments

Phenomenon of the adaptive stabilization of sarcoplasmic and nuclear structures in myocardium
Meerson, F.Z., I.Y.U. Malyshev, A.B. Shneider 205

Cardioprotection: endogenous protective mechanisms promoted by prostacyclin
Szekeres, L., J. Pataricza, Z. Szilvássy, É. Udvary, Á. Végh 215

Long-term treatment in arterial hypertension for protecting hypertrophic myocardium
Vogt, M., W. Motz, B.E. Strauer 223

Subject Index 235

Part I: Chronic Reactions of the Heart to Overload: Hypertrophy and Dilatation

The functional ambivalence of adaptive processes – Considerations based on the example of the hemodynamically overloaded heart

R. Jacob

Physiologisches Institut II, Universität Tübingen, FRG

Summary: Cardiac hypertrophy and neuro-humoral reactions in hemodynamic overload are employed as examples to show that adaptive processes, while in principle enabling the whole organ to cope with increased load, as a rule also include unfavorable components. This is primarily due to competition between different demands with respect to, for instance, mechanical or energetic parameters. An impressive demonstration of the ambivalence of adaptive processes can be seen in the functional consequences of myocardial mass increase, eccentric configurational changes, and the alteration of the myocardium towards a "slower muscle". It can be demonstrated that, due to structural modifications in the heart, unfavorable effects occur at the level of the whole organ as well as in macromolecular dimensions from the very beginning, and not only as a consequence of qualitatively and quantitatively inappropriate adaptation. Thus, a clear-cut distinction between "physiological" and "pathological" processes is almost impossible. In the clinic, the unfavorable effects of the process of hypertrophy are often emphasized and the reduction of hypertrophy is declared the principal therapeutic aim. However, in the individual case the extent to which vascular alterations participate in, or are even mainly responsible for the unfavorable effects occurring in pressure hypertrophy should be clarified. In any case, reduction of hemodynamic overload should be the focus of therapeutic concern.

Key words: Cardiac adaptation; cardiac hypertrophy; cardiac failure; ventricular geometry; myosin isoenzyme pattern; neuro-humoral reactions

Introduction

What do we call "pathological"?

The terms "health" and "disease" have found widely differing definitions in the past, and they still do today. The World Health Organization defines health as "a state of complete physical, mental, and social well-being, and not merely the absence of disease or infirmity". Here the main stress lies on the patient's subjective sense of health. Such a definition, however, is not very helpful from a scientific viewpoint. Other definitions of "health" and "disease," or of "physiological" and "pathological" processes, respectively, are based rather more on objective criteria such as deviation from the norm, deterioration in objective performance or failure of functional adaptation (35). A really comprehensive definition is hardly possible, and as scientific knowledge and insights continue to grow, basic difficulties arise in setting up general principles of pathology or a really coherent theory on all forms of illness.

In the following discourse a certain aspect shall be discussed, namely, the relationship between "adaptive" and "pathological" processes. In literature the question is often discussed as to whether a certain process or alteration should be classified as "adaptive" or "pathological", which means that the two terms are regarded as opposites, hence, necessarily excluding each other. It can clearly be demonstrated on the basis of cardiac and neuro-endocrine alterations under the conditions of hemodynamic overload, however, that this question is not adequate, i.e., the adaptive character of a process does not exclude unfavorable or so-called pathological consequences. Above all, it is obvious that not only inappropriate or failing adaptation is detrimental, but also the normal course of adaptive processes as a rule involves negative components.

Definition of cardiac hypertrophy

Hypertrophy is defined as an increase in size of an organ or a certain region due to enhanced cell growth, triggered, as a rule, by increased functional load. In contrast to connective tissue cells, hyperplasia in myocytes, i.e., an increase in number of these cells, plays a significant role only at an early postnatal stage. The term hypertrophy does not, however, cover all aspects of alterations at the macroscopic level and the level of cell organelles and biochemical structures (13). Both ventricular configuration and macromolecular expression can show greatly different patterns, depending on the nature of the underlying overload and/or humoral conditions. Therefore, it does not seem adequate, for instance, to regard all alterations in receptor density or in myosine isoenzyme pattern as an expression of the process of hypertrophy. Moreover, especially in later stages, many alterations cannot be considered primary reactions at the level of the myocytes, but rather secondary effects of vascular changes or inadequate blood perfusion.

Bearing these limitations in mind, the ambivalence of adaptive processes will be discussed based mainly on the example of the hypertrophied heart.

Animal models and clinical cases

The following discourse is principally based on investigations in several animal models: Rats with chronic swim training; spontaneously hypertensive rats (SHR); stroke-prone rats (SHR SP); rats with renal hypertension (Goldblatt II); with supravalvular aortic stenosis; with aorto-caval fistula; with aorto-caval fistula and additional unilateral renal artery coarctation; with experimental hyper- and hypothyroidism. Reference is also made to an analysis of ventricular function in patients with dilative cardiomyopathy [for details, see (12, 13)].

Favourable effects of cardiac hypertrophy and accompanying chronic cardiac reactions

Cardiac mechanics

Cardiac hypertrophy due to pressure or volume overload leads to an augmentation of ventricular working capacity, thus enabling the heart to cope with the increased load, as a rule, without the necessity of enhanced systolic wall stress. It can be seen from the P-V diagram of Goldblatt rats at the 8-week stage (20) that without hypertrophy, the ventricle would at this stage not be able to produce the systolic pressure required for overcoming the increased peripheral resistance. Furthermore, it can be derived from these diagrams that an increase in end-diastolic pressure and the corresponding change in ventricular dynamics could not compensate for the enhanced systolic pressure load. In other models, e.g., some cases of experimental supravalvular aortic stenosis (2), it can be concluded from the P-V diagram that, in the absence of hypertrophy, the required stroke volume could be maintained via the Frank-Starling mechanisms, though at the expense of increased end-diastolic pressure with corresponding congestive effects, as well as the necessity of enhanced systolic stress development and a correspondingly increased energy demand per unit of muscle mass (13).

The example of experimental aorto-caval fistula (27) shows that the required increase in systolic stress does not necessarily lead to pumping failure of the heart within a period of a few weeks. This, however, does not conflict with the basic significance of hypertrophy in cardiac mechanics.

Cardiac energetics

In the pressure or volume loaded heart of smaller laboratory animals a redistribution of the myosine isoenzyme pattern towards V-3 occurs with consequently reduced ATPase activity and an improved economy of tension development, while shortening velocity is reduced, and, due to the increased mass, total heart oxygen consumption is increased (1, 21, 31). In human myocardium, two myosin components could be detected which seem not to be related to α and β chains. The ratio of the two components depends on the hemodynamic load and account for an altered ATPase activity (32). An increase in the level of the 200 KD β-MHC as described in the case of the pressure loaded baboon heart (9) may also be of relevance for the ATPase activity in higher mammals and human patients (1). However, one should be careful not to overestimate the quantitative significance of alterations at the level of contractile proteins for cardiac energetics. In the rat model, even an extreme redistribution towards V-3 cannot counterbalance the energetically unfavorable effects of structural dilatation (38).

Unfavorable consequences of cardiac hypertrophy and accompanying cardiac and neuro-humoral reactions

Although functionally unfavorable components are an integral part of chronic cardiac reactions from the onset, they do not become effective, as a rule, until hypertrophy becomes more pronounced or the hemodynamic overload is at an advanced stage. Such negative components involve cardiac mechanics, energetics, and electrophysiology. In cases of considerable training-induced hypertrophy, arrhythmias are basically the only unfavorable effects of clinical relevance.

Cardiac mechanics

At given ventricular dimensions, a marked increase in wall thickness causes reduced *ventricular compliance,* i.e., a (relatively) steeper end-diastolic pressure-volume curve. This may have consequences for diastolic inflow and, thus, atrial and venous pressure. As in the case of idiopathic hypertrophy, an extreme thickening of the ventricular wall will necessarily impede diastolic ventricular filling.

Furthermore, reduced compliance influences the end-diastolic fiber strain. At a given end-diastolic pressure, wall stress and, thus, sarcomere length of the hypertrophied myocardial cell is shorter than in the non-hypertrophied tissue. Due to changes in fiber arrangement, diastolic sarcomere length is reduced even at a given diastolic stress (7). Reduced diastolic sarcomere length will, however, influence systolic myocardial function, i.e., stroke volume (with minor consequences for ejection fractions). Fibrosis and reduced sarcoplasmic reticulum Ca^{2+}-transport will impair diastolic ventricular function independently of the geometrical conditions.

Another aspect which should be briefly discussed in this context concerns the functional significance of the velocity of ventricular filling as measured by echocardiography. In the clinic, considerable significance has been ascribed to this parameter in evaluating "diastolic ventricular function". If, however, end-diastolic ventricular pressure is increased – as often occurs in cases of pressure-induced hypertrophy, even without systolic failure – then a higher velocity of ventricular filling would not be of any advantage. Inflow congestion would not be reduced, nor would an increase in inflow velocity have significant consequences for diastolic fiber strain as the end-diastolic filling in this case has reached the steep part of the end-diastolic pressure-volume curve.

As a rule, at an early stage, *the contractile properties* of the hypertrophied heart are not altered in such a way that cardiac pumping function is impaired.

In close relation to the alterations in the myosine isoenzyme pattern the unloaded shortening velocity of the hypertrophied myocardium is found to be reduced in the pressure or volume-loaded ventricle and increased in the myocardium of swim-trained or hyperthyreotic rats (12, 13). In the given context, interest focuses principally on the performance of the chronically overloaded heart. Even within this group, mechanical parameters vary. For instance, in contrast to models involving arterial hypertension, in aortic stenosis, isovolumically developed stress is not elevated at an early stage. At later stages of overload, shortening velocity as well as isometric myocardial force development are reduced. Due to additional alterations such as fibrosis, the previously close correlation between shortening velocity and isoenzyme pattern is no longer present, i.e., shortening velocity is slower than would be expected from the V_1/V_3 ratio. Although insufficient rat hearts, as a rule, display an essentially homogeneous myosine V-3 pattern, in view of the findings in skinned fibers (5) and experimental hypothyreodism (19), the isoenzyme redistribution and the consequent decrease in shortening velocity do not seem to be the decisive factor for heart failure. It is certainly not adequate to assess the contractile properties of the myocardium exclusively on the basis of velocity parameters. The pressure-loaded heart is not equipped for high velocity contraction: tractors or trucks, not racing cars are used for transporting heavy loads.

Alterations in the field of electromechanical coupling, above all, reduced sarcoplasmic reticulum calcium transport due to reduced density of the Ca^{2+}-pump molecules (34, 37), have a significant influence, both on the rate of relaxation and on contractility of the hypertrophied myocardium. In Goldblatt rats, the rate of pressure decline (dP/dt_{min}) related to the rate of pressure rise (dP/dt_{max}) is already affected at the compensatory stage of hypertrophy (18). These alterations could be interpreted in the context of a development towards a "slower" muscle, parallel to changes in the contractile apparatus.

Cardiac energetics. In the hemodynamically overloaded hypertrophied heart, the demands on mechanical function and energy supply compete with each other at various levels of the organ. Overproportional increase in contractile material at the expense of the mitochondria (41), reduced vascular density with elongated vessel tracks (24), increased and more variable intercapillary distances (29) and arterial media hyperplasia in the pressure loaded heart (24, 25) worsen the energetic situation, particularly for the subendocardial layers (10). Coronary reserve is reduced and, of course, further impaired by arteriosclerosis. Configurational changes in the heart towards eccentric hypertrophy with inadequate increase in wall thickness is deleterious from an energetical point of view, because of the necessity of an increased systolic wall stress and thus increased energy demand (23, 38). Besides other reasons (28, 30), an energy deficit also is an important factor in the pathogenesis of arrhythmias.

Alterations in late stages of cardiac overload

The numerous morphological and biochemical alterations found at later stages of hemodynamic overload are partly consequences of adaptive processes and partly degenerative processes. Out of the variety of alterations (13, 15), only fibrosis and configurational changes in the sense of structural dilatation shall briefly be discussed in the given context.

To some extent, fibrosis is a result of a stimulation of the connective tissue accompanying the hypertrophy of the myocytes, a process in which humoral factors (angiotensine II, aldosterone) seem to play a role (40). Furthermore, fibrosis can occur in the course of "repair" processes. In our animal models, we found that fibrosis [accompanied by an increased type III content (25)] was expressed differently, i.e., stronger in hypertensive rats than in experimental aortic stenosis (2). Development of fibrosis is reduced by interventions that lower blood pressure, for instance, dietary interventions, such as a diet rich in linseed oil, fish oil or garlic (3, 13, 14).

In assessing the effects, one has to distinguish between interstitial fibrosis and perivascular fibrosis, the latter possibly being less significant for mechanical parameters. The connective tissue can interfere with diffusion processes. Furthermore, it diminishes the relative content of contractile material in the myocardial tissue and thus impairs myocardial mechanics. Doubtlessly, the mechanical effects are particularly significant with respect to the "diastolic function", since the end-diastolic fiber strain is reduced further for a given end-diastolic pressure and, thus, the compensating function of the Frank-Starling mechanism is impaired. Analyzing ventricular dynamics in hypertensive rats as well as in patients suffering from dilative cardiomyopathy on the basis of model calculations (16, 17), we found a surprisingly strong influence of this factor on stroke volume in many cases (4, 15, 16).

As our investigations in SHR at later stages show, pronounced fibrosis is not a prerequisite for substantial configurational changes in the sense of dilatation with comparatively insufficient increase in wall thickness (13). The geometrical conditions under dilatation per se, i.e., the unfavorable myocardial mechanics according to the law of Laplace, as a rule cannot be regarded as the direct cause for a decrease in stroke volume (17). If we only considered stroke volume, an increase in ventricular size could be judged as a favorable adaptive process even in the case of insufficient ventricular wall growth. Under energetic aspects, however, dilatation is fundamentally detrimental due to increased systolic stress requirement. Furthermore, reduced myocardial contractility and distensibility (as well as increased pressure load and insufficient hypertrophy) depress the stroke volume-enddiastolic volume relation so that the adverse effects of dilatation are manifested already at smaller ventricular dimensions (16, 17). Thus, ventricular configuration must be taken into account in considering interventions aiming at the regression of cardiac hypertrophy.

Inhibition of an eccentric configurational change can be achieved experimentally in spontaneously hypertensive rats treated with various antihypertensive diets involving fish oil, linseed oil or high doses of garlic (3, 13). In experimental aortic stenosis, particularly Ca^{2+} entry blockers seem to inhibit the tendency towards structural dilatation (2).

The negative consequences of *neuro-endocrine reactions* essentially characterize the clinical symptomatology of congestive cardiac failure. From a teleological point of view, stimulation of the renin-angiotensin-aldosterone system with an increase in circulating blood volume can be regarded as an attempt of the organism to prevent a decrease in cardiac output and organ perfusion. However, the consequences are certain to be mainly detrimental (8). In the model of combined aortic-caval fistula and renal hypertension of the Goldblatt II type (26), it can be shown that hydropic symptoms can occur which cannot be explained on the basis of impaired cardiac function. In this model of so-called high-output failure with increased stroke volume and cardiac output, the peripheral effects of the aortic-caval fistula including neuro-endocrine reactions are certainly decisive for the development of the congestive symptoms, which means that the symptomatology of pumping failure is imitated in this model. Here the causes for the change in the water and electrolyte balance are, however, essentially of peripheral origin (17). Reactive increase in sympathetic tone with a chronically elevated level of plasma catecholamines are the main cause for reduced myocardial responsiveness to catecholamines. Receptor down-regulation and alterations at the level of G proteins impair compensatory effects of sympathetic drive in addition to reduced presynaptic noradrenaline concentration.

Conclusions

Table 1 summarizes some particularly striking examples demonstrating the ambivalence of adaptive processes. The increase in muscle mass and in wall thickness is favorable for ventricular working capacity and the constancy of systolic wall stress, but is potentially unfavorable for energy supply, diastolic inflow, and myocardial fiber strain, at least in cases of severe hypertrophy. Eccentric hypertrophy as such increases stroke volume, even in the presence of a moderate increase in the radius/wall-thickness ratio (6, 17). But such a change in ventricular geometry has negative consequences for systolic wall stress and, thus, energy demand per unit cardiac mass. The changes at the level of contractile proteins are favorable for the economy of stress development, but diminish shortening velocity and myocardial power. Salt and water retention could be interpreted as a means of supporting the Frank Starling mechanism. In the final analysis, however, it is mainly

Table 1. Functional ambivalence of adaptive processes

Increase in myocardial mass	Ventricular working capacity	↑	Coronary reserve	↓
			Ventricular compliance	↓
			Arrhythmias	
Eccentric hypertrophy	Stroke volume	↑	Systolic wall stress, energy demand	↑
			Arrhythmias	
Redistribution of the myosin isoenzyme pattern → V_3	Economy of stress development	↑	Shortening velocity, myocardial power	↓
Increase in circulating blood volume	Frank Starling mechanism	↑	Congestion	
			Energy demand	↑
			Myocardial component of coronary resistance	↑
			Arrhythmias	

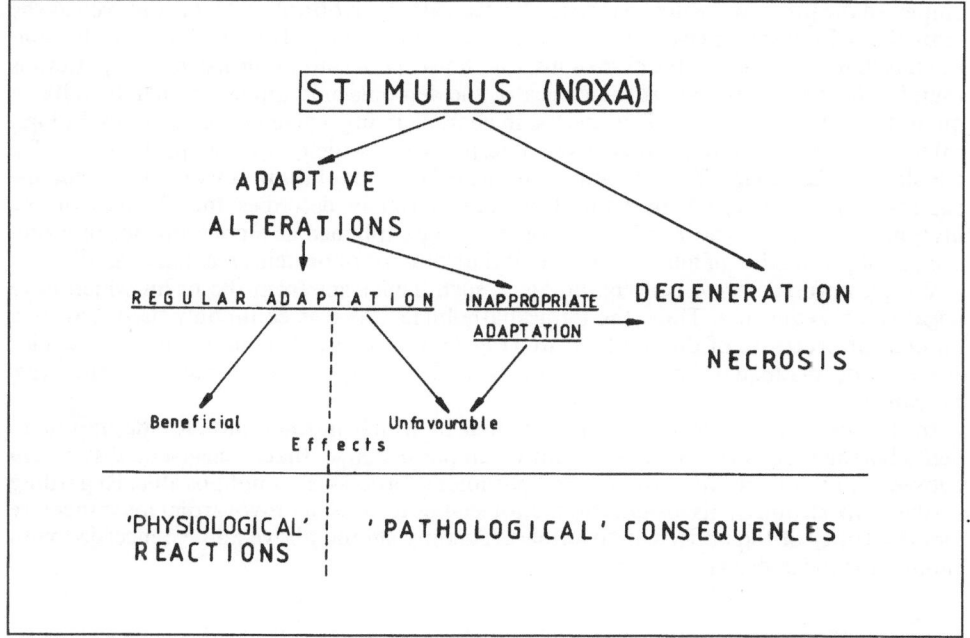

Fig. 1

unfavorable by inducing congestion, high energy demand, increase in the myocardial component of coronary resistance and arrhythmias.

Thus, besides the favorable effects of adaptation which enable the heart to cope with altered loading conditions, unfavorable consequences are inherent even in the normal course of the underlying adaptation processes (Fig. 1). This is principally the result of competition between various functional needs. In the case of hypertrophy, this aspect concerns the increase in cell size as well as myocardial alteration towards a slower muscle, and alterations in ventricular configuration.

Adaptation to some extent means specialization and thus implies a reduction in the spectrum of functional possibilities. In an earlier paper, Krayenbuehl chose the image of the Janus-face to describe the ambivalence of the hypertrophic process (22). This ambivalence is manifested at various levels of the organ and, apparently, is an inherent aspect of most adaptive processes. As a rule, potentially detrimental components which are present from the onset do not impair the performance of the organ as a whole until later stages. Of course, the functional consequences also depend on the circumstances, as in the case of cardiac hypertrophy, on the level of hemodynamic overload and on the magnitude of neuroendocrine reactions.

Furthermore, adaptation can prove to be quantitatively or qualitatively inappropriate. The response of the genetic apparatus to a certain stimulus is stereotyped, be the consequences favorable or detrimental. It can be assumed that molecular biology will provide a more exact distinction between the consequences of normal adaptation and quantitatively or qualitatively inappropriate adaptation from those of degenerative changes due to insufficient energy supply. The contributions which a detailed causal analysis can make to a definition of the term "pathologic" are, however, limited. For example: In the pressure loaded ventricle, the decrease in myofibrillar ATPase as well as the reduction of the sarcoplasmic Ca^{2+}-ATPase activity are involved in changing the contractile characteristics. In the case of myosin, however, a shift in the isoenzyme pattern is found, whereas the transport molecules of the sarcoplasmic reticulum merely suffer a quantitative reduction (37). This means: in characterizing a given process as "pathological", we ultimately remain tied to an interpretation which, strictly speaking, is of a teleological character. The same applies to the term of adaptation. It would be worth discussing, for instance, whether this term appropriately describes the changes of the myosin isoenzymes, whose redistribution could be explained as a consequence of a predominant production of fetal isoenzymes if the synthesis of proteins is enhanced.

We are accustomed to call "pathologic" such deviations from the norm which have negative consequences. Thus, the term "pathologic", as it is commonly used, covers a number of processes of different nature (Fig. 1): unfavourable consequences of regular adaptation, inadequate adaptive changes and, finally, unequivocally degenerative processes.

In any case, we have to consider an area in which normal cardiac adaptation to hemodynamic overload involves negative components so that a clear-cut distinction between "physiologic adaptation" and "pathologic processes" is not possible. Regarding cardiac hypertrophy, this insight should not lead us to consider myocardial mass increase independently of the underlying overload. Therapy should above all be concerned with eliminating the underlying causes.

References

1. Alpert NR, Mulieri LA (1982) Increased myothermal economy of isometric force generation in compensated cardiac hypertrophy induced by pulmonary artery constriction in the rabbit. Circ Res 50:491–500
2. Brändle M (1990) Einfluß der adrenergen Stimulation und des transmembranären Ca^{2+}-Influx auf Geometrie und Pumpfunktion des chronisch druckbelasteten Herzens. Dissertation, University of Tübingen
3. Brändle M, Jacob R (1990) Effects of a diet rich in Omega-3 fatty acids on left ventricular geometry and dynamics in spontaneously hypertensive rats. Europ J appl Physiol, Occupat Physiol 61:177–181
4. Dierberger B, Gülch RW, Jacob R (1990) Quantitative analysis of cardiac dynamics based on Frank's diagram and computer simulation. Significance of mathematical models. Pflügers Arch 415 (Suppl 1):186
5. Ebrecht G, Rupp H, Jacob R (1982) Alterations of mechanical parameters in chemically skinned preparations of rat myocardium as a function of isoenzyme pattern of myosin. Basic Res Cardiol 77:220–234
6. Gülch RW, Jacob R (1988) Geometric and muscle physiological determinants of cardiac stroke volume as evaluated on the basis of model calculations. Basic Res Cardiol 83:476–485
7. Hamrell BB, Hultgren PB, Dale L (1983) Reduced auxotonic sarcomere shortening in pressure-overloaded cardiac hypertrophy: subcellular cardiac compensation. In: Alpert NR (ed) Myocardial Hypertrophy and Failure, Perspective in Cardiovasc Res. Raven Press, New York, pp 311–322
8. Harris P (1983) Evolution and the cardiac patient. Cardiovasc Res 17 (No 6):313–319; 17 (No 7):373–378; 17 (No 8):437–445
9. Henkel RD, Vande Berg JL, Shade RE, Leger JJ, Walsh RA (1989) Cardiac beta myosin heavy chain diversity in normal and chronically hypertensive baboons. J Clin Invest 83:1487–1493
10. Holtz J, Restorff W v, Bard P, Bassenge E (1977) Transmural distribution of myocardial blood flow and of coronary reserve in canine left ventricular hypertrophy. Basic Res Cardiol 72:286–292

11. Jacob R (1983) Chronic reactions of myocardium at the myofibrillar level. Reflexions on "adaptation" and "disease" based on the biology of long-term cardiac overload. In: Jacob R, Gülch RW, Kissling G (eds) Cardiac Adaptation to Hemodynamic Overload, Training and Stress. Steinkopff, Darmstadt, pp 3–24
12. Jacob R (1986) Cardiac responses to experimental chronic pressure overload. In: Zanchetti A, Tarazi RC (eds) Handbook of Hypertension, vol 7 (Pathophysiology of Hypertension – Cardiovascular Aspects). Elsevier Science Publishers BV, pp 59–83
13. Jacob R, Brändle M, Dierberger B, Rupp H (1991) Functional consequences of cardiac hypertrophy and dilatation. In: Smits JFM, DeMey JGR, Daemen MJAP, Struyker Boudier HAJ (eds) Pharmacology of Cardiac and Vascular Remodeling. Steinkopff Verlag Darmstadt, pp 113–130
14. Jacob R, Brändle M, Dierberger B, Ohkubo T, Rupp H (1990) Antihypertensive und kardioprotektive Effekte verschiedener Öldiäten. In: Mall G, Ganten D (eds) Herz-Kreislauf-Regulation, Organprotektion und Organschäden. Stuttgart, Schattauer-Verlag, pp 25–46
15. Jacob R, Dierberger B, Gülch RW, Rupp H, Voelker W (1990) Factors contributing to the transition from cardiac hypertrophy to heart failure. Cardiol Angiol Bulletin 27:1–9
16. Jacob R, Dierberger B, Gülch RW, Mall G, Voelker W, Karsch KR (1990) Significance of myocardial and geometric factors for ventricular dynamics. Analysis demonstrated on the example of idiopathic dilative cardiomyopathy. In: Jacob R, Seipel L, Zucker I (eds) Cardiac Dilatation. Fischer, Stuttgart New York, pp 99–108
17. Jacob R, Gülch RW (1988) Functional significance of ventricular dilatation. Reconsideration of Linzbach's concept of chronic heart failure. Basic Res Cardiol 83:461–475
18. Jacob R, Kissling G, Ebrecht G, Holubarsch Ch, Medugorac I, Rupp H (1983) Adaptive and pathological alterations in experimental cardiac hypertrophy. Advanc Myocardiol 4:55–77
19. Jacob R, Kissling G, Ebrecht G, Jörg E, Rupp H, Takeda N (1984) Cardiac alterations at the myofibrillar level: is a redistribution of the myosin isoenzyme pattern decisive for cardiac failure in hemodynamic overload? Europ Heart J 5 (Suppl F):13–26
20. Kissling G, Gassenmaier T, Wendt-Gallitelli MF, Jacob R (1977) Pressure-volume relations, elastic modulus, and contractile behaviour of the hypertrophied left ventricle of rats with Goldblatt II hypertension. Pflügers Arch 369:213–221
21. Kissling G, Rupp H, Malloy L, Jacob R (1982) Alterations in cardiac oxygen consumption under chronic pressure overload. Significance of the isoenzyme pattern of myosin. Basic Res Cardiol 77:255–269
22. Krayenbuehl HP (1977) Effects of hypertrophy on contractile function in man. Basic Res Cardiol 72:184–189
23. Linzbach AJ (1960) Heart failure from the point of view of quantitative anatomy. Am J Cardiol 5:370–382
24. Mall G, Mattfeldt T (1990) Capillary growth patterns in cardiac hypertrophy and normal growth. A stereological study on papillary muscles. In: Jacob R, Seipel L, Zucker IH (eds) Cardiac Dilatation. Fischer, Stuttgart New York, pp 51–67
25. Medugorac I, Jacob R (1983) Heterogenity of collagen in the normal and hypertrophied left ventricle of the rat. In: Jacob R, Gülch RW, Kissling G (eds) Cardiac Adaptation to Hemodynamic Overload, Training and Stress. Steinkopff, Darmstadt, pp 349–353
26. Noma K, Brändle M, Jacob R (1988) Evaluation of an experimental model of congestive heart failure due to combined arteriovenous shunt and renal hypertension. Basic Res Cardiol 83:58–64
27. Noma K, Brändle M, Rupp H, Jacob R (1990) Left ventricular performance in rats with chronic cardiac overload due to arterio-venous shunt. Heart and Vessels 5:65–70
28. Nordin Ch (1989) Abnormal Ca^{2+} handling and the generation of ventricular arrhythmias in congestive heart failure. Heart Failure 5:143–154
29. Rakusan K, Turek Z (1986) Oxygen sources and sinks in myocardial hypertrophy. In: Dhalla NS, Singal P, Beamish RE (eds) Pathophysiology of Heart Disease. Nijhoff Publishing, Boston Dordrecht Lancaster, pp 83–92
30. Reiter MJ (1989) Pathophysiology of ventricular arrhythmias in patients with congestive heart failure. Heart Failure 5:155–166

31. Rupp H (1987) Polymorphic myosin as the common determinant of myofibrillar ATPase in different haemodynamic and thyroid states. Basic Res Cardiol 77:34–46
32. Rupp H, Fenchel G, Jacob R (1991) Human ventricular myosin exists in two components which are influenced by the hemodynamic load. To be submitted
33. Rupp H, Jacob R (1986) The autonomic nervous system of the heart: adaptation, deadaptation and impaired nervous control of heart performance. In: Rupp H (ed) The Regulation of Heart Function – Basic Concepts and Clinical Applications. Thieme, New York, pp 53–70
34. Rupp H, Wahl R, Jacob R (1986) Remodelling of the myocyte at a molecular level – relationship between myosin isoenzyme population and sarcoplasmic reticulum. In: Dhalla NS, Pierce GN, Beamish RE (eds) Heart Function and Metabolism. Nijhoff Publishing, Boston Dordrecht Lancaster, pp 307–318
35. Sandritter W, Beneke G (1986) Allgemeine Pathologie. Schattauer, Stuttgart New York
36. Strauer BE, Mahmoud MA (1985) Coronary hemodynamics in hypertensive heart disease: basic concepts and clinical consequences. J Cardiovasc Pharmacol 7:S62–S69
37. Swynghedauw B (1990) Heart failure: a disease of adaptation. Heart Failure 6:57–62
38. Vogt M, Jacob R, Kissling G, Rupp H (1987) Chronic cardiac reactions II. Mechanical and energetic consequences of myocardial transformation versus ventricular dilatation in the chronically pressure loaded heart. In: Jacob R, Just Hj, Holubarsch Ch (eds) Cardiac Energetics. Steinkopff, Darmstadt, Springer, New York, pp 147–159
39. Vogt M, Motz W, Strauer BE (1989) Decreased coronary vasodilator reserve and left ventricular hypertrophy in hypertensive patients. Circ 80 (Suppl II):595
40. Weber KT, Brilla CG, Janicki JS, Reddy HK, Campbell SE (1991) Myocardial fibrosis: role of ventricular systolic pressure, arterial hypertension, and circulating hormones. Basic Res Cardiol 86 (Suppl 3):25–31
41. Wendt-Gallitelli MF, Ebrecht G, Jacob R (1979) Morphological alterations and their functional interpretation in the hypertrophied myocardium of Goldblatt hypertensive rats. J Molec Cell Cardiol 11:275–287

Author's address:

Prof. Dr. R. Jacob
Physiologisches Institut II
Universität Tübingen
Gmelinstraße 5
W-7400 Tübingen, FRG

Experimental congestive heart failure due to myocardial infarction: Sarcolemmal receptors and cation transporters *

N. S. Dhalla, I. M. C. Dixon, H. Rupp **, and J. Barwinsky

Division of Cardiovascular Sciences, St. Boniface General Hospital Research Centre and Departments of Physiology and Surgery, Faculty of Medicine, University of Manitoba, Canada

Summary: Rats, subsequent to loss of a large amount of left ventricular free wall due to surgically-induced myocardial infarction, form a good model of congestive heart failure. Since depressed cardiac pump function is the hallmark of heart failure, it is suspected that decreased influx of Ca^{2+} into the cardiac cell is responsible for depressed contractile function. Because Ca^{2+} movements in the sarcolemmal membrane are known to involve Ca^{2+}-channels, Na^+-Ca^{2+} exchange, Ca^{2+}-pump, Na^+-K^+ ATPase, β-adrenoceptors and α-adrenoceptors directly or indirectly, the status of these mechanisms was examined by employing rats at different degrees of congestive heart failure. The left coronary artery was ligated and hearts were examined 4, 8, and 16 weeks later; sham-operated animals served as controls. The number of Ca^{2+} channels in the myocardium was depressed in moderate and severe stages of heart failure. Furthermore, depressions in sarcolemmal Na^+-Ca^{2+} exchange activity and β-adrenoceptor number were associated with the development of early stages of heart failure, whereas sarcolemmal Na^+-K^+ ATPase activity was decreased and the number of α-adrenoceptors was increased at moderate and severe stages. The Ca^{2+}-pump activities were not altered in failing hearts. Thus it appears that changes in Na^+-Ca^{2+} exchange as well as β-adrenoceptors and Ca^{2+} channels may contribute towards decreasing Ca^{2+} influx at early and moderate stages of congestive heart failure, respectively. On the other hand, changes in α-adrenoceptors and Na^+-K^+ ATPase may act as compensatory mechanisms for maintaining Ca^{2+} influx at moderate and late stages of congestive heart failure.

Key words: $\underline{Ca}^{2+}$-channels; $\underline{a}$drenoceptors; $\underline{Na}^+$-K^+ ATPase; $\underline{Na}^+$-Ca^{2+} exchange; $\underline{Ca}^{2+}$-pump; $\underline{f}$ailing $\underline{h}$eart

Introduction

It is estimated that about 1.5% of the total North American population has congestive heart failure, but this figure escalates to $>10\%$ of the population over the age of 75 years (8, 36, 37). Approximately 500000 people develop congestive heart failure every year and the 5-year mortality from the time of diagnosis is about 60% in men and about 45% in women. It is commonly held that increasing prevalence of congestive heart failure is due to the aging population as well as to improvements in therapy which have allowed patients with cardiovascular disease to live longer. Etiological studies of congestive heart failure reveal that the most prevalent cause of this pathophysiologic state is the presence of coronary artery disease followed by incidence of systemic hypertension, valvular heart disease, cardiomyopathy and congenital heart disease (36). The best example of a patient

* The research work reported in this study was supported by a grant from the Manitoba Heart and Stroke Foundation.
** Dr. Heinz Rupp was a visiting Professor from the Institute of Physiology II, University of Tübingen, Tübingen, F.R. Germany.

with congestive heart failure is one with coronary artery disease who has had one or more heart attacks with subsequent loss of cardiac muscle.

As congestive heart failure has become one of the most common serious disorders and is one of the most common causes of death, many different experimental models of heart failure have been developed to aid in the assessment of biochemical changes during the development of cardiac dysfunction and to investigate various modes of treatment of the failing heart. However, there are very few reliable models of congestive heart failure secondary to myocardial infarction (42) and one noted example in this regard is provided by Johns and Olson (28), who published the first comprehensive description of surgical ligation of the left coronary artery in rats. These investigators initiated their study to find an alternative model of infarction to the canine model as the infarct size and mortality in dogs due to coronary occlusion was "unpredictable", presumably due to collateral blood supply and differences among various breeds. By successful mapping of the arterial network of hearts from these small animals, establishing the indicence of mortality as a result of coronary occlusion and achieving a high incidence of infarction in rats, these investigators set the stage for further studies of experimentally produced myocardial infarction where congestive heart failure was noted by the presence of peripheral edema in some rats. Several years later a group lead by Selye found that larger myocardial infarct due to coronary occlusion and increased survival of the experimental animals can be achieved with some modification of earlier techniques (47). This rat model was used to study morphologic features of evolving infarcts, and to assess the effect of various interventions on infarct size (5, 15, 29, 31). This model of myocardial infarction was also used in the assessment of metabolic and mechanical adaptations in these hearts (6).

Rat heart as a model for congestive heart failure

Although the rat heart lacks collateral capillaries and is therefore dissimilar from human heart, the rat model of infarction was useful by virtue of the reproducibility of infarct size. The nature of the inflammatory response of the myocardium was studied during a 21-day period following coronary occlusion (18). Following a brief inflammatory response at the margin of the necrotic myocardium, chronic inflammation, vascular and collagenous proliferation and resorption of necrotic tissue progressed until 21 days, whereupon scar formation was complete. Recently, the process of scar reabsorption has been carefully assessed by morphometric techniques in rat heart and it was shown that these processes are responsible for a 59% shrinkage of the necrotic myocardium in both small and large infarcts over the first 40 days (2). Although measurement of scar size is a valuable relative indicator of extent of damage to the myocardium, the first study to assess the left ventricular function in rats with large myocardial infarction appeared in 1979, wherein in vivo measurements of baseline and intravenous volume loaded hemodynamics were made in rats 21 days following coronary occlusion (41). Little change of the baseline hemodynamics or peak indices of cardiac pumping or pressure generating ability was observed in experimental animals with small left ventricular infarct (4–30%) when compared to control. Experimental animals with moderate myocardial infarction (31–45%) had normal baseline hemodynamics, but cardiac pump function was reduced upon volume overload. Rats with large infarcts (>45%) had overt heart failure characterized by elevated filling pressures, reduced cardiac output and low capacity to respond to preload and afterload stress. Subsequent work from this group indicated that coronary ligation in the rat provided an experimental model of graded left ventricular dysfunction, whose magnitude was closely related to the extent of the healed myocardial infarction (19, 20).

A parameter used in forming the prognosis for survival of post-infarct patients is the presence and extent of left ventricular dilatation (17). Left ventricular distention and dilatation were illustrated by upward and rightward movement on the pressure-volume relationship of experimental animals when compared to control (19, 20). It was suggested that increased ventricular volume aided maintenance of peak stroke volume despite the linear reduction of ejection fraction index with increasing infarction size in animals 3–4 weeks after the induction of myocardial infarction. A study of the time course (4, 7, 10, 20, and 35 weeks) of hemodynamic changes in rats with healed severe myocardial infarction revealed that at 4 weeks, peak left ventricular blood pressure, left ventricular maximum rate of contraction, diastolic blood pressure and systemic vascular resistance were decreased when compared to control (11). Furthermore, the left ventricular end-diastolic pressure was increased by 313% in these experimental animals. These investigators found no further significant deviation in diastolic blood pressure, left ventricular end-diastolic pressure, peak left ventricular blood pressure, and maximum rate of left ventricular contraction after 4 weeks. The cardiac output and systemic vascular resistance progressively decreased and increased, respectively; these changes were accompanied by decreased blood flow to liver, stomach, brain and kidney in the period from 7–35 weeks, which suggested that progressive cardiac decompensation was present in these animals (11). Recent use of this model for investigation of pharmacological tolerance to nitrate therapy has revealed that the rapid reduction of left ventricular end diastolic pressure caused by glyceryl trinitrate resembles that seen in man, and therefore could be used as a model for examining the mechanisms of nitrate action and tolerance (4). In humans, the most common cause of right-sided cardiac failure and pulmonary hypertension is the left-sided cardiac failure (7, 36). Likewise, right ventricular hypertrophy was consistently present in experimental rats showing elevated left ventricular filling pressures and, in fact, a close relationship between left ventricular end-diastolic pressure and right ventricular systolic pressure was observed (19, 20, 41). Thus it appears that the left ventricular dysfunction may eventually cause severe right ventricular overload and dysfunction such that the right ventricle becomes a limiting factor in heart failure in rats with chronic coronary occlusion.

The incidence of myocardial hypertrophy after myocardial infarction has long been thought to be beneficial as a nonspecific compensatory mechanism for increasing mass and thereby functional capacity of these hearts (45). While the validity of this concept remains to be established, some research on cellular processes associated with the incidence of hypertrophy in infarcted rat heart has yielded some useful information (2, 3). An early report of cardiac hypertrophy in experimental rat hearts 12 weeks after the induction of myocardial infarction suggested that overall cardiac hypertrophy was about 170% when compared to control (34); no normalization for loss of the infarcted myocardium was incorporated in this estimate. Recent work has shown in hearts of rats sacrificed 5 weeks after coronary occlusion with so-called medium (>15–30%) or large (>30%) infarct size that myocytes had undergone significant hypertrophy (43). In a study of the morphometry of the right ventricle in rat hearts 4 weeks after occlusion of the left coronary artery, the weight of the right ventricle had increased by 30%, with 17% ventricular wall thickening and 13% greater diameter of myocytes (3). Inadequate growth of the microvasculature that supports tissue oxygenation was evidenced by relative decreases in capillary luminal volume density (25%), capillary luminal surface density (20%) and by an increase in the average maximum distance from the capillary wall to the mitochondria of myocytes (20%). These authors suggested that inadequate compensation of the coronary bed in the right ventricle may result in alterations in oxygen availability, diffusion and transport which may be detrimental to the myocardial tissue. A report of these parameters in viable left ventricular myocardium of rat hearts 5 weeks after the induction of myocardial infarction revealed about 80% expansion of the spared myocardium which was found to be insufficient in restoration of ventricular tissue; infarcts affecting an average of 20% of the left ventricle were characterized by a 25% hypertrophic growth of the remaining myocardium (2). Hearts with large infarcts were shown to have 25%, 30%, and 30% reduction in the absolute amounts of capillary lumen, surface and length per ventricle, respectively; these changes indicated that the surviving ventricle may be vulnerable to additional ischemic episodes.

As the rat model of congestive heart failure became established, and because it is generally believed that the function of the scarred ventricle would depend not only on size and location of the infarct but also on evolving changes in neurohumoral influences, systemic vascular resistance and venous compliance, recent research has been directed toward description of these parameters in an attempt to clarify whether these animals are in a compensated or decompensated state. For example, marked changes in systemic and renal microcirculatory dynamics in congestive heart failure patients (48) may reflect, in part, significant increases in plasma renin and aldosterone levels. Plasma atrial natriuretic peptide levels in experimental rats 4 weeks after induction of infarction were shown to be elevated when compared to control (25), as in humans with congestive heart failure (9), however plasma renin and aldosterone levels were unchanged. Ventricular levels of norepinephrine were decreased in experimental animals when compared to control (25). Thus, while the neurohormonal status of these experimental animals is altered to some extent 4 weeks after myocardial infarction, not all of the criterion for congestive heart failure in humans are met at this stage of failure. However, plasma atrial natriuretic peptide concentration was found to vary directly with size of myocardial infarction in rats (32), and atrial content of atrial natriuretic peptide mRNA was increased in animals with large infarct versus those control animals (9). Although the exact significance of increased plasma atrial natriuretic factor is not clear, injection of monoclonal antibodies specific for atrial natriuretic factor into rats with large myocardial infarction and high baseline plasma atrial natriuretic factor was associated with a specific increase in the systemic vascular resistance (14). Venous capacitance, inferred by effective vascular compliance, was decreased in rats 3 weeks after the induction of large myocardial infarction (22); it has been suggested that elevated plasma atrial natriuretic factor levels affect central hemodynamics by reducing venous pressure and possibly by arterial dilatation. Since chronic treatment with captopril, an angiotensin-converting enzyme inhibitor, was shown to maintain normal left ventricular filling pressure and cardiac output, reduce ventricular hypertrophy and prolong survival in rats 3–12 months after induction of myocardial infarction, it seems logical that there is a pathophysiologic role for elevated levels of angiotensin in this model (21, 38–40, 43, 44). In this regard, reduced glomerular plasma flow rate and single nephron glomerular filtration rate, as well as increased single nephron filtration fraction, efferent arteriolar resistance and fractional proximal tubule fluid reabsorption in rats with large myocardial infarction were normalized by treatment of these animals with teprotide, an angiotensin-converting enzyme inhibitor (27). As Na^+ excretion was shown to be impaired in rats with either large or small infarcts at 3–4 weeks, defective renal function was present in these animals (26, 27).

Biochemical alterations in failing hearts

Relatively little is known of biochemical parameters such as myofibrillar ATPase activity, myosin isozyme composition, myocardial high-energy phosphate content, sarcoplasmic reticular function, mitochondrial function and sarcolemmal function in the viable myocardium of rat heart with myocardial infarction, especially in later stages of congestive heart failure. Myofibrillar ATPase activity was found to be 20% lower in both sedentary and exercised infarct groups 11 weeks post-myocardial infarction when compared to sham-operated control animals (24). A shift in the myosin heavy chain isozyme content from V_1 toward V_3 is known to occur in viable myocardium of the infarcted hearts (33). Furthermore, although actomyosin APTase activity and the percent V_1 myosin heavy-chain isozyme were shown to be decreased in all viable regions of the infarcted hearts by 3 weeks, some regional variation was noted as greater depression of V_1 myosin in the left ventricle and papillary muscle when compared to the right ventricular free wall and septum V_1 content from the same hearts (23). Two days following infarction, the ATP content of viable myocardium was found to be significantly lower than control; intravenous ribose administration attenuated this decrease and was associated with an improvement of cardiac pump function (50). These investigators also found that ATP content of the nonischemic portion of the myocardium was not different from control 4 days after occlusion of the left coronary artery. While other investigators also showed that ATP and total adenine nucleotide contents were normal in viable tissue of hearts 1 or 3 weeks after the induction of large myocardial infarction, tissue concentrations of creatine phosphate and free creatine were decreased (16). Sarcoplasmic reticular Ca^{2+} uptake and Ca^{2+} ATPase activities in purified vesicle preparations were depressed in the viable left ventricular myocardium in experimental animals 16 weeks after induction of myocardial infarction (1). Very few studies to directly or indirectly assess sarcolemmal function have been attempted with this model of myocardial infarction, and none have assessed sarcolemmal function in decompensated stages of heart failure. One week after coronary occlusion, sensitivity of the surviving myocardium to verapamil was increased when compared to control (16). Accordingly, it was demonstrated that sensitivity to extracellular Ca^{2+} was decreased in viable tissue 1 or 3 weeks after myocardial infarction, and it was suggested that inward Ca^{2+} channel activity was depressed in the infarcted hearts (16).

Myocardial noradrenaline content was shown to be reduced and a small increase in dihydroalprenolol binding site density was noted in rats 3 weeks after coronary occlusion, but the responsiveness of the nonischemic myocardium to isoprenaline was not changed in these animals (10). Nonetheless, these studies indicate that virtually nothing is known about sarcolemmal changes during the development of congestive heart failure secondary to myocardial infarction.

Sarcolemmal changes in congestive heart failure

Data from studies of the rat model of congestive heart failure secondary to myocardial infarction carried out in our laboratory confirm the presence of heart dysfunction in experimental animals (13). We have arbitrarily designated experimental animals at 4, 8, and 16 weeks after induction of myocardial infarction as those in early failure stage, moderate failure stage and severe stage, based on general and hemodynamic characteristics as this classification scheme is useful in comparison of clinical and hemodynamic changes with biochemical parameters. A study of left ventricle, right ventricle, scar weight, left ventricle body weight ratio, appearance of abdominal ascites and lung weight revealed significant differences between experimental (16 weeks after coronary occlusion) and sham-operated animals (Table 1). Evidence of cardiac hypertrophy in experimental animals was noted by the increased normalized mass of the left ventricle as well as right ventricular myocardium. Left ventricular/body weight ratio was increased

Table 1. Alterations in general characteristics of experimental rats 4, 8, and 16 weeks after induction of myocardial infarction

Parameters	4 weeks	8 weeks	16 weeks
Left ventricle (LV) wt	94 ± 12	137 ± 17*	140 ± 13*
Normalized hypertrophy	135 ± 7*	197 ± 11*	201 ± 9*
Right ventricle (RV) wt	133 ± 17*	160 ± 17*	158 ± 16*
LV wt/body wt	105 ± 13	141 ± 14*	151 ± 15*
Lung wet wt	103 ± 12	141 ± 8*	162 ± 9*
Lung dry wt	95 ± 14	106 ± 17	113 ± 8
Lung wet wt/dry wt ratio	107 ± 13	134 ± 8*	142 ± 6*

Data are expressed as mean ± SEM of eight experiments. Left ventricular weight indicated for experimental animals does not include scar tissue. For the determination of degree of hypertrophy, the percent of the infarcted left ventricle was estimated 3 weeks after coronary ligation by plonimetic techniques; this percentage was extrapolated to the respective experimental groups. All values expressed in percent of sham control. * = $p < 0.05$.

Table 2. Alterations in hemodynamic characteristics of experimental rats 4, 8, and 16 weeks after myocardial infarction

Group	MAP	LVSP	LVEDP	+ dP/dt	− dP/dt	HR	Total mechanical energy
4 weeks	90 ± 10	84 ± 7	307 ± 32*	81 ± 4*	69 ± 8*	92 ± 7	78 ± 5*
8 weeks	77 ± 5*	88 ± 6	361 ± 40*	82 ± 3*	75 ± 4*	91 ± 3	83 ± 4*
16 weeks	56 ± 3*	68 ± 5*	412 ± 23*	65 ± 4*	56 ± 6*	64 ± 2*	43 ± 3*

Data are expressed as means ± SEM of eight experiments. All measurements were made on Beckman dynograph by using a Millar microcatheter; the catheter was inserted into the left ventricle via cannulation of the right carotid artery. MAP = mean arterial pressure; LVSP = left ventricular systolic pressure; LVEDP = left ventricular end diastolic pressure; HR = heart rate; + dP/dt = rate of contraction; − dP/dt = rate of relaxation; Total mechanical energy = HR × LVSP. All data are expressed as percent of control values. * = $p < 0.05$.

and the accumulation of fluid in the abdominal cavity was evident in 16-week experimental animals. Congestion of lungs in 16-week experimental animals was noted by increased wet lung weight and wet/dry lung weight ratio. Although no difference in liver weight or wet/dry liver weight ratio between sham-operated and 16 week experimental animals was seen, the livers of experimental animals had rounded edges and yellowish colorations. Signs of clinical congestive heart failure were also evident in experimental rats 8 weeks following infarction and the extent of normalized hypertrophy of the left ventricles of these hearts was only slightly less than those of the 16 week experimental group. No difference in the scar weights of the left ventricular free wall was seen among the 4, 8 or 16 week experimental groups. At a period of 4 weeks after surgery, the experimental animals were not significantly different from the sham-operated animals in any of the parameters indicated above except the development of ascites (Table 1).

Assessment of hemodynamic performance of the 16-week experimental group revealed decreases in mean arterial pressure, left ventricular systolic pressure, rate of contraction, rate of relaxation, heart rate and the total mechanical energy output of these hearts

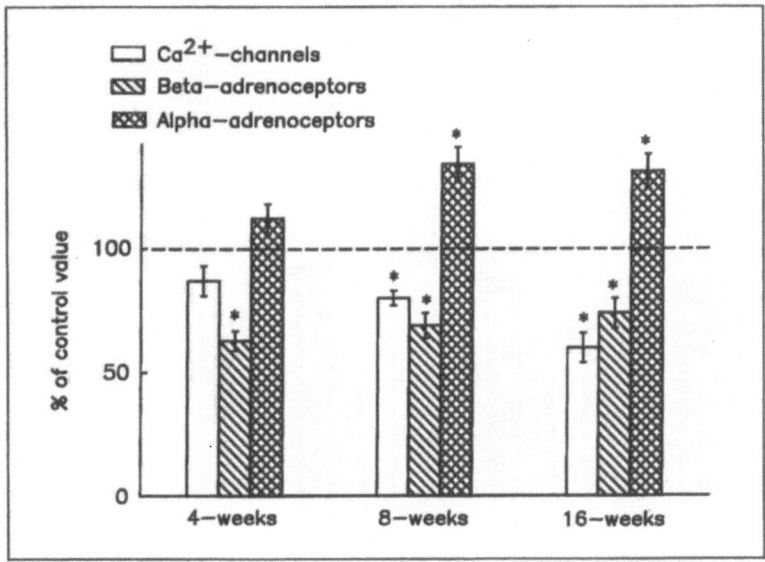

Fig. 1. Alterations in sarcolemmal Ca^{2+}-channels, β-receptors and α-receptors during the development of congestive heart failure in rats subsequent to myocardial infarction. The data are expressed as % of control values for number of the respective Ca^{2+}-channels and adrenoceptors and are mean $\pm$S.E. of 6 to 8 experiments. $*=p<0.05$

(Table 2) as compared to sham-operated animals. The left ventricular end-diastolic pressure in the 4-, 8-, and 16-week experimental animals was significantly elevated when compared to control values. Although the 8-week experimental group did show significant reductions in many hemodynamic parameters as observed in the 16-week experimental group, these changes were lesser in magnitude. Mean arterial pressure, heart rate and left ventricular systolic pressure were unchanged in the 4-week experimental group; however, left ventricular diastolic pressure, rate of contraction, rate of relaxation and total mechanical energy output were reduced.

Since disturbances in myocardial Ca^{2+} metabolism are suspected to be involved in heart failure, and because the sarcolemmal membrane plays an important role in excitation-contraction coupling, we assessed different aspects of cardiac sarcolemmal function in animals with congestive heart failure secondary to myocardial infarction. Biochemical ligand binding techniques with [3H]-nitrendipine have allowed us to estimate the number of Ca^{2+}-channels in crude membrane or purified sarcolemmal membrane preparations prepared from viable left ventricular myocardial tissue (13), and we have reported that the specific binding of [3H]-nitrendipine was significantly reduced in samples from 8- and 16-week experimental animals (Fig. 1). Scatchard plot analysis of [3H]-nitrendipine binding revealed that the B_{max} of specific binding sites was reduced in these experimental groups with no changes in K_d, or the affinity binding. Furthermore, we found that these changes were independent of incident hypertrophy of the remaining viable myocardium. Since alterations in cardiac pump function were evident in 4-week experimental animals, and since many other sarcolemmal mechanisms are known to regulate cellular Ca^{2+} metabolism, we examined the status of cardiac adrenoceptor

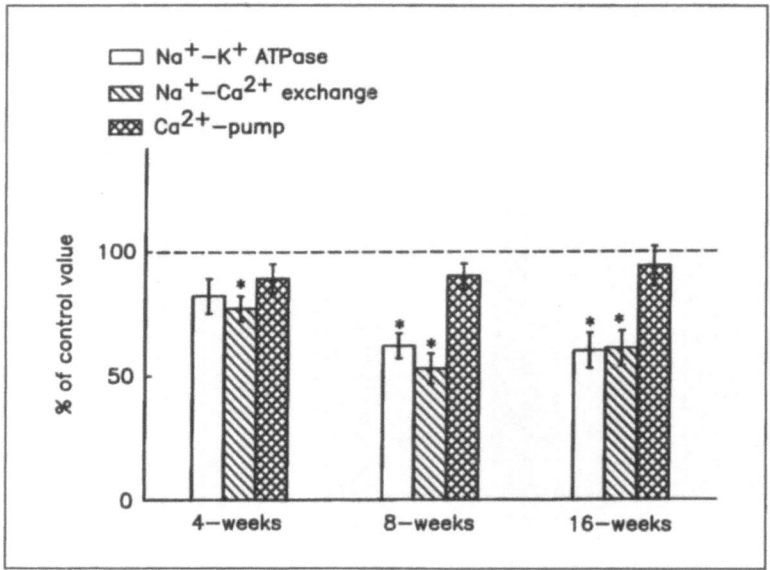

Fig. 2. Alterations in sarcolemmal Na^+-K^+ ATPase, Na^+-Ca^{2+} exchange and Ca^{2+}-pump activities during the development of congestive heart failure in rats subsequent to myocardial infarction. The data are expressed as % of control values for the respective parameter and are mean ±S.E. of 6 to 8 experiments. *=p<0.05

systems by ligand binding techniques. A summary of results (Fig. 1) indicates that cardiac sarcolemmal β-adrenoceptor number, measured by specific binding of [³H]-dihydroalprenolol, was decreased in 4-, 8-, and 16-week experimental groups, with no changes in the values of K_d. On the other hand, the number of cardiac α-adrenoceptors was increased in samples of 8- and 16-week experimental groups (Fig. 1).

Abnormalities in Ca^{2+} channels and adrenoceptors in the failing heart would be taken to suggest that there is a generalized defect in the sarcolemmal membrane. Accordingly, it is possible that other sarcolemmal functions such as Na^+-K^+ pump, Na^+-Ca^{2+} exchange and Ca^{2+}-pump may also become defective in congestive heart failure; the results of experiments carried out to assess these activities are summarized in Fig. 2. It can be seen that the activity of sarcolemmal Na^+-K^+ ATPase is significantly depressed in samples prepared from viable left ventricular myocardium in 8- and 16-week experimental animals, when compared to control values. Na^+-dependent Ca^{2+} uptake in sarcolemmal vesicles was depressed in samples of 4-, 8-, and 16-week experimental groups, whereas sarcolemmal Ca^{2+}-pumping ATPase activities (measured as either ATP-dependent Ca^{2+} accumulation in vesicle preparations or Ca^{2+}-stimulated ATPase activity) were unchanged in samples from 4-, 8-, and 16-week experimental animals when compared to control values (Fig. 2).

As sarcolemma is thought to be functionally coupled to sarcoplasmic reticulum in both delivery and removal of Ca^{2+} ions to and from the myoplasm in the cardiac excitation and relaxation phases (12), any defect in sarcolemmal Ca^{2+}-translocation could conceivably contribute to disruption of myocardial Ca^{2+} homeostasis and abnormalities in the development of cardiac contractile force. Reduced numbers of sarcolemmal Ca^{2+}-

channels and β-adrenoceptors may directly and indirectly contribute to a reduction in Ca^{2+} permeation across the sarcolemma upon excitation of the myocardium, and the resultant intracellular Ca^{2+} deficiency may lead to depressed cardiac contractility seen in experimental animals. Mediation of Ca^{2+}-influx across the sarcolemmal membrane by Na^+-Ca^{2+} exchange has been shown recently to be involved in the release of sarcoplasmic reticular stores of Ca^{2+} (30). Depression of cardiac sarcolemmal Na^+-dependent Ca^{2+} uptake in experimental animals suggests that release of Ca^{2+} from sarcoplasmic reticulum may be decreased in hearts of experimental animals. Thus depression of this mechanism may also contribute to reduction in the delivery of Ca^{2+} for myocardial contraction. It is pointed out that the activity of sarcoplasmic reticular Ca^{2+}-stimulated ATPase is depressed in 16-week experimental animals (1). Therefore, the Ca^{2+}-sequestering ability of this intracellular storage site is depressed in the failing myocardium, which can be seen to lead to a reduction of stored intracellular Ca^{2+} and, therefore, less available Ca^{2+} for release to the contractile machinery upon excitation of the myocardium. It is pointed out that since the sarcolemmal Ca^{2+}-pump activities are normal in all stages of heart failure, other changes in sarcolemmal function do not appear to be due to some generalized defect in the sarcolemmal membrane. The alterations in sarcolemmal β-adrenoceptors and Na^+-Ca^{2+} exchange activity occur at all stages of heart failure subsequent to myocardial infarction, and may represent primary defects in the genesis of this pathophysiologic state. Although a decrease in the number of sarcolemmal Ca^{2+}-channels does not occur until 8 weeks after induction of myocardial infarction, this defect can be viewed as a contributing factor to intracellular Ca^{2+}-deficiency. On the other hand, increased α-adrenoceptor number and decreased Na^+-K^+ ATPase activity may be compensatory changes in the myocardium to increase the levels of intracellular Ca^{2+} in moderate (8-week) an severe (16-week) stages of congestive heart failure subsequent to myocardial infarction. The former mechanism may act to increase intracellular Ca^{2+} by the inositol trisphosphate-dependent release of sarcoplasmic reticular stores in the heart (35), and the latter mechanism may operate to increase intracellular Ca^{2+} levels similar to that effected by the application of cardiac glycosides (46). Support for the notion regarding partially compensated alterations in intracellular Ca^{2+}-metabolism is given by the fact that rates of contraction and relaxation of viable myocardium were equally depressed in the 4- and 8-week experimental groups. Furthermore, the 16-week experimental group did not show a dramatic depression in the rates of contraction and relaxation compared to 4- and 8-week experimental groups.

References

1. Afzal N, Dhalla NS (1989) Depressed sarcoplasmic reticular Ca^{2+}-transport in congestive heart failure secondary to myocardial infarction. J Mol Cell Cardiol 21 (SII):S 49
2. Anversa P, Beghi C, Kikkawa Y, Olivetti G (1986) Myocardial infarction in rats. Infarct size, myocyte hypertrophy, and capillary growth. Circ Res 58:26–37
3. Anversa PC, Beghi C, McDonald SL, Levicky V, Kikkawa Y, Olivetti G (1984) Morphometry of right ventricular hypertrophy induced by myocardial infarction in the rat. Am J Pathol 116:504–513
4. Bauer JA, Fung HL (1990) Effects of chronic glyceroyl trinitrate on left ventricular haemodynamics in a rat model of congestive heart failure: demonstration of a simple animal model for the study of in vivo tolerance. Cardiovasc Res 24:198–203
5. Bajusz E, Jasmin GJ (1964) Histochemical studies on the myocardium following experimental interference with coronary circulation. I. Occlusion of the coronary artery. Acta Histochem 18:222–237

6. Bester AJ, Bajusz E, Lochner AL (1972) Effect of ischaemia and infarction on the metabolism and function of the isolated perfused rat heart. Cardiovasc Res 6:284–294
7. Bloomfield RA, Lauson HD, Cournand A, Breed ES, Richards Jr DW (1946) Recording of right heart pressures in normal subjects and in patients with chronic pulmonary disease and various types of cardio-circulatory disease. J Clin Invest 25:639–664
8. Braunwald E (1982) Historical overview and pathophysiologic considerations. In: Braunwald E, Mock MB, Watson J (eds) Congestive Heart Failure: Current Research and Clinical Applications. Grune and Stratton Inc, New York, pp 3–9
9. Burnett J, Kako P, Hu D, Heser D, Heublein D, Granger J, Opgenorth T, Reeder G (1985) Atrial natriuretic peptide elevation in congestive heart failure in the human. Science 231:1145–1147
10. Clozel J-P, Holck M, Osterrieder W, Burkard W, Da Prada M (1987) Effects of chronic myocardial infarction on responsiveness to isoprenaline and the state of myocardial beta adrenoceptors in rats. Cardiovasc Res 21:688–695
11. Defelice A, Frering A, Horan P (1989) Time course of hemodynamic changes in rats with healed severe myocardial infarction. Am J Physiol 257:H289–H296
12. Dhalla NS, Pierce GN, Panagia V, Singal PK, Beamish RE (1982) Calcium movements in relation to heart function. Basic Res Cardiol 77:117–139
13. Dixon IMC, Lee SL, Dhalla NS (1990) Nitrendipine binding in congestive heart failure due to myocardial infarction. Circ Res 66:782–788
14. Drexler H, Hirth C, Stasch H-P, Lu W, Neuser D, Just H (1990) Vasodilatory action of endogenous atrial natriuretic factor in a rat model of chronic heart failure as determined by monoclonal ANF antibody. Circ Res 66:1371–1380
15. Dusek J, Rona G, Kaher DS (1971) Healing process in the marginal zone of an experimental myocardial infarct: findings in the surviving cardiac muscle cells. Am J Pathol 62:321–338
16. Fellenius E, Hansen CA, Mjos O, Neely JR (1985) Chronic infarction decreases maximum cardiac work and sensitivity of heart to extracellular calcium. Am J Physiol 249:H80–H87
17. Feild BJ, Russel Jr RO, Moraski RE (1974) Left ventricular size and function and heart size in the year following myocardial infarction. Circulation 50:331–339
18. Fishbein MC, Maclean D, Maroko PR (1978) Experimental myocardial infarction in the rat. Qualitative and quantitative changes during pathologic evolution. Am J Pathol 90:57–70
19. Fletcher PJ, Pfeffer JM, Pfeffer MA, Braunwald E (1981) Left-ventricular diastolic pressure-volume relations in rats with healed myocardial infarction: effects on systolic function. Circ Res 49:618–626
20. Fletcher PJ, Pfeffer JM, Pfeffer MA, Braunwald E (1982) Effects of hypertension on cardiac performance in rats with myocardial infarction. Am J Cardiol 50:488–496
21. Fouad FM, Tarazi RC (1986) Restoration of cardiac function and structure by converting enzyme inhibition: possibilities and limitation of long-term treatment in hypertension and heart failure. J Cardiovasc Pharmacol 8 (51):S53–S57
22. Gay R, Wool S, Paquin M, Goldman S (1986) Total vascular pressure-volume relationship in conscious rats with chronic heart failure. Am J Physiol 251:H483–H489
23. Geenen DL, Malhotra A, Scheuer J (1989) Regional variation in rat cardiac myosin isoenzymes and ATPase activity after infarction. Am J Physiol 256:H745–H750
24. Geenen DL, White TP, Lampman RM (1987) Papillary mechanics and cardiac morphology of infarcted rat hearts after training. J Appl Physiol 63 (1):92–96
25. Hodsman GP, Kohzuki M, Howes LG, Sumithran E, Tsunoda K, Johnston CI (1988) Neurohumoral responses to chronic myocardial infarction in rats. Circulation 78:376–381
26. Hostetter TH, Pfeffer JM, Pfeffer MA, Dworkin DL, Braunwald E, Brenner BM (1983) Cardiorenal hemodynamics and sodium excretion in rats with myocardial infarction. Am J Physiol 245:H98–H103
27. Ichikawa I, Pfeffer JM, Pfeffer MA, Hostetter TH, Brenner BM (1984) Role of Angiotensin II in the altered renal function of congestive heart failure. Circ Res 55:669–675
28. Johns TNP, Olson BJ (1954) Experimental myocardial infarction. I. A method of coronary occlusion in small animals. Ann Surg 140:675–682
29. Kaufman N, Gavan TL, Hill RW (1959) Experimental myocardial infarction in the rat. Arch Pathol 67:482–488

30. Leblanc N, Hume JR (1990) Sodium current-induced release of calcium from cardiac sarcoplasmic reticulum. Science 248:372–376
31. Maclean D, Maroko PR, Fishbein MC, Braunwald E (1977) Effects of corticosteroids on myocardial infarct size and healing following experimental coronary occlusion. Am J Cardiol 39:280
32. Mendez RE, Pfeffer JM, Ortola FV, Bloch KD, Anderson S, Seidman JG, Brenner BM (1987) Atrial natriuretic peptide transcription, storage, and release in rats with myocardial infarction. Am J Physiol 253:H1449–H1455
33. Mercadier JJ, Lopmpre AM, Wisnewsky C, Samuel J-L, Bercovici J, Swynghedauw B, Schwartz K (1981) Myosin isoenzymic changes of several models of rat cardiac hypertrophy. Circ Res 49:525–532
34. Norman T, Coers CR (1960) Cardiac hypertrophy after coronary artery ligation in rats. Arch Pathol 69:181–184
35. Otani H, Otani H, Das DK (1988) α-adrenergic-mediated phosphoinositide breakdown and inotropic response in rat left ventricular papillary muscles. Circ Res 62:8–17
36. Parmley WW (1985) Pathophysiology of congestive heart failure. Am J Cardiol 55:9A–14A
37. Parmley WW (1989) Pathophysiology and current therapy of congestive heart failure. J Am Coll Cardiol 13:771–785
38. Pfeffer J, Pfeffer M (1988) Angiotensin converting enzyme inhibition and ventricular remodeling in heart failure. Am J Med 84:37–44
39. Pfeffer JM, Pfeffer MA, Braunwald E (1985) Influence of chronic captopril therapy on the infarcted left ventricle of the rat. Circ Res 57:84–95
40. Pfeffer J, Pfeffer M, Braunwald E (1987) Hemodynamic benefits and prolonged survival with long-term captopril therapy in rats with myocardial infarction and heart failure. Circulation 75:I149–I155
41. Pfeffer MA, Pfeffer JM, Fishbein MC, Fletcher PJ, Spadaro J, Kloner RA, Braunwald E (1979) Myocardial infarct size and ventricular function in rats. Circ Res 44:503–512
42. Pfeffer JM, Pfeffer MA, Fletcher PJ, Braunwald E (1984) Ventricular performance in rats with myocardial infarction and failure. Am J Med 76:99–103
43. Pfeffer M, Pfeffer J, Steinberg C, Finn P (1985) Survival after an experimental myocardial infarction: Beneficial effects of long-term therapy with captopril. Circulation 72:406–412
44. Raya TE, Gay RG, Aguirre M, Goldman S (1989) Importance of venodilatation in prevention of left ventricular dilatation after chronic large myocardial infarction in rats: a comparison of captopril and hydralazine. Circ Res 64:330–337
45. Rubin SA, Fishbein MC, Swan HJC (1983) Compensatory hypertrophy in the heart after myocardial infarction in the rat. J Am Cell Cardiol 1:1435–1441
46. Schwartz A, Lindenmayer GE, Allen JC (1975) The sodium-potassium adenosine triphosphate: pharmacological, physiological and biochemical aspects. Pharmacol Rev 27:3–134
47. Selye H, Bajusz E, Grasso S, Mendell P (1960) Simple techniques for the surgical occlusion of coronary vessels in the rat. Angiology 11:398–407
48. Stanton RC, Brenner BM (1986) Role of the kidney in congestive heart failure. Acta Med Scand (S) 707:21–25
49. Tsunoda K, Hodsman GP, Sumithran E, Johnston CI (1986) Atrial natriuretic peptide in chronic heart failure in the rat: a correlation with ventricular dysfunction. Circ Res 59:256–261
50. Zimmer H-G, Martius PA, Marschner G (1989) Myocardial infarction in rats: effects of metabolic and pharmacologic interventions. Basic Res Cardiol 84:332–343

Authors' address:

Prof. Dr. Naranjan S. Dhalla
Division of Cardiovascular Sciences
St. Boniface General Hospital Research Centre
351 Tache Avenue
Winnipeg, Manitoba
Canada R2H 2A6

Myocardial fibrosis: role of ventricular systolic pressure, arterial hypertension, and circulating hormones *

K. T. Weber, C. G. Brilla, J. S. Janicki, H. K. Reddy, and S. E. Campbell

Division of Cardiology, University of Missouri, Columbia, Missouri, USA

Summary: The myocardium contains myocyte and non-myocyte cells. A disproportionate growth of the nonmyocyte cell population can alter myocardial structure and lead to pathologic hypertrophy. Myocardial fibrosis, the result of cardiac fibroblast growth or abnormal accumulation of fibrillar collagen within the interstitial space, can adversely influence myocardial stiffness and ultimately ventricular function. We have examined the relative importance of ventricular systolic and arterial pressures and the effector hormones of the renin-angiotensin – aldosterone system in mediating this reactive fibrous tissue response in the hypertensive left and normotensive right ventricles in various experimental models of arterial hpertension. To date, our findings implicate arterial hypertension, together with an elevation in plasma aldosterone, as being contributory to the fibrosis in renovascular hypertension that creates tissue heterogeneity in either ventricle and impaired diastolic function. The endocrine properties of aldosterone in this nonclassical mineralocorticoid target tissue, the myocardium, requires further investigation.

Key words: Myocardial fibrosis; diastolic stiffness; cardiac hypertrophy; aldosterone; hypertension

Introduction

It is well recognized that the myocardium is composed of cardiac myocytes. Less well appreciated is its population of nonmyocyte cells (1). The growth of myocyte and non-myocyte cells, such as may occur with cardiovascular disease, must be balanced if myocardial structure is to remain normal (1). Myocyte hypertrophy is expressed as an increase in cell length or width. It is the common denominator to the increment in myocardial mass that defines ventricular hypertrophy irrespective of cause. Myocyte hypertrophy and accordingly, ventricular hypertrophy are adaptive responses that accompany exercise training and enhance cardiac performance. Myocyte hypertrophy also occurs in many different disease states, where left ventricular hypertrophy (LVH) is oftentimes the primary risk factor associated with the appearance of myocardial failure (2). Why is it then, that in the athlete myocyte growth and LVH prove adaptive, while in the patient they often lead to myocardial failure? Perhaps, it is the growth of nonmyocyte cells, rather than myocyte hypertrophy that accounts for pathologic LVH in the patient with cardiovascular disease.

Nonmyocyte cells include endothelial and vascular smooth muscle cells, cardiac fibroblasts, macrophages, and mast cells. Their growth, or the consequences of their growth, can adversely alter myocardial structure. For example, the growth of endothelial and smooth muscle cells, expressed as an increment in their number (i.e., hyperplasia) and/or size (i.e., hypertrophy) can lead to intimal and medial thickening of in-

* This work was supported in part by NIH grant R01-31701 and Deutsche Forschungsgemeinschaft Br-1029-2.

tramyocardial coronary arteries and arterioles, respectively. The consequences of fibroblast growth, represented by a mitogenic response with cell proliferation, can account for the accumulation of type-I and type-III fibrillar collagens in the interstitium and adventitia of intramural vessels. Hence, the relative proportions of myocyte and nonmyocyte cell growth will determine whether a departure in normal myocardial structure occurs which is expressed as tissue heterogeneity. It has been previously suggested that it is the loss of tissue homogeneity, created by disproportionate growth between myocyte and nonmyocyte cells, that distinguishes adaptive from pathologic myocardial hypertrophy (3). In the postmortem hypertrophied human left ventricle that accompanies hypertension, a significant increase in myocardial collagen concentration has been observed (4, 5). This disproportionate accumulation of collagen was evident within the cardiac interstitium and was not simply scar tissue.

Over the past decade, this laboratory has addressed the role of the cardiac interstitium, or extracellular space of the myocardium, in mediating pathologic hypertrophy. The interstitium, by definition, contains the nonmyocyte cell population of the myocardium. It can be a dynamic participant in the hypertrophic remodeling of the myocardium seen in various disease states (4–6) as evidenced by the disproportionate accumulation of fibrillar collagen that creates tissue heterogeneity. The consequences of this fibrosis are to adversely raise myocardial diastolic stiffness (7–9) and to eventuate in ventricular dysfunction (10). The pathogenetic basis of myocardial fibrosis is therefore of considerable interest. Various hemodynamic and/or hormonal factors may be involved in mediating the fibrous tissue response. Herein, we review a series of experimental studies (11–13) that addressed these issues and suggest that ventricular systolic pressure is the major determinant of myocyte growth, while arterial hypertension, together with an elevation in circulating aldosterone (ALDO), are associated with myocardial fibrosis.

Myocardial fibrosis: role of elevations in ventricular systolic and arterial pressures and circulating renin-angiotensin-aldosterone system

A reactive myocardial fibrosis (vis a vis a reparative fibrosis that presents after myocyte necrosis as an in-series addition of scar tissue between viable myocytes) has been observed in the hypertrophied left ventricle in the nonhuman primate and rat with renovascular hypertension (7–9, 14–16). The associated rise in collagen volume fraction, or collagen concentration, was found to begin within the adventitia of intramyocardial coronary arteries and subsequently extend into the interstitial space. The resultant perivascular and interstitial fibrosis was found to be progressive over time (17, 18) and to raise the stiffness of myocardial tissue (18) and the diastolic stiffness of the intact ventricle (7, 8).

These findings prompted us to examine whether a) the hypertrophic process that accompanied arterial hypertension was itself responsible for the fibrous tissue response or, alternatively, b) renovascular hypertension (RHT), which represented an elevation in ventricular systolic and coronary perfusion pressures, together with an activation of the renin-angiotensin-aldosterone (RAA) system, was a special circumstance. Thus the relative importance of the elevation in left ventricular systolic pressure, arterial hypertension, and the activation of the RAA system remained to be determined. Toward this end, we undertook several in vivo studies in the rat, where the contribution of these variables could be addressed.

In the first study, Brilla et al. (11) reasoned that these issues could be addressed by considering the *in-series* and *in-parallel* arrangements of the right and left ventricles. On one

Table 1. Arterial hypertension, left ventricular hypertrophy, myocardial fibrosis, and circulating angiotensin II and aldosterone in various experimental models

Model	HT/LVH	FIB	A II/ALDO
RHT	++/+	+	↑/↑
IRB	++/+	−	→/→
ALDO/hi Na+	++/+	+	↓/↑
Unineph/hi Na+	−/+	−	→/→
ALDO/lo Na+	−/−	−	↑↑/↑↑
RHT+C	−/−	−	↓/↓
RHT+S	+/+	−	↑/↑

Notation: Animal models abbreviated as in the text. HT = hypertension, defined as a significant rise in systolic and mean arterial pressures over control; LVH = left ventricular hypertrophy, based on the left to right ventricular weight ratio being statistically greater than control and where right ventricular weight was no different from control in all experimental groups; FIB = interstitial and perivascular fibrosis defined as a statistically significant rise in collagen volume fraction over control; A II and ALDO = plasma angiotensin II and aldosterone concentrations, respectively; ++ = systolic blood pressure >180 mm Hg while + = 150–160 mm Hg; ↑↑ = plasma aldosterone >100 ng/dl while ↑ = 60–100 ng/dl; ↓ = plasma level <20 ng/dl (normal = 20–30 ng/dl).

hand, the right and left ventricles are connected to each other by the pulmonary circulation. This *in-series* configuration would distinguish the role of ventricular systolic pressure in arterial hypertension, where the normotensive right ventricle serves as a negative internal control compared to the hypertensive left ventricle. Alternatively, their common coronary circulation creates an *in-parallel* configuration to the ventricles, making each susceptible to elevations in coronary perfusion pressure and plasma concentrations of angiotensin II (AII) and/or ALDO.

This logic was applied to the following experimental models of arterial hypertension: a) abdominal aorta banding with unilateral renal ischemia, or RHT; b) infrarenal abdominal aortic banding (IRB); and c) the chronic administration of ALDO (0.75 mg/kg/sc by osmotic minipump) in previously uninephrectomized animals maintained on enhanced dietary sodium. As a control to this latter group with hyperaldosteronism, uninephrectomized animals were placed on a high sodium diet, but the implanted minipump did not contain ALDO. Plasma concentrations of AII and ALDO were quite different in each of these models (see Table 1): in RHT, each was increased; with IRB their plasma concentrations remained normal; with ALDO administration, plasma AII was suppressed while plasma ALDO was increased; and with uninephrectomy and high dietary sodium, where ALDO administration was withheld, plasma AII and ALDO were each normal.

We found comparable elevations in arterial pressure associated with an equivalent degree of LVH in the RHT, IRB, and ALDO models. A modest degree of LVH was seen in uninephrectomized animals on high sodium diet without ALDO in their minipumps; these animals, however, remained normotensive despite the associated circulatory overload. Right ventricular weight was unchanged in each of these models and comparable to unoperated controls.

In the hypertrophied left ventricle that accompanied RHT and hyperaldosteronism, we found an abnormal rise in interstitial and perivascular collagen volume fraction. This was not the case for IRB or the ALDO control group, where myocardial collagen concentration remained normal. Of particular interest, the reactive myocardial fibrosis was also found in the normotensive, nonhypertrophied right ventricle in RHT and ALDO; this was not the case with IRB or the ALDO control model. Thus, collagen accumulation can occur in the absence of myocyte hypertrophy.

The findings of this study led us to conclude that ventricular systolic pressure was responsible for myocyte growth and LVH, which was found in each model of arterial hypertension. Given that right ventricular weight was unchanged in all models, we further concluded that elevations in coronary perfusion pressure did not cause myocyte hypertrophy in the right ventricle, despite previous inferences drawn from studies of myocardial protein synthesis in the isolated heart (19). Finally, it was clear that elevations in either left ventricular systolic or coronary perfusion pressures were not responsible for the abnormal fibrous tissue response unless there was an associated activation of the RAA system. Hence, we suggested that arterial hypertension, together with elevations in plasma AII and/or ALDO, were involved in mediating the interstitial and perivascular fibrosis that appeared in the nonhypertrophied right and hypertrophied left ventricles in unilateral renal ischemia and hyperaldosteronism.

Myocardial fibrosis: role of elevations
in circulating angiotensin II vs. aldosterone

In a subsequent in vivo study, Brilla et al. (12, 13) and Jalil et al. (20) sought to distinguish the relative importance of arterial hypertension from the elevation in circulating AII and/or ALDO, as well as to differentiate the role of AII and ALDO. The following models were created in uninephrectomized rats to address these issues: a) chronic administration of ALDO, with the hypertension that accompanies hyperaldosteronism dissociated from the elevation in circulating ALDO by providing one group of animals with enhanced dietary sodium while another received a restricted sodium diet (ALDO/low Na^+); b) rats with RHT pretreated with the angiotensin converting enzyme (ACE) inhibitor captopril (C; 100 mg/kg po); and c) rats with RHT pretreated with the ALDO antagonist spironolactone (S; 20 mg/kg/day sc).

Comparable levels of arterial hypertension and LVH were found when ALDO or DOCA administration included supplemental dietary sodium (see Table 1). This was not the case for the ALDO-treated animals on a sodium-restricted diet or the animals with RHT pretreated with C, where arterial hypertension and LVH were not seen. For the dose of S selected, S-treated animals with RHT had only a modest reduction in arterial pressure, and as a result, we did not prevent LVH in this group.

A diverse profile in plasma AII and ALDO concentrations was purposefully created in these models (see Table 1). Plasma ALDO was elevated in the high-sodium diet group receiving ALDO and rose even further in those given ALDO together with a low-sodium diet, while circulating AII was suppressed in the former and increased in the letter. Plasma AII and ALDO were both suppressed following DOCA administration and with C pretreatment in RHT; each of these hormones remained elevated in the RHT group pretreated with S.

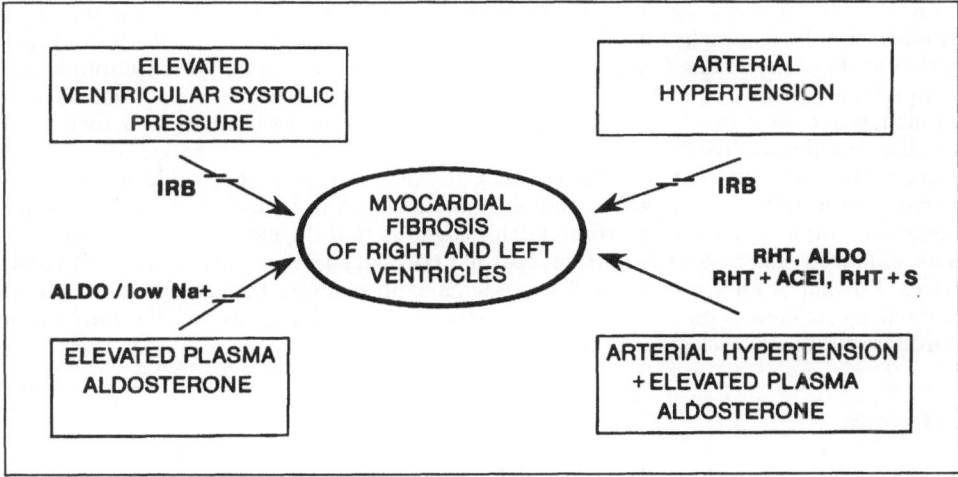

Fig. 1. Various hemodynamic and hormonal factors, acting alone or in combination, may lead to myocardial fibrosis of the ventricles. This interstitial fibrosis and perivascular fibrosis of intramyocardial coronary arteries, however, has only been observed in animal models where arterial hypertension is accompanied by an elevation in plasma aldosterone. Therefore, we would conclude that elevations in ventricular systolic pressure, arterial pressure, or plasma angiotensin II or aldosterone alone are not responsible. The various models which have led us to this conclusion are identified next to each variable. (Abbreviations are defined in the text.)

Interstitial and perivascular fibrosis were observed in the hypertrophied left ventricle that accompanied ALDO administration with enhanced dietary sodium. Collagen volume fraction due to this reactive fibrosis was not elevated in normotensive animals receiving ALDO under conditions of sodium deprivation, or in RHT groups pretreated with C or S.

These findings, therefore, have led us to conclude that arterial hypertension, together with an elevation in plasma ALDO, was responsible for the interstitial and perivascular fibrosis (see Fig. 1). Elevations in plasma ALDO alone, without hypertension, did not lead to the abnormal fibrous tissue response. These recent findings would require us to modify our previous supposition regarding the importance of circulating AII (21). However, the importance of plasma AII remains to be clarified, particularly since previous reports from other laboratories indicate that AII can alter endothelial cell structure and permeability of intramyocardial and systemic arteries (22–26).

Arterial hypertension and hydrostatic pressure within intramyocardial coronary arteries and the microcirculation

The importance of arterial hypertension on the intramural coronary circulation is frequently debated. Unlike systemic arterioles, it has been presumed (22, 23) that elevations in arterial pressure are not transmitted to the intramural coronary circulation because of their compression by myocardial contraction. It is of interest, however, that Laine (27) observed an increase in coronary permeability in the dog with renovascular hypertension. Given our view that hypertension (and hormones) is in some manner contributory to myocardial fibrosis, we have chosen to explore this issue more fully. In preliminary studies, Reddy has measured cardiac lymph flow and protein concentration during pharmacologically-induced elevations in arterial pressure. Based on the assumption that lymph is in dynamic equilibrium with the interstitial space and its tissue fluid, this approach was selected to address whether arterial hypertension would lead to an increment in microcirculatory hydrostatic pressure and, thereby, alter fluid exchange between the intravascular and interstitial compartments. It was observed that a 1–2 h increment in mean arterial pressure was associated with an elevation in lymph flow without an increase in lymph protein concentration. This suggests that the elevation in arterial pressure is indeed transmitted to intramyocardial coronary arteries, arterioles, and capillaries. Further studies are required to systematically address the long-term effects of arterial hypertension on coronary microvascular permeability, as well as intramural coronary endothelial cell structure and function.

References

1. Weber KT, Brilla CG, Pick R, Janicki JS, Silver MA (1991) Cell biology of myocardial remodeling: contribution of nonmyocyte cells. J Vas Med Biol (in press)
2. Kannel WB (1989) Epidemiological aspects of heart failure. In: Weber KT (ed) Congestive Heart Failure. Cardiol Clin 7:1–9
3. Weber KT, Clark WA, Janicki JS, Shroff SG (1987) Physiologic versus pathologic hypertrophy and the pressure-overload myocardium. J Cardiovasc Pharmacol 10:537–549
4. Pearlman ES, Weber KT, Janicki JS, Pietra G, Fishman AP (1982) Muscle fiber orientation and connective tissue content in the hypertrophied human heart. Lab Invest 46:158–164
5. Huysman JAN, Vliegen HW, Van der Laarse A, Eulderink F (1989) Changes in nonmyocyte tissue composition associated with pressure overload of hypertrophic human hearts. Pathol Res Pract 184:577–581
6. Weber KT (1989) Cardiac interstitium in health and disease: the fibrillar collagen network. J Am Coll Cardiol 13:1637–1652
7. Doering CW, Jalil JE, Janicki JS, Pick R, Aghili S, Abrahams C, Weber KT (1988) Collagen network remodeling and diastolic stiffness of the rat left ventricle with pressure overload hypertrophy. Cardiovasc Res 22:686–695
8. Jalil JE, Doering CW, Janicki JS, Pick R, Shroff SG, Weber KT (1989) Fibrillar collagen and myocardial stiffness in the intact hypertrophied rat left ventricle. Circ Res 64:1041–1050
9. Jalil JE, Doering CW, Janicki JS, Pick R, Clark WA, Weber KT (1988) Structural vs contractile protein remodeling and myocardial stiffness in hypertrophied rat left ventricle. J Mol Cell Cardiol 20:1179–1187
10. Weber KT, Janicki JS, Pick R, Capasso J, Anversa P (1990) Myocardial fibrosis and pathologic hypertrophy in the rat with renovascular hypertension. Am J Cardiol 65:1G–7G
11. Brilla CG, Pick R, Tan LB, Janicki JS, Weber KT (1990) Remodeling of the rat right and left ventricle in experimental hypertension. Circ Res 67:1355–1364
12. Brilla CG, Pick R, Janicki JS, Weber KT (1990) Myocardial fibrosis in either renovascular or mineralocorticoid hypertension (abstract). Clin Res 38:588A
13. Brilla CG, Pick R, Janicki JS, Weber KT (1990) Myocardial fibrosis in experimental hypertension: potential role of fibroblast corticoid receptors (abstract). J Hypertens (Suppl 3):S8
14. Abrahams C, Janicki JS, Weber KT (1987) Myocardial hypertrophy in macaca fascicularis: structural remodeling of the collagen matrix. Lab Invest 56:676–683
15. Weber KT, Janicki JS, Shroff SG, Pick R, Chen RM, Bashey RI (1988) Collagen remodeling of the pressure-overloaded, hypertrophied nonhuman primate myocardium. Circ Res 62:757–765
16. Pick R, Janicki JS, Weber KT (1989) Myocardial fibrosis in nonhuman primate with pressure overload hypertrophy. Am J Pathol 135:771–781
17. Silver MA, Pick R, Brilla CG, Jalil JE, Janicki JS, Weber KT (1990) Reactive and reparative fibrosis in the hypertrophied rat left ventricle. Cardiovasc Res 24:741–747

18. Thiedemann KU, Holubarsch C, Medugorac I, Jacob R (1983) Connective tissue content and myocardial stiffness in pressure overload hypertrophy. A combined study of morphologic, morphometric, biochemical and mechanical parameters. Basic Res Cardiol 78:140–155
19. Morgan HE, Gordon EE, Kira Y, Siehl DL, Watson PA, Chua BHL (1985) Biochemical correlates of myocardial hypertrophy. Physiologist 28:18–27
20. Jalil JE, Janicki JS, Pick R, Weber KT (1991) Coronary vascular remodeling and myocardial fibrosis in the rat with renovascular hypertension: response to captopril. Am J Hypertens (in press)
21. Weber KT, Janicki JS (1989) Angiotensin and the remodeling of the myocardium. Br J Clin Pharmacol 28:141S–150S
22. Giacomelli F, Anversa P, Wiener J (1976) Effect of angiotensin-induced hypertension on rat coronary arteries and myocardium. Am J Pathol 84:111–125
23. Bhan RD, Giacomelli F, Wiener J (1978) Ultrastructure of coronary arteries and myocardium in experimental hypertension. Exp Mol Pathol 29:66–81
24. Engler E, Matthias D, Becker CH (1980) Pathomorphological reactions of myocardium and intramural vessels of rats in the course of hypertension induced by depot angiotensin. Autoradiographic, light and electron microscopic investigations. Exp Pathol 18:37–51
25. Wiener J, Lattes RG, Meltzer BG, Spiro D (1969) The cellular pathology of experimental hypertension. IV. Evidence for increased vascular permeability. Am J Pathol 54:187–207
26. Wiener J, Giacomelli F (1973) The cellular pathology of experimental hypertension. VII. Structure and permeability of the mesenteric vasculature in angiotensin-induced hypertension. Am J Pathol 72:221–240
27. Laine GA (1988) Microvascular changes in the heart during chronic arterial hypertension. Circ Res 62:953–960

Authors' address:

Prof. Dr. K. T. Weber
Division of Cardiology
Room 432 Medical Science Building
University of Missouri, Columbia
Columbia, MO 65212
USA

Effects of nifedipine and moxonidine on cardiac structure in spontaneously hypertensive rats (SHR) - Stereological studies on myocytes, capillaries, arteries, and cardiac interstitium *

G. Mall, D. Greber, H. Gharehbaghi, G. Wiest, K. Amann, and T. Mattfeldt

Department of Pathology, University of Heidelberg, FRG

Summary: Light and electron microscopic stereological studies were performed on the myocardium of spontaneously hypertensive rats (SHR) before and after treatment with nifedipine (27 mg/kg b.w./day) and the sympatholytic agent moxonidine (8 mg/kg b.w./day). The treated groups were compared with nontreated SHR and normotensive WKY (n = 10 in each group).

When the therapy was started in 6-month old male SHR, blood pressure was increased and left ventricular hypertrophy had developed. On the other hand, pathologic changes of myocardial structure were not observed. After 3 months, the nontreated hypertensive rats showed cardiac fibrosis (volume density of fibrosis +45%), activation and proliferation of interstitial cells (volume density of nonvascular interstitium +240%), media hypertrophy of small arteries (total volume of arterial media in the left ventricle +180%), reduced capillarization (length density of capillaries −11%), as well as focal degeneration of myocytes at the ultrastructural level.

Both treatments showed similar effects on blood pressure, degree of hypertrophy, and cardiac structure. Blood pressure as well as degree of hypertrophy were significantly reduced (relative left ventricular weights: −25% and −16%). As far as myocardial fibrosis, capillarization, and regressive changes of myocytes are concerned a complete normalization was observed. Microarteriopathy and activation of nonvascular interstitial cells (first step in development of interstitial myocardial fibrosis) were significantly suppressed by therapy (total media volume −40%, volume density of nonvascular interstitium −38%), but the normal level of the normotensive control could not be maintained (+70%, +111% vs WKY). This may be due to the slightly elevated systolic blood pressure despite therapy (+25%, vs WKY) or to hormonal factors in SHR which are independent of blood pressure.

Since nifedipine and moxonidine are pharmacologically different drugs with different effects on sympathetic activity, one may cautiously conclude that increase in blood pressure itself is an important determinant of arterial, interstitial as well as myocellular alterations which are related to the pathogenesis of hypertensive heart muscle disease.

Key words: Spontaneously hypertensive rat; cardiac fibrosis; capillarization; nifedipine; moxonidine

Introduction

Arterial hypertension is a frequent disorder in modern industrial societies and contributes significantly to the high cardiovascular mortality (34).

Pathomorphological changes of hypertensive hearts are not only caused by coronary atherosclerosis, but also by pathologic reactions of the myocytes, capillaries, arteries, and the endomysial collagenous network (19, 21, 28, 30, 45, 47, 51). Therefore, antihypertensive therapy should not only consider the decrease in blood pressure, but also cardiac structure. Since arterial hypertension is the result of a complex dysfunction of blood pressure regulation, drug-induced lowering of blood pressure will not necessarily prevent from hypertensive heart muscle disease.

---

* With support of the "Deutsche Forschungsgemeinschaft" (ma-912/1–3) and Fa. Giulini.

Recent clinical investigations of hypertensive patients showed a decrease of left ventricular mass after antihypertensive treatment with Ca-antagonists, ACE-inhibitors, sympatholytic agents as well as β-blockers (12–14, 17, 40, 48).

Treatment of spontaneously hypertensive rats (SHR) with Ca-antagonists and ACE-inhibitors showed a reduction of myocardial fibrosis (7, 35, 42).

The present study was assigned in order to compare the effects of a Ca-antagonist (nifedipine) and a new sympatholytic agent (moxonidine). Cardiac structure was analyzed by means of new quantitative stereological techniques.

Experimental model of hypertrophy regression

Six-month-old male spontaneously hypertensive rats (SHR) were treated either with the Ca-antagonist nifedipine or with the new sympatholytic agent moxonidine for 3 months.

Both drugs were added to food-pellets from Altromin (Lage, FRG). The dosage was 27 mg/kg b.w. nifedipine/day and 8 mg/kg b.w. moxonidine/day. Systolic blood pressure was determined plethysmographically under slight ether narcosis. Age-matched normotensive male Wistar-Kyoto-rats (WKY) were introduced as control group.

Quantitative morphologic investigations of the hearts were performed after fixation by perfusion via the aorta abdominalis on paraffin sections and plastic sections (Epon-Araldite). For electron microscopy, ultrathin sections were used as described elsewhere (29, 30). Paraffin sections were stained with SIRIUS-red for collagen and with a modified silver-enhancement technique for arterial walls (52), and the semithin sections were stained with methylene blue and basic fuchsin.

Quantitative stereological investigations were done according to standard techniques. In addition, some new methods, which had been recently developed in our laboratory, were employed (20, 29, 33, 52).

Volumes and lengths of the following myocardial structures were determined (referred to the left ventricle including septum ventriculorum):
– Total volume of myocytes (V_{myo});
– total length of intramyocardial arteries (L_{art});
– total media volume of intramyocardial arteries (V_{med});
– total volume of fibrosis (V_{fib});
– total volume of nonvascular interstitium (V_{int}).

The following stereological parameters of myocardial structure were determined:
– Volume density (volume per unit reference volume, symbol V_V) of nonvascular interstitium, myofibrils, mitochondria, and free sarcoplasm;
– length density (length per unit reference volume, symbol L_V) of capillaries and of intramyocardial arteries.

In addition, V_V fibrosis was obtained by means of an automatic image-analyzing system (IBAS II, Kontron, Eching, FRG) using Sirius red-stained paraffin sections.

Results

Two animals of the non-treated SHR-group died from cerebral hemorrhage, whereas in the treated group and in the normotensive control croup there were no deaths. Systolic blood pressure was decreased by both treatments (Tables 1 and 2), and the degree of hypertrophy was reduced (decreased left ventricular weight, reduced total volume of left ventricular myocytes).

Table 1. Systolic blood pressure, heart- and body weights

Variables before treatment

Group	SP mmHg	BW (g)	HW (g)	HW/BW (mg/g)	LVW (g)	LVW/BW (mg/kg)	LVW/HW (%)
SHR	228	255	1.34	5.30	1.09	4.30	81
	± 31	± 32	±0.10	±0.36	±0.08	±0.31	± 2
WKY	116*	367*	1.48*	4.03*	1.10	3.00*	74*
	± 16	± 21	±0.12	±0.14	±0.06	±0.09	± 4

Arithmetic mean ± standard deviation; *: $p < 0.05$, Student's t-test.
SP: systolic blood pressure; BW: body weight; HW: heart weight; HW/BW: heart weight/body weight; LVW: left ventricular weight; LVW/BW: left ventricular weight/body weight; LVW/HW: left ventricular weight/heart weight.

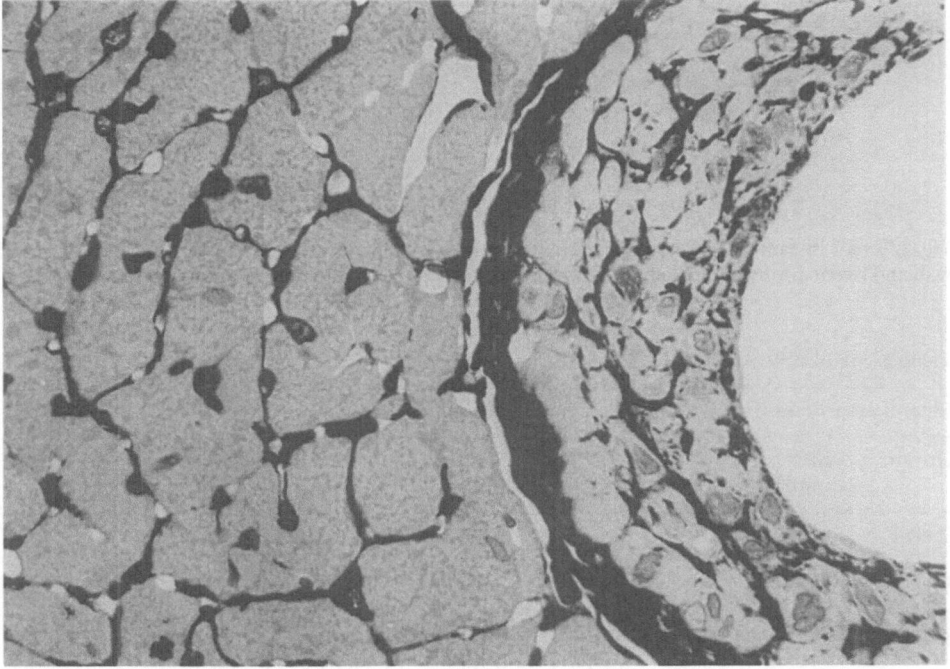

Fig. 1. Silver-stained paraffin section of the myocardium of a spontaneously hypertensive rat with media thickening and hypertrophy of smooth muscle cells (*microarteriopathy*). Light microscopic magnification 600 : 1

In nontreated hypertensive animals the media of intramyocardial arteries was considerably thickened (Figs. 1, 2), interstitial myocardial fibrosis had developed, and myocardial scarring (Figs. 3, 4) was occasionally detected.

Quantitative stereological parameters provided evidence that microarteriopathy (total media volume of the left ventricle) and myocardial fibrosis (volume density of fibrosis,

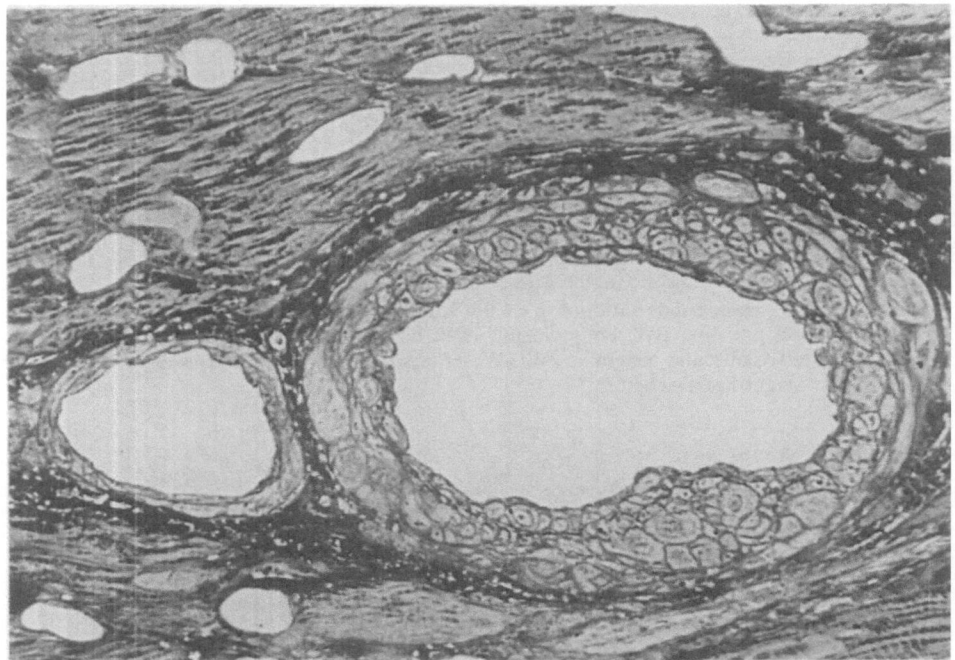

Fig. 2. Small intramural artery of a spontaneously hypertensive rat with thickening of the arterial wall and hypertrophy of media cells. Semithin section (1 µm), light microscopic magnification 640:1

Table 2. Systolic blood pressure, heart- and body weights

Figures after treatment (4 groups)

Group	SP mmHg	BW (g)	HW (g)	HW/BW (mg/g)	LVW (g)	LVW/BW (mg/kg)	LVW/HW (%)
SHR-K	193+	308+	1.55+	5.03+	1.25+	4.06+	81+
	± 39	± 24	±0.13	±0.26	±0.1	±0.97	± 3
SHR-N	144*+	308+	1.27*	4.15*	1.07*	3.48*+	84+
	± 21	± 32	±0.09	±0.23	±0.08	±0.19	± 2
SHR-M	144*+	310+	1.32*	4.16*	1.04*	3.36*+	79+
	± 14	± 12	±0.09	±0.26	±0.05	±0.12	± 5
WKY	116*	367*	1.37*	3.73*	0.97*	2.64*	71*
	± 16	± 53	±0.18	±0.29	±0.14	±0.09	± 4

Arithmetic mean $\pm$ standard deviation; *: $p < 0.05$ vs SHR-K (Scheffe test); +: $p < 0.05$ vs WYK (Scheffe test).

SP: systolic blood pressure; BW: body weight; HW: heart weight; HW/BW: heart weight/body weight; LVW: left ventricular weight; LVW/BW: left ventricular weight/body weight; LVW/HW: left ventricular weight/heart weight.

SHR-K: nontreated hypertensive rats; SHR-N: Nifedipine-treated hypertensive rats; SHR-M: Moxonidine-treated hypertensive rats; WKY: normotensive WKY group.

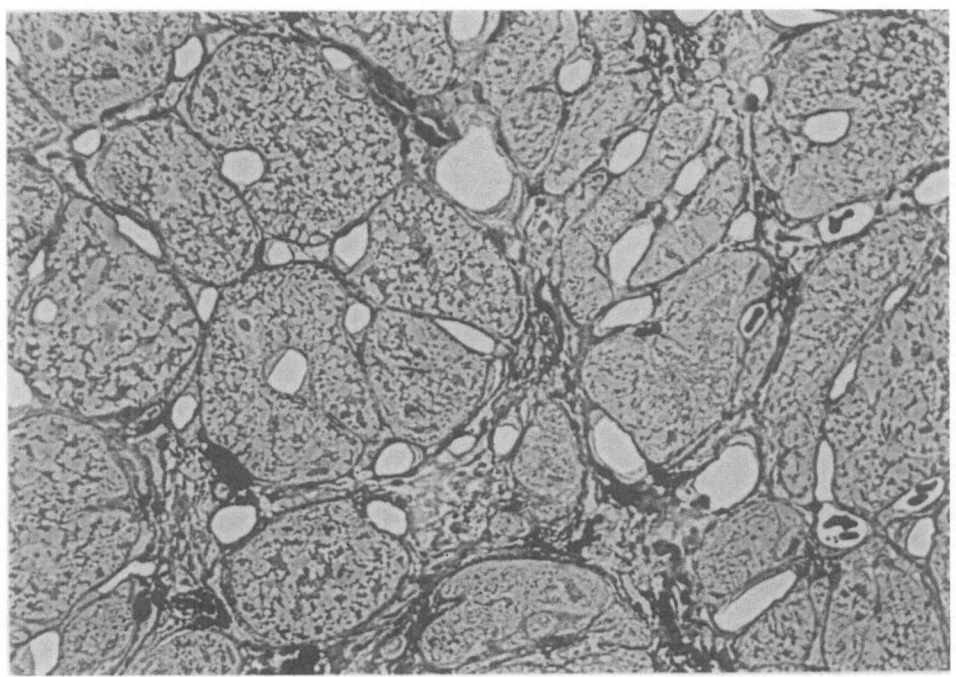

Fig. 3. Interstitial myocardial fibrosis of a spontaneously hypertensive rat. Fibrosis is locally pronounced and causes atrophy of some myocytes. Semithin section, magnification 950:1

Table 3. Stereological parameters at the beginning of the study

Fibrosis, myocellular volume, capillarization (2 groups)

Group	$V_V$int (mm^3/mm^3)	$L_V$cap (mm/mm^3)	V myocytes (mm^3)	V interstitium (mm^3)
SHR	0.028	3321	952	30
	±0.008	± 309	± 74	± 9
WKY	0.023	3344	961	24
	±0.008	± 124	± 56	± 8

Arithmetic mean ± standard deviation; no significant differences (Student's t-test).
Lack of significant differences in capillarization are explained by missing differences in left ventricular weights (see Table 1) (resulting from the different body weights of SHR and WKY).
$V_V$int : volume density of nonvascular interstitium; $L_V$cap: length density of capillaries; V myocytes: total volume of myocytes in the left ventricle; V interstitium: total volume of nonvascular interstitium in the left ventricle.

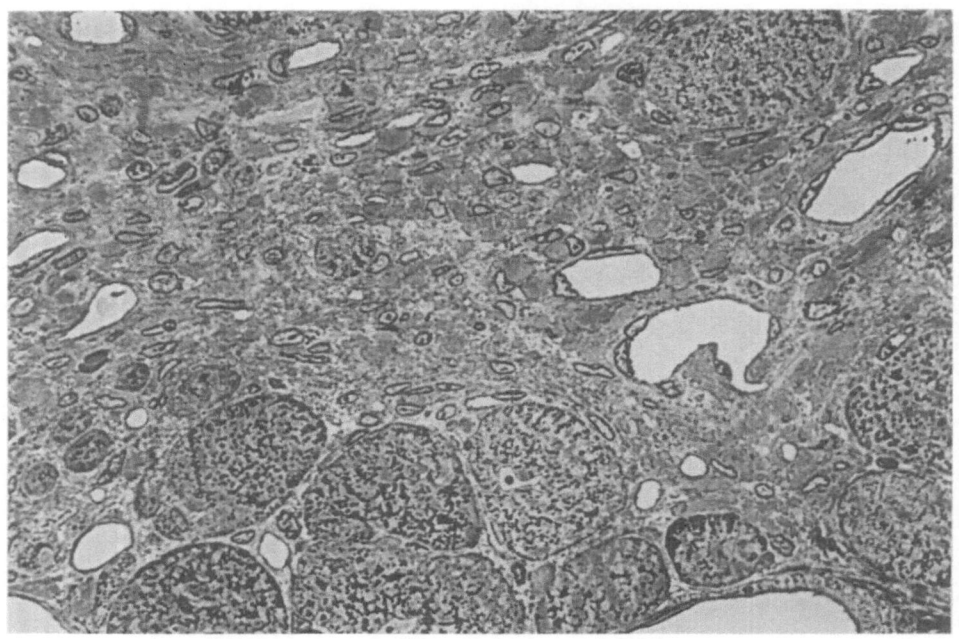

Fig. 4. Extensive myocardial scarring of a spontaneously hypertensive rat. Reparative fibrosis is indicated by the granulation tissue. Semithin section, magnification 950:1

Table 4. Myocytes and interstitium after therapy

Group	V_{myo} (mm³)	V_{int} (mm³)	V_{fib} (mm³)	V_V int (mm³/mm³)	V_V fib (mm³/mm³)
SHR-K	1 022	93	32	0.088	0.026
	± 64	±38	± 8	±0.034	±0.007
SHR-N	912[+]	58[+]	20[+]	0.056[+]	0.019[+]
	± 60	±18	± 3	±0.015	±0.003
SHR-M	884[+]	53[+]	20[+]	0.053[+]	0.019[+]
	± 43	±13	± 3	±0.013	±0.003
WKY	894[+]	26[+]	17[+]	0.026[+]	0.018[+]
	± 80	± 6	± 4	±0.004	±0.004

Arithmetic mean ± standard deviation.
Multiple comparisons according to Dunnett (11): [+] $p < 0.05$ vs. SHR-K.
V_{myo}: total volume of myocytes of left ventricle; V_{int}: total volume of nonvascular interstitium of left ventricle; V_{fib}: total volume of fibrosis of left ventricle; V_V int: volume density of nonvascular interstitium; V_V fib: volume density of fibrosis.
SHR-K: nontreated hypertensive rats; SHR-N: Nifedipine-treated hypertensive rats; SHR-M: Moxonidine-treated hypertensive rats; WKY: normotensive WKY group.

Table 5. Vascular parameters after therapy

Group	L_V cap (mm/mm^3)	V media (mm^3)	L art (mm)	L_V art (mm/mm^3)
SHR-K	2787	1.68	4780	3.88
	± 250	±0.68	± 527	±0.27
SHR-N	3648[+]	1.01[+]	4130[+]	3.88
	± 354	±0.46	± 344	±0.29
SHR-M	3364[+]	1.03[+]	4092[+]	3.97
	± 251	±0.36	± 268	±0.21
WKY	3127[+]	0.53[+]	4029[+]	4.16
	± 261	±0.17	± 678	±0.49

Arithmetic mean ± standard deviation.
Multiple comparisons according to Dunnett (11): [+] p < 0.05 vs. SHR-K.
L_V cap: length density of capillaries; V media: total volume of arterial media in the left ventricle; L art: total length of arteries in the left ventricle; L_V art: length density of arteries.
SHR-K: nontreated hypertensive rats; SHR-N: Nifedipine-treated hypertensive rats; SHR-M: Moxonidine-treated hypertensive rats; WKY: normotensive WKY group.

volume density of nonvascular interstitium) were significantly reduced after therapy (Tables 4, 5). Furthermore, capillary supply (length density of capillaries) was normalized (Tables 5). It should be emphasized that media hypertrophy of intramural arteries was not associated with a pathological increase in the total length of arteries (Table 5). Elongation of the arterial tree in nontreated SHR did not exceed the physiologic growth of arteries during adolescence.

If SHR and WKY are compared, the left ventricular weights do not indicate the degree of hypertrophy, since WKY grow faster, resulting in significant differences of body weights of age-matched animals. Therefore, the degree of hypertrophy was assessed by the ratio of left ventricular weight to body weight (relative left ventricular weight). At the beginning of the study, a +44% left ventricular hypertrophy was found and at the end of the experiment a +54% hypertrophy. Oral therapy with nifedipine and moxonidine reduced the degree of hypertrophy to +30% (Tables 1, 2). Since myocardial collagen, especially in cases of fibrosis, contributes to left ventricular weights, total volume of left ventricular myocytes/100 g b.w. was used as an additional indicator of hypertrophy. However, even this parameter established the above-mentioned conclusions.

If the total media volume of the arteries and the volume density of nonvascular interstitium before and after drug therapy are compared with the control group, both parameters were slightly increased despite therapy (Tables 4, 5). It should be emphasized that volume density of nonvascular interstitium was normal in the SHR-group at the beginning of the study and that arteries showed a regular morphology at this point of time.

Volume density of myocardial fibrosis and length density of capillaries ("capillarization") were completely normalized by therapy (Table 4, 5). Furthermore, capillary supply tended to be increased after nifedipine-treatment when compared with the normotensive control.

Ultrastructure of myocytes was grossly normal in SHR with and without drug therapy. In nontreated SHR a focal degeneration of myocytes with atrophy and loss of myofibrils was observed (Fig. 5), but not in treated SHR. This corresponds to the slightly decreased volume density of myofibrils in nontreated SHR (data not shown in detail).

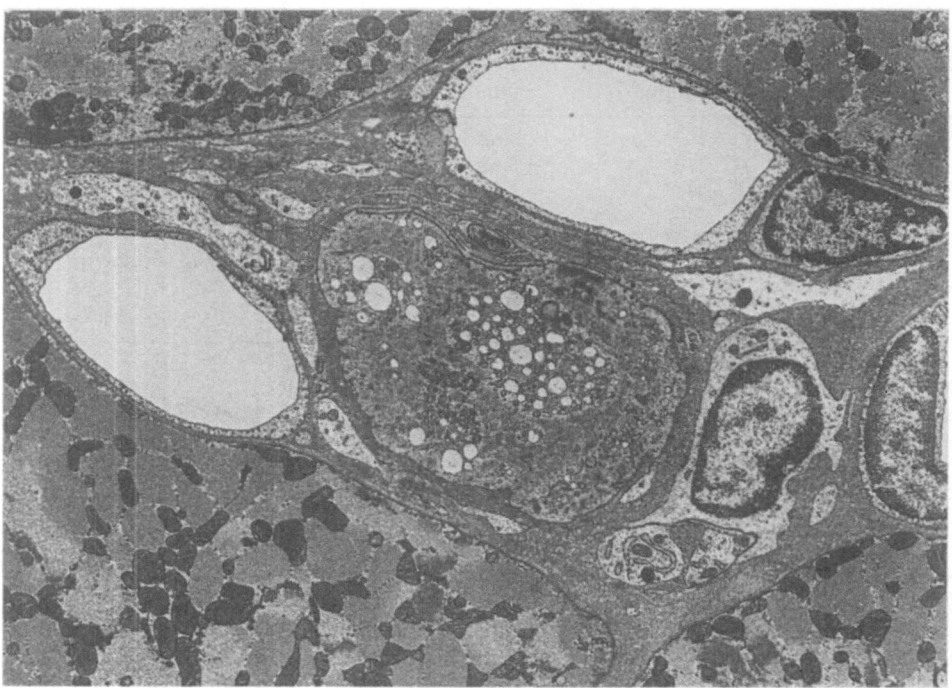

Fig. 5. Myocardial cross-section of a spontaneously hypertensive rat. At the edges of the electron micrograph regular myocytes are observed. In the middle capillaries, mesenchymal cells (pericytes, fibroblasts, fibrosis) as well as an atrophic myocyte are seen (note the vesiculation of the sarcoplasm). Electron microscopic magnification 4000 : 1

Furthermore, the stereological parameters indicate absence of myocellular edema in all groups. This supports the conclusion that decrease in left ventricular weights is due to a true hypertrophy regression and not to prevention from edema.

Discussion

Antihypertensive treatment with nifedipine and moxonidine leads, not only to a reduction in blood pressure and a reduction in the degree of myocardial hypertrophy, but also to a significant protection of myocardial structure. Beneficial influences on fibrosis, interstitial cell activation, media hypertrophy of arteries, and capillary supply could be established with quantitative stereological methods.

It is remarkable that both drugs induced a similar extent of blood-pressure reduction which was associated with comparable effects on the degree of cardiac hypertrophy and on myocardial structure. This is surprising because of the different pharmacology of the drugs. Ca-antagonists tend to activate the sympathetic system indirectly via drug-induced vasodilatation, whereas moxonidine decreases sympathetic activity. The similar protective effects of both drugs support the hypothesis that the level of blood pressure itself is one important determinant of hypertensive heart muscle disease. However, a complete protection of myocardial structure was not observed despite therapy. For example, the nonvascular interstitial space was slightly expanded. It is suggested that this finding corresponds to the first step in developing interstitial fibrosis (31, 32).

On the other hand, "true" cardiac fibrosis, which was assessed on SIRIUS-red stained sections, was completely prevented by therapy. Thus, our data agree with reports on biochemically determined hydroxyproline (collagen) levels after nifedipine (35) therapy and after lisinopril application (7). In contrast, development of myocardial fibrosis could not be inhibited after blood pressure reduction with hydralazine (37). Interstitial fibrosis should be distinguished from reparative fibrosis (scarring) after myocyte necrosis (2, 51). However, progressive thickening of collagen bundles also induces myocyte atrophy, necrosis, and scarring. Another possible mechanism which may cause myocardial scarring in hypertension is the disturbed microcirculation due to microarteriopathy. Severe myocardial fibrosis enhances systolic and diastolic stiffness of the heart (22, 37, 47, 50). At final stages of hypertensive heart muscle disease structural dilatation with left ventricular systolic dysfunction may occur (8, 9).

With respect to media hypertrophy of arteries and the activation of nonvascular interstitium which both could not completely be prevented by therapy, different possible mechanisms should be considered:

1) Since systolic blood pressure and degree of hypertrophy remain slightly increased despite therapy, it cannot be precluded that the changes are related to the persistent blood-pressure elevation. However, recent experiments on rats with mild renovascular hypertension provided evidence that significant interstital changes (28) did not occur even after 6 months.

2) It cannot be precluded that genetic differences exist between SHR and WKY (23).

3) The reactions of the interstititum may be modified by systemic and local factors such as angiotensin II or aldosterone (6, 7). This point of view is supported by recent experimental and autoptic findings that the hypertensive myocardial fibrosis occurs even in right ventricles where hemodynamic overload (16) is absent.

In order to introduce a reliable quantitative characterization of microarteriopathy, we determined the total volume of intramural arteries as well as the total arterial length in the left ventricle. These stereological parameters seem to be superior to the frequently described ratio of wall thickness to lumen diameter which is influenced by the tone of the media smooth muscle cells. According to qualitative morphological observations the increase in media volume is caused by hypertrophy of media cells. Whether there also exists hyperplasia, as shown for mesenteric vessels in SHR (36), is not yet known for intramyocardial coronary arteries.

Eisenlohr and coworkers (15) found a positive effect of nifedipine-treatment on the degree of media hypertrophy in SHR, too. Even application of ACE-inhibitors protected from microarteriopathy as well as from decreased capillary supply (10). At present, numerous investigations have been published on the interactions of blood pressure and arterial walls. These studies indicate that pathologic changes of arteries are not strongly correlated with the blood pressure, and one should consider the experimental model of hypertension as well as the anatomical site of the arteries under study. For example, ACE-inhibitors completely normalize the morphology of the carotids in rats with renovascular hypertension, but not in SHR (25).

In contrast to the excessive increase in media volume in nontreated SHR the length increase of arteries was similar to the physiologic growth of arteries in adolescent rats (52). With respect to capillaries, nifedipine treatment tends to increase capillarity beyond normal levels. This may result from nifedipine-induced dilatation of resistance vessels. The protective effects of therapy on the structure of microvessels corresponds to clinical and experimental findings that microcirculatory disturbances (38, 44) can be prevented with antihypertensive drugs, e.g., nifedipine and ACE-inhibitors (10, 41).

In summary, both drugs led to a similar reduction of systolic blood pressure and regression of hypertrophy as well as to normalization of capillary supply and prevention of fibrosis. The development of microarteriopathy and the activation of nonvascular interstitial cells (presumably the first step of interstitial fibrosis) were significantly suppressed. All pathological alterations of myocardial structure in nontreated SHR were beneficially influenced by therapy.

References

1. Aalkjaer C, Eiskjaer H, Mulvany MJ, Jespersen B, Kjaer T, Sorensen SS, Pedersen EB (1989) Abnormal structure and function of isolated subcutaneous resistance vessels from essential hypertensive patients despite antihypertensive treatment. J Hypertension 7:305–310
2. Abrahams C, Janicki JS, Weber KT (1987) Myocardial hypertrophy in Macaca fascicularis – Structural remodeling of the collagen matrix. Lab Invest 56:676–683
3. Agabiti-Rosei E, Muiesan ML, Geri A, Romanelli G, Beschi M, Castellano M, Muiesan G (1988) Long-term antihypertensive treatment may induce normalization of left ventricular mass before complete regression of vascular structural changes: consequences for cardiac function at rest and during stress. J Hypertension 6:94–96
4. Anderson PG, Bishop SP, Digerness SB (1989) Vascular remodeling and improvement of coronary reserve after hydralazine treatment in spontaneously hypertensive rats. Circ Res 64:1127–1136
5. Anderson PG, Bishop SP, Digerness SB (1988) Coronary vascular function and morphology in hydralazine treated DOCA salt rats. J Mol Cell Cardiol 20:955–976
6. Brilla CG, Pick R, Janicki JS, Weber KT (1990) Myocardial fibrosis in experimental hypertension: potential role of fibroblast corticoid receptors. J Hypertension 8:IC 31 (abstract)
7. Brilla CG, Janicki JS, Weber KT (1990) Kardioprotektive Effekte von Lisinopril bei arterieller Hypertonie. Z Kardiol 79 (suppl 1):130
8. Capasso JM, Robinson TF, Anversa P (1989) Alterations in collagen cross-linking impair myocardial contractility in the mouse heart. Circ Res 65:1657–1664
9. Capasso JM, Palackal T, Olivetti G, Anversa P (1990) Left ventricular failure induced by long-term hypertension in rats. Circ Res 66:1400–1412
10. Clozel J-P, Kuhn H, Hefti F (1989) Effects of chronic ACE inhibition on cardiac hypertrophy and coronary vascular reserve in spontaneously hypertensive rats with developed hypertension. J Hypertension 7:267–275
11. Dunnett CW (1955) A multiple comparison procedure for comparing several treatments with a control. J Amer Statist Assoc 54:613–621
12. Dzhumagulova AS, Abdykadyrov UD, Mirrakhimov MM (1989) Comparison of selective beta-blockers and calcium antagonists in essential hypertension. Cardiovasc Drugs 3 (suppl 2):583 (abstract)
13. Eichstaedt H, Richter W, Baeder M, Cordes M, Langer M, Felix R, Schmutzler H (1989) Demonstration of hypertrophy-regression with magnetic resonance tomography under the new adrenergic inhibitor moxonidine. Cardiovasc Drugs 3 (suppl 2):583 (abstract)
14. Eichstaedt H, Richter W, Baeder M, Cordes M, Felix R, Schmutzler H (1989) Darstellung der Hypertrophie-Regression unter Gabe des neuen adrenergen Inhibitors Moxonidin durch magnetische Resonanztomographie (MR). Z Kardiol 78:61 (abstract)
15. Eisenlohr H, Klepzig M, Schmiebusch H, Strauer BE (1989) Hypertensive koronare Mikroangiopathie – Therapieinduzierte Regression der Mediahypertrophie in koronaren Widerstandsgefäßen. Cor Vas 3:72–77
16. Fein FS, Cho S, Zola BE, Miller B, Factor SM (1989) Biventricular damage with right ventricular predominance. Am J Pathol 134:1159–1166

17. Fouad FM, Nakashima Y, Tarazi RC, Salcedo EE (1982) Reversal of left ventricular hypertrophy in hypertensive patients treated with methyldopa. Am J Cardiol 49:795–801
18. Harper SL (1987) Antihypertensive drug therapy prevents cerebral microvascular abnormalities in hypertensive rats. Circ Res 60:229–237
19. Jacob R (1976) Different fractions in the normal and hypertrophied rat ventricular myocardium: an analysis of two models of hypertrophy. Basic Res Cardiol 71:608–623
20. Jalil JE, Doering CW, Janicki JS, Pick R, Shroff SG, Weber KT (1989) Fibrillar collagen and myocardial stiffness in the intact hypertrophied rat left ventricle. Circ Res 64:1041–1050
21. Klepzig M, Eisenlohr H, Steindl S, Schmiebusch H, Strauer B (1987) Media hypertrophy in hypertensive coronary resistance vessels. J Cardiovasc Pharmacol 10:97–102
22. Krayenbühl HP, Hess OM, Monrad ES, Schneider J, Mall G, Turina M (1989) Left ventricular myocardial structure in aortic valve disease before, intermediate and late after aortic valve replacement. Circulation 79:744–755
23. Kurtz TW, Morris RC (1987) Biological variability in Wistar-Kyoto rats. Implications for research with the spontaneously hypertensive rat. Hypertension 10:127–131
24. Laine GA (1988) Microvascular changes in the heart during chronic arterial hypertension. Circ Res 62:953–960
25. Levy BI, Michel J-B, Salzmann JL, Azizi M, Poitevin P, Camilleri JP, Safar ME (1988) Arterial effects of angiotensin converting enzyme inhibition in renovascular and spontaneously hypertensive rats. J Hypertension 6 (suppl 3):23–25
26. Liu J, Bishop SP, Overbeck HW (1988) Morphometric evidence for non-pressure-related arterial wall thickening in hypertension. Circ Res 62:1001–1010
27. Stacy DL, Prewitt RL (1989) Effects of chronic hypertension and its reversal on arteries and arterioles. Circ Res 65:869–879
28. Mall G, Mattfeldt T, Hasslacher C, Mann J (1986) Morphologic reaction patterns in experimental cardiac hypertrophy. Basic Res Cardiol 81:193–201
29. Mall G, Schikora I, Mattfeldt T, Bodle R (1987) Dipyridamole-induced capillary neoformation in the rat heart – a quantitative stereological study on papillary muscles. Lab Invest 57:86–93
30. Mall G, Klingel K, Hasslacher C, Mann J, Mattfeldt T, Baust H, Waldherr R (1987) Synergistic effects of diabetes mellitus and renovascular hypertension on the rat heart – stereological investigations on papillary muscles. Virchow's Archiv A 411:531–542
31. Mall G, Rambausek M, Neumeister A, Kolmar S, Vetterlein F, Ritz E (1988) Myocardial interstitial fibrosis in experimental uremia – potential implications for cardiac compliance. Kidney Int 33:804–811
32. Mall G, Huther W, Schneider J, Lundin P, Ritz E (1990) Diffuse intermyocardiocytic fibrosis in uremic patients. Nephrol Dial Transplant 5:39–44
33. Mattfeldt T, Mall G, Gharehbaghi H, Möller P (1990) Estimation of surface area and length with the orientator. J Microsc 159:301–317
34. McKee PA, Castelli WP, McNamara PM, Kannel WB (1971) The natural history of congestive heart failure: the Framingham study. N Eng J Med 285:1441–1446
35. Motz W, Strauer BE (1989) Left ventricular function and collagen content after regression of hypertensive hypertrophy. Hypertension 13:43–50
36. Mulvany MJ, Baandrup U, Gundersen HJG (1985) Evidence for hyperplasia in mesenteric resistance vessels of spontaneously hypertensive rats using a 3-dimensional disector. Circ Res 57:794–800
37. Narayan S, Janicki JS, Shroff SG, Pick R, Weber KT (1989) Myocardial collagen and mechanics after preventing hypertrophy in hypertensive rats. Am J Hypertens 2:675–682
38. Opherk D, Mall G, Zebe H, Schwarz F, Weihe E, Manthey J, Kübler W (1984) Reduction of coronary reserve: a mechanism for angina pectoris in patients with arterial hypertension and normal coronary arteries. Circulation 69:1–7
39. Plunkett WC, Overbeck HW (1988) Arteriolar wall thickening in hypertensive rats unrelated to pressure or sympathoadrenergic influence. Circ Res 63:937–943
40. Ram CVS (1989) Regression of left ventricular hypertrophy in hypertension with alpha-adrenergic blockade: physiological basis and therapeutic implications. J Hypertension 7 (suppl 6):98–99

41. Reed VR, Tuma RF (1986) The effects of nifedipine on regional vascular resistance and blood flow in the spontaneously hypertensive rat. Clin Exper Theor Pract A8:963–979
42. Sen S, Bumpus FM (1979) Collagen synthesis in development and reversal of cardiac hypertrophy. Am J Card 44:954–958
43. Smeda JS, Lee RM, Forrest JB (1988) Prenatal and postnatal hydralazine treatment does not prevent renal vessel wall thickening in SHR despite the absence of hypertension. Circ Res 63:534–542
44. Strauer BE (1983) Das Hochdruck-Herz. Springer, Berlin Heidelberg New York
45. Tanaka M, Fujiwara H, Onodera T, Wu D-J, Hamashima Y, Kawai C (1986) Quantitative analysis of myocardial fibrosis in normals, hypertensive hearts, and hypertrophic cardiomyopathy. Br Heart J 55:575–581
46. Tomanek RJ, Schalk KA, Marcus ML, Harrison DG (1989) Coronary angiogenesis during long-term hypertension and left ventricular hypertrophy in dogs. Circ Res 65:352–359
47. Thiedemann K-U, Holubarsch C, Medugorac I, Jacob R (1983) Connective tissue content and myocardial stiffness in pressure overload hypertrophy – a combined study of morphologic, morphometric, biochemical, and mechanical parameters. Basic Res Cardiol 78:140–155
48. Tsoporis J, Leenen FHH (1988) Effects of arterial vasodilators on cardiac hypertrophy and sympathetic activity in rats. Hypertension 11:376–386
49. Vial JH, Boyd GW (1989) Histometric assessment of renal arterioles during DOCA and post-DOCA hypertension and hydralazine treatment in rats. J Hypertension 7:203–209
50. Weber KT, Janicki JS, Shroff SG, Pick R, Chen RM, Bashey RI (1988) Collagen remodeling of the pressure-overloaded, hypertrophied nonhuman primate myocardium. Circ Res 62:757–765
51. Weber KT (1989) Cardiac interstitium in health and disease: the fibrillar collagen network. J Am Coll Cardiol 13:1637–1652
52. Wiest G (1990) Die Längenzunahme der arteriellen Gefäße im Rattenherzen während des physiologischen Wachstums. Inaug Diss Heidelberg

Authors's address:
Professor Dr. G. Mall
Pathologisches Institut
Im Neuenheimer Feld 220/221
W-6900 Heidelberg, FRG

Principal considerations on the stroke volume-heart size relationship based on different heart models

R. W. Gülch, B. Dierberger, and M. Brändle

Physiologisches Institut II der Universität Tübingen, FRG

Summary: The aim of the present study was to show by hemodynamic investigations in a rat heart and by theoretical considerations based on different heart models that a chronic enlargement of the heart does not necessarily lead to an impairment of the stroke volume. In the experiments performed on rat hearts of various sizes, in situ pressure-volume diagrams were obtained which clearly demonstrate that, in principle, larger hearts are able to eject larger stroke volumes despite the fact that for geometrical reasons, they have to develop higher wall stress. These findings are supported by calculations of stroke volume-heart size relations being based on the assumption of different geometrical models for the left ventricle. By means of these relations, when applying them to pressure-volume data of a dilated or failing heart, it is in principle possible to differentiate between effects of altered geometry and of altered contractility. A simple lever-pump system is introduced which is appropriate to simulate transmission aspects in the transformation of myocardial shortening into ventricular ejection for hearts of variable size.

Key words: Stroke volume; heart size; heart model; rat heart; dilatation

Introduction

The influence of ventricular geometry on cardiac output as a result of chronic change in ventricular size is one feature of cardiac dynamics which has been ignored for quite a long time and which is now slowly finding increasing significance in connection with studies or discussions about chronic alterations in heart size. In this context, the opinion has become firmly established (especially in the clinic) that according to Linzbach's concept (9), a chronic enlargement of the heart without a sufficient increase in wall thickness must necessarily lead to impaired cardiac performance. This conclusion is based on the generally accepted fact that, for constant filling pressure, the wall stress increases with increasing ventricular volume. As a first approximation this can already be predicted with the simple Laplace relationship originally derived for a thin-walled sphere. But even on the basis of more sophisticated heart models, this fundamental statement is still valid (10, 11, 13, 14). Thus, enlarged ventricles, without sufficient increase in wall thickness, can develop a given pressure only with higher wall stress. Consequently, this means that the shortening capability of the myocardium must be reduced in the chronically enlarged hearts and that, at first sight, the enlarged ventricles will eject a reduced stroke-volume against normal aortic pressure. Referring to the ejection fraction, any enlargement of the ventricle must be considered to be even more detrimental from a clinical point of view. The present study is intended to fundamentally revise this opinion on the basis of theoretical considerations and experimental facts.

Methods

Model calculations

On the basis of different heart models (3), the aim of the calculations is to arrive at relationships between stroke volume and ventricular volume for hearts of various sizes and geometry, but under defined constant conditions of contraction. The calculations are based on left ventricular pressure-volume diagrams being obtained from hemodynamic measurements (Fig. 1 a). The end-systolic pressure-volume relations were mathematically converted into end-systolic length-tension curves, using different heart models such as a thick-walled sphere (4), rotational ellipsoid with uniform wall-thickness (12) or rotational ellipsoid with nonuniform wall-thickness (16) (Fig. 1 b). A unique end-systolic length-tension relation results for hearts of different size, but defined contractile state if all volume and length values are normalized with respect to a standard heart under optimum filling corresponding to maximum isometric pressure development. For any end-systolic wall stress being a function of ventricular volume and of intraventricular pressure, the corresponding circumferential shortening can be predicted by means of this relation. Knowing the systolic shortening of the myocardium for any heart size, one is able to calculate the resulting stroke volume to arrive finally at the stroke volume-heart size relation.

Animal experiments

All hemodynamic investigations were performed on male normotensive Wistar rats at 12 months of age, under urethane anesthesia (1.2 g urethane/kg body weight intraperitoneally). The left ventricular pressure and aortic flow were simultaneously recorded under open-chest conditions. For this purpose, the left ventricle was cannulated at the apex with a fine cannula which was connected to a fluid-filled pressure transducer. In addition, an electromagnetic flow probe was placed around the ascending aorta. The end-diastolic volume was derived from the end-diastolic pressure-volume relation which could be registered at the end of each experiment [for further details see (1, 15)].

Results and discussion

The simplified interpretation that any chronic enlargement of the heart under unchanged end-diastolic wall stress is detrimental because of a reduction in stroke-volume due to higher wall stress can be refuted by measurements demonstrated in Fig. 1. The results shown were obtained in two normotensive rats of the same age, but of different body weights and heart sizes, and the results are plotted in the form of pressure-volume diagrams, including a working loop for each heart. In both registrations, constancy of end-diastolic wall stress, wall thickness, and of contractile state have been adjusted or could be presumed. In spite of higher wall stress, the chronically enlarged heart was able to eject a greater stroke volume although the absolute and relative myocardial shortenings were reduced, as shown in the length-tension diagrams of Fig. 1 b and 1 c. Both diagrams have been calculated from the original pressure-volume relations using the formula of thick-walled sphere. Of course, the choice of the heart model is of paramount importance in this context. Calculations using more sophisticated procedures such as the Finite Element Method (FEM) are more generally applicable (2, 5) and will yield more

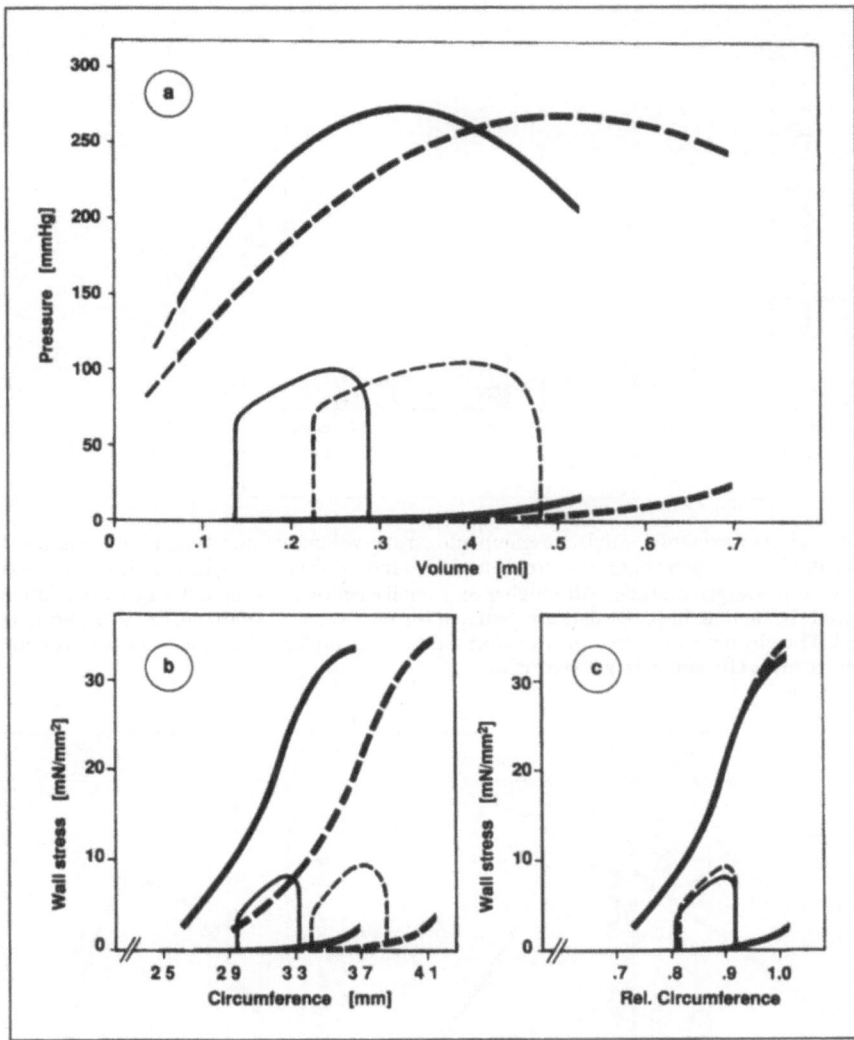

Fig. 1. Mathematical transformation of the pressure-volume diagram (a) into circumference-wall stress diagram (b) and normalized length-wall stress diagram (c). The pressure-volume diagram consisting of the end-diastolic pressure-volume relation, the curve of isovolumic maxima and a working loop is obtained from hemodynamic measurement on two quite differently sized hearts of rats of the same age. Note the enhanced stroke-volume of the larger heart under otherwise almost constant contractile conditions (dashed curves). The normalization in diagram (c) is related to the smallest heart in the whole group

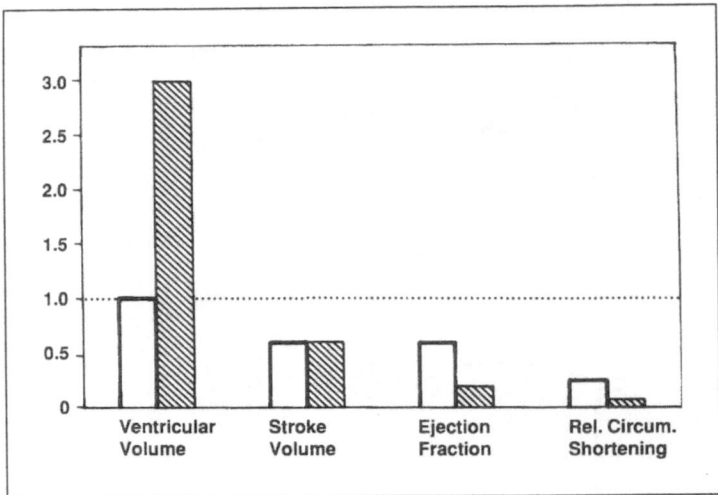

Fig. 2. Transmission of circumferential shortening into stroke-volume demonstrated for a rotational ellipsoidal ventricle. The open columns correspond to a standard ventricle of volume 1, the hatched ones to a three-times larger ventricle. Although a very small ejection fraction and very small relative circumferential shortening, in particular, are assumed for the oversized ventricle, its stroke volume is unchanged. Thereby it is shown that the transformation of circumferential shortening into volume changes is much more efficient in larger ventricles

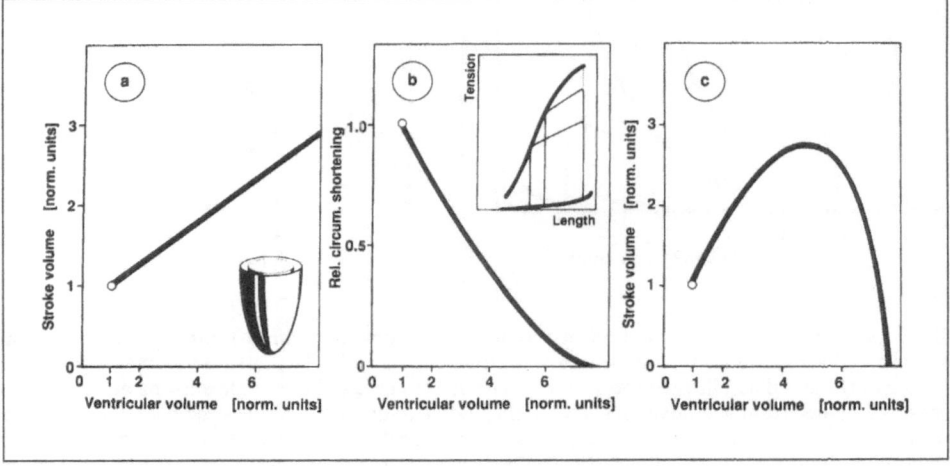

Fig. 3. Schematic illustration of two principally opposing effects on the stroke volume-heart size relation shown in diagram (c). In diagram (a) the improved transformation of a given degree of circumferential shortening into stroke volume leads to inceased stroke volumes with growing heart size. Under the assumption of constant end-systolic pressure, a reduction in circumferential shortening with increasing heart size must result due to increased wall stress (diagram b). In the inset this fact is shown in the form of a length-tension diagram with two contraction loops under different systolic wall stress conditions

reliable results. By this method, wall stress and deformation in every wall element can be calculated in the same manner, irrespective of how complex the heart geometry. We are currently carrying out these calculations.

If the length-tension diagram in Fig. 1 b is normalized with respect to a standard heart, which we selected as the heart with the smallest size in this series, the normalized length-tension diagram in Fig. 1 c results. In this case, both isometric maxima curves coincide, verifying that both hearts are in the same state of contractility. That means that a myocardial strip of identical length of either heart shows the same contractile behavior, independent of ventricular size.

The question now arises of why, in principle, larger hearts – even despite increased wall stress and, thus, limited shortening capability – are able to eject a larger stroke volume. The answer should become clear from Fig. 2. Independent of the cardiac model under consideration, one can generally deduce that a larger ventricle is in a better position to transform any circumferential shortening into volume displacement. For a sphere – but also valid for a rotational ellipsoid – shortening is calculated under the assumption of constant stroke volume. Hearts enlarged up to three times their normal size were able to eject an identical stroke volume, even with minimal circumferential shortening. Of course, the ejection fraction of the enlarged heart is also markedly reduced despite unchanged stroke volume. In the clinic a reduction in this index is often interpreted as indicating a reduced contractility which underlines once again how unreliable this index is.

It can therefore be stated that (Fig. 3):
– Larger hearts are able to more favorably transform circumferential shortening, i.e., wall displacements, into volume changes. Presuming constant relative shortening $\Delta L/L$, the stroke volume will increase with increasing ventricular volume, as shown in the diagram of Fig. 3 a.
– Chronic enlargement of the heart, however, basically leads to an increase in wall stress under constant pressure load, resulting in reduced circumferential shortening and, thus, reduced stroke volume. In the diagram of Fig. 3 b this tendency is expressed for constant endsystolic pressure.

This means in mathematical terms that any physical entity which is determined by two effects counteracting each other will exhibit a maximum. Hence, based on diagram (a) and (b), we obtain the typical stroke volume-heart size relation of Fig. 3 c. All values are normalized with respect to a standard heart size. Ascending in the range of moderate ventricular volume the relation reaches a maximum, then falls abruptly in the range of large chronic volumes. For geometrical reasons, dilatation may have a deleterious effect on stroke volume, but only in the range of the descending branch. Presuming constant wall thickness or at least insufficient increase in wall thickness and constant end-diastolic and end-systolic pressure as well as constant contractility, any further enlargement of heart size will further reduce the stroke volume in this range in the sense of a vicious circle.

The theoretical considerations can be supported impressively by the experimental findings illustrated in Fig. 4. Stroke volumes of normotensive rats of the same age are plotted as a function of their heart size expressed by the end-diastolic left ventricular volume. Each solid point represents data of a single heart. The normal biological scattering of heart size within the homogeneously aged group shows a variation of a factor of about two. As predicted by calculation, the hearts with larger ventricular volume eject larger stroke volumes. The solid curve drawn through the squared points was additionally calculated with the aid of a spherical model using the measured pressure-volume data of the whole experimental group in order to be able to extrapolate the relation to the range of higher ventricular volumes. The lower diagram shows a magnification of the volume range of interest in this series.

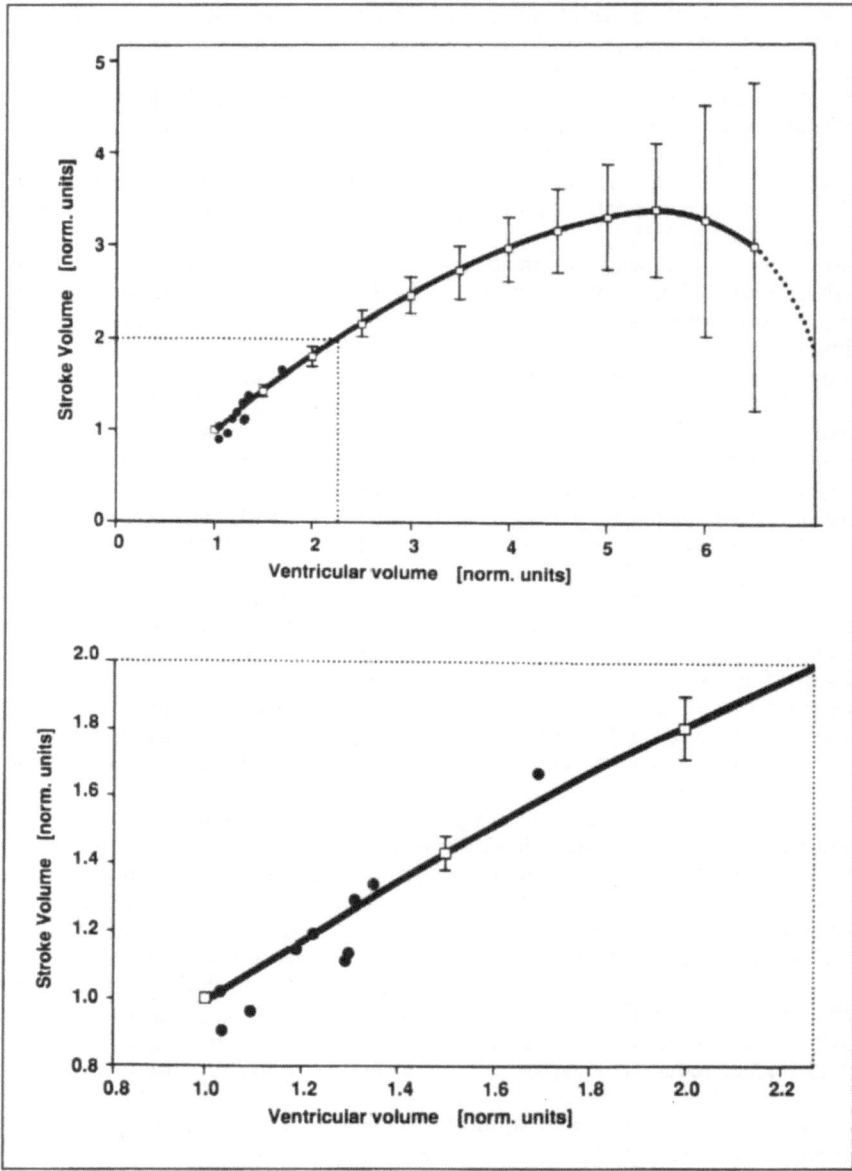

Fig. 4. Stroke volume-heart size relation based on directly measured data on normotensive rats of the same age. The solid curve is calculated on the basis of the measured data, allowing the extrapolation to larger ventricular volumes. The vertical bars symbolize the standard deviation which increases with progressive extrapolation. In the lower diagram a magnification of the volume range of interest is presented

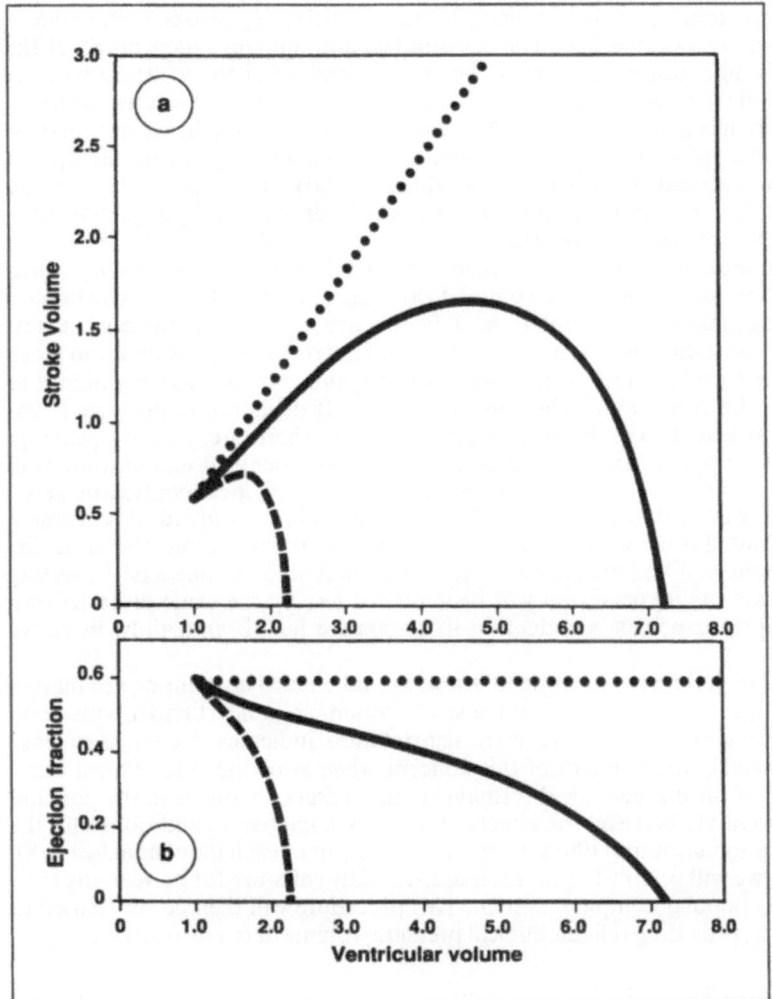

Fig. 5. The effect of wall thickness on the stroke volume-heart size relation (a) and on the ejection fraction-heart size relation (b). Three typical cases are exhibited: ——— constancy of wall thickness; ········ harmonic growth corresponding to a constant ratio of wall thickness to ventricular radius; ————dilatation characterized by constant wall volume

The degree to which wall thickness influences the stroke volume-heart size relation can be documented by the following three special cases illustrated in Fig. 5. The stroke volume is plotted as a function of ventricular volume in diagram (a), the ejection fraction in diagram (b). Under the assumption of constant wall thickness the solid lines were obtained. The stroke volume-heart size relation exhibits, as expected, a clear maximum which occurs at a radius of about 1.7 in that case. The ejection fraction decreases from the beginning. On the other hand, harmonic growth, corresponding to a constant ratio of wall thickness to ventricular radius, leads to a linearly ascending stroke volume-heart size relation plotted as a dotted line. The ejection fraction remains independent of the heart size. Typical dilatation characterized by an enlargement of the ventricle without sufficient increase in wall volume and, thus, in wall thickness generally results, however, in a considerably reduced stroke volume. The dashed stroke volume-heart size relation was calculated under the assumption of constant wall volume. In this case the critical radius of 1.2 will be reached very easily, above which any further increase will lead to an enhanced deterioration of cardiac output. The extremely dramatic fall in ejection fraction underscores this behavior in particular.

The central question with respect to clinical application of this concept is, which further factors will influence the stroke volume-heart size relations (6)? In the calculation of a single-stroke volume-heart-size relation, all factors acutely affecting the cardiac output are to be held constant. Thus, it is assumed that all hearts under consideration work against the same systolic pressure. As is well known, any pressure increase would lead to a depression in stroke volume and, thus, of the relation. If deviation in pressure is unavoidable, it can at least be corrected mathematically. Furthermore, strictly speaking, the calculation of a single relationship should be based on identical enddiastolic wall stresses to ensure identical sarcomere lengths and hence an identical contractile state. The conclusion, however, that identical wall stress corresponds to identical sarcomere length is only permitted if the wall material of the different hearts exhibits the same distensibility. For example, if fibrotic processes lead to an enhanced steepness of the resting length-tension curve, the myocardium will be stretched less by the same diastolic wall stress. The consequence will be a reduction in sarcomere length and, thus, in active shortening (8).

If all the factors or influences mentioned above are taken into account or are mathematically corrected, then any deviation in the stroke volume of a heart under consideration from the normal stroke volume-heart size relation indicates a change in contractility. This is exactly the strength of this concept when applying it to clinical questions: with the aid of the mathematical formalism outlined above, one is in the position to be able to differentiate between the effects of altered geometrical conditions and the effects of any alteration in contractile state on cardiac output of each individual heart (8). In the near future, we will be able to provide a user-friendly software for performing such calculations on any popular computer system. This procedure will then be very suited to clinical applications, providing reliable clinical pressure-volume data are available.

Conclusions

With the aid of the concept of stroke volume-heart size relations, it was intended to correct the general opinion that chronic enlargement of the heart combined with a reduction in ejection fraction should automatically be evaluated as impaired cardiac performance. Although under unfavorable energetic conditions, a chronically enlarged heart is, nevertheless, quite well in a position to eject an elevated stroke volume. The evaluation of its performance requires a much more sophisticated view to differentiate between geometrical and myocardial factors. For this reason, the mathematical formalism presented in this study seems to be a very useful instrument.

To visualize the alterations in the mechanical operation of enlarged hearts more easily, a rather simple lever-pump system is presented in Fig. 6 which is appropriate for simulating the transformation of myocardial contraction into ventricular ejection. A transmission of force S_1, i.e., of wall stress, and of displacement ΔL_1, i.e., of shortening into a dis-

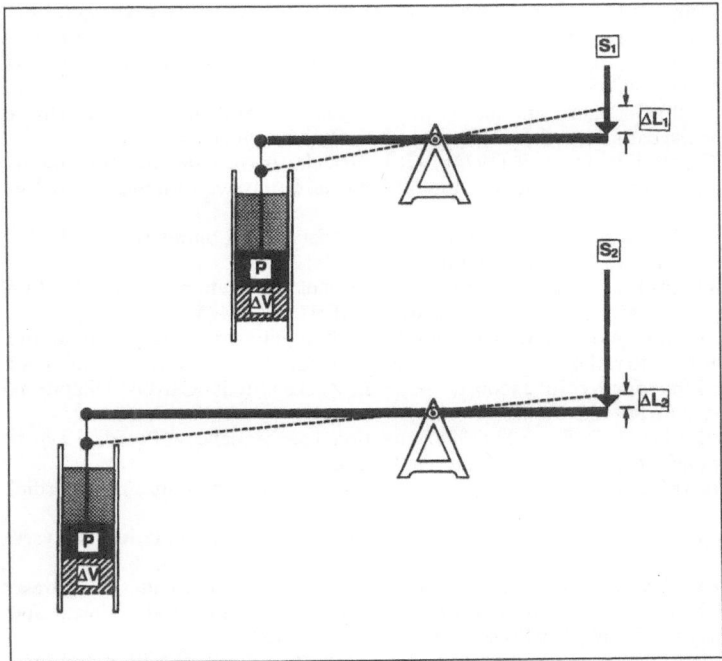

Fig. 6. Simple lever system allowing the transmission of wall stress S and shortening ΔL into pressure P and volume change ΔV. The lower case illustrates the reduction in the displacement ΔL_2 and the parallel increase in wall stress S_2 in order to displace the same volume ΔV against the same pressure P if the load arm is doubled

placement of volume ΔV against the pressure P can be accomplished by the double-armed lever. Lengthening the load arm (i.e., in our analogy equivalent to increasing ventricular radius) means, on the basis of the lever principle, that the same displacement of volume ΔV against the same pressure P requires a higher force S_2, but a reduced lever displacement ΔL_2. Thus, any enlargement of the ventricle under constant wall thickness may be interpreted as a change in the transmission characteristic of the cardiac pump:
- small-sized hearts correlate with low wall stress, but considerable shortening;
- large-sized hearts correlate with high wall stress, but little shortening.

Furthermore, the force arm of the lever can be considered to represent the influence of wall thickness. For a given pressure, any increase in wall thickness will lead to a reduction in wall stress, as would be the case with the lever force if the force arm were to be lengthened.

References

1. Brändle M (1990) Einfluß der adrenergen Stimulation und des transmembranären Ca^{2+}-Influx auf Geometrie und Pumpfunktion des chronischen druckbelasteten Herzens. PhD Thesis, Tübingen

2. Chen CJ, Kwak BM, Rim K, Falsetti HL (1980) A model for an active left ventricle deformation – Formulation of a nonlinear, quasi-steady finite element analysis for orthotropic, threedimensional myocardium. Proceeding of the International Conference on Finite Elements in Biomechanics, University of Arizona, Tucson, pp 639–655
3. Gülch RW, Jacob R (1988) Geometric and muscle physiological determinants of cardiac stroke volume as evaluated on the basis of model calculations. Basic Res Cardiol 83:476–485
4. Hepp A, Hansis M, Gülch RW, Jacob R (1974) Left ventricular isovolumic pressure-volume relations, "diastolic tone", and contractility in the rat heart after physical training. Basic Res Cardiol 5:516–532
5. Horowitz A, Perl M, Sideman S (1986) Comprehensive model for the Simulation of the left ventricular mechanics. Med Biol Comp 24:150–156
6. Jacob R, Gülch RW (1988) Functional significance of ventricular dilatation. Reconsideration of Linzbach's concept of chronic heart failure. Basic Res Cardiol 83:461–475
7. Jacob R, Gülch RW, Mall G, Voelker W, Karsch KR (1990) Significance of myocardial and geometrical factors for ventricular dynamics. Analysis demonstrated on the example of idiopathic dilative cardiomyopathy. In: Jacob R, Seipel L, Zucker I (eds) Cardiac Dilatation. Fischer Verlag, Stuttgart, pp 99–108
8. Jacob R, Brändle M, Dierberger B, Rupp H (1991) Functional consequences of cardiac hypertrophy and dilatation. Basic Res Cardiol 86 (Suppl 1):113–130
9. Linzbach AJ (1960) Heart failure from the point of view of quantitative anatomy. Am J Cardiol 5:379–382
10. Mirsky I (1973) Ventricular and arterial wall stresses based on large deformation analyses. Biophys J 13:1141–1159
11. Mirsky I (1974) Review of various theories for the valuation of the left ventricular wall stress. In: Mirsky I, Ghista DN, Sandler H (eds) Cardiac Mechanics: Physiological, Clinical and Mathematical Considerations. J Wiley & Sons, New York, pp 381–409
12. Mirsky I (1979) Elastic properties of the myocardium: a quantitative approach with physiological and clinical applications. In: Berne RM (ed) Handbook of Physiology, sec 2, The Cardiovascular System. Washington, DC, Amer Physiol Soc, pp 497–531
13. Sandler H, Dodge HT (1963) Left ventricular tension and stress in man. Circ Res 13:91–104
14. Streeter DD, Vaishnav RN, Patel DJ, Spotnitz HM, Ross J Jr, Sonnenblick EH (1970) Stress distribution in the canine left ventricle during diastole and systole. Biophys J 10:345–363
15. Vogt M, Jacob R (1985) Myocardial elasticity and left ventricular distensibility as related to oxygen deficiency and right ventricular filling. Analysis in a rat heart model. Basic Res Cardiol 80:537–547
16. Wong AYK, Rautaharju PM (1968) Stress distribution within the left ventricular wall approximated as a thick ellipsoidal shell. Am Heart J 75:649–662

Authors' address:

Prof. Dr. R. W. Gülch
Physiologisches Institut II
der Universität Tübingen
Gmelinstraße 5
W-7400 Tübingen, FRG

Part II: Biochemical, Molecular-biological and Immunological Aspects of Heart Failure

The role of adrenergic system in regulation of cardiac myosin heavy chain gene expression

M. P. Gupta [1], M. Gupta [1], and R. Zak [1,2,3]

Departments of Medicine [1], Organismal Biology & Anatomy [2]
and The Pharmacological & Physiological Sciences [3],
The University of Chicago, Illinois, USA

Summary: The cardiac phenotype exhibits considerable plasticity, being under the regulation of numerous factors, such as developmental stage, functional load, as well as nutritional and hormonal states of the animal. Several lines of evidence indicate that the adrenergic nervous system plays an important role in the redistribution of myosin isoforms in the heart. For example, chemical sympathectomy favors the expression of V_3 isomyosin at the expense of V_1. In this study, we have examined the effect of adrenergic pathways on the expression of cardiac myosin heavy chain (MHC) genes. The level of cAMP was modulated by either adding forskolin or 8-bromo-cAMP to primary cultures of embryonic (18 d) cardiac myocytes. We have found that the level of mRNA coding for MHC-α was increased two- to three-fold. The effect was dose- and time-dependent and was potentiated further when the 8-Br-cAMP was given together with a phosphodiesterase inhibitor. The same changes were found in KCl arrested cells, indicating independence of contractile activity. Treatment of cells known to activate the protein kinase C (TPA) and inositol triphosphate pathways has increased the level of β-MHC mRNA while that of α-MHC remained unchanged. These data lend strong support to direct effect of the adrenergic system on activity of cardiac genes.

Key words: Adrenergic system; cAMP; cardiac myosin; myosin isoforms; myosin heavy chain mRNA

Introduction

All the constituents of cardiac myocytes, except the nuclear RNA, are continuously turning over. The half-lives of individual proteins and of their mRNAs (6) differ widely, according to some as yet not deciphered rules. The ability of a cell to turn over, i.e., to degrade and resynthesize its constituents, is the basis for phenotypic adaptations that takes place in altered physiological and pathological states of the heart. The plasticity of muscle phenotype has its basis in multiple molecular variants of its constituting proteins (isoforms) that differ slightly in their primary structure and, in some cases, also in their functional parameters. At any given moment, the muscle cells express only a subset of its existing isoforms. Such a selection of a particular set of isoforms apparently represents one of the adaptive strategies of the myocardial cells to cope with altered demands.

The phenotypic transitions in the heart have been, so far, most extensively studied in the case of myosin which exists in three isoforms, V_{1-3}, composed of dissimilar heavy chains (MHC), α and β, that are encoded by two separate genes (19). The isoforms V_1 and V_3 are α and β MHC homodimers while the V_2 is α-β heterodimer. Multiple regulators of the MHC expression have been identified, such as thyroid hormone and hemodynamic load (3). In addition, several lines of evidence indicate that the neuroendocrine system also might play an important modulatory role. Thus, chemical sympathectomy (16), bilateral stellar ganglionectomy (8), and β-adrenergic blockade (16) favor the V_3 expression, while the V_1 is increased following injection of adrenergic agonists (4) and swimming exercise that is associated with a high adrenergic drive (16). Moreover, in nonworking heterotopically transplanted rat heart, swimming-induced increase in V_1 isoform can be prevented by pretreatment of rats with atenolol (1). That these in vivo effects of adrenergic system have, as its component, a direct effect on myocardial cells is indicated by studies of cultured cells in which β-adrenergic agonist was found to induce the expression of V_1 isoform (17) and the amount of α-MHC mRNA (22).

In contrast to the above well-documented effects, very little is known about the mechanisms by which the adrenergic system regulates cardiac gene expression. It is known, however, that organisms as diverse as bacteria and man contain genes that are transcriptionally induced in response to increased intracellular concentration of cAMP. Most of these genes share conserved DNA sequences, identified as cAMP-responsive elements, and multiple DNA binding transcription factors have been found that bind to them. Their role in cAMP-induced gene expression, however, has not yet been elucidated.

Materials and methods

Primary cultures of cardiac myocytes were prepared as described (11), with the following modifications. Hearts from 18-day-old fetal rats (Sprague-Dawley) were washed and rinsed in phosphate-buffered saline supplemented with 0.1% glucose. Minced tissue was incubated with the above solution containing 0.25% trypsin, 0.025% collagenase, 4% chicken serum, and 0.02% pancreatin. Minced hearts were digested twice, 15 min each time, and the digests discarded. Finally, the dispersed cells were collected, treated with DNase I, and resuspended in culture medium consisting of Ham's F-12 medium plus 5% calf serum. Nonmyocytes were depleted by preplating the cells suspension two times for 30 min each. Unattached cells were pelleted and resuspended in the above culture medium. Cultures generally consisted of more than 90% myocytes, as determined by staining with antimyosin antibody.

Total cellular RNA was isolated by CsCl gradient method, the final RNA pellet was resuspended in RNase-free distilled water, and its absorbance measured at 260 nm. Aliquots of RNA were immobilized on nitrocellulose filters using standard slot-blot manifold. Synthetic oligonucleotide probes complementary to isoform specific 3'-nontranslated sequences of rat α- and β-MHC mRNAs were labeled at the 5' end with ^{32}ATP and T4 polynucleotide kinase. The relative hybridization was determined after exposure to Kodak XAR film using densitometric scanning. The hybridization signal was normalized to a signal obtained with rehybridization of the filters to a 28 S ribosomal cDNA probe (human 28 S rRNA cDNA was a gift from Dr. S. Gorsk, University of Michigan).

Results

To study the effect of cAMP on the regulation of α- and β-MHC gene, we have used primary cultures of myocytes derived from hearts of 18-day-old rat fetuses. These cells predominantly expressed β-MHC, as determined both by myosin isoform electrophoretic analysis under non-denaturing conditions (17), and by measurements of mRNA. The myosin phenotype of these cells thus corresponds to that of fetal hearts (5). When the cells are treated with 10 μM forskolin or 1 mM 8-bromo-cAMP, the amount of α-MHC mRNA relative to nontreated cells was increased 300% and 200%, respectively

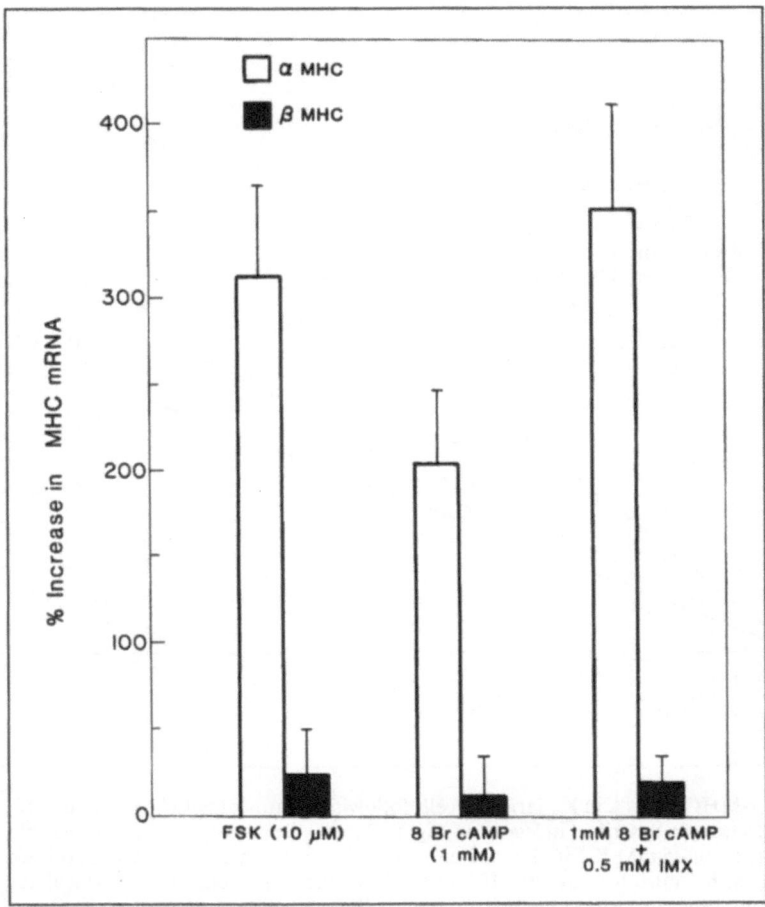

Fig. 1. Effect of different cAMP-inducing agents on the expression of α- and β-MHC mRNAs. The cells were plated at a density of 3×10^6 cell per plate into 90-mm Petri dishes that had been precoated with 0.1% gelatin. More than 90% of the cells began to contract spontaneously within 24 h after plating. The cells were cultured in Ham's F-12 medium supplemented with 5% calf serum. Forskolin was prepared as $2000 \times$ stock in absolute ethanol, 8-bromo-cAMP as $100 \times$ stock in culture medium, and 3-isobutyl-1-methylxanthine (IMX) as $500 \times$ stock in dimethylsulfoxide. Cells were grown in control and experimental media for 48 h. Total cellular RNA was prepared and analyzed by slot blot analysis using oligonucleotide probes. Values are expressed as the percentage changes from the untreated control plates. Each bar represents the mean $\pm$ S.E. cf three different experiments

(Fig. 1). The up-regulation of α-MHC mRNA steady-state level was further potentiated when 8-bromo-cAMP was present along with 0.5 mM 3-isobutyl-1-methylxanthine, a phosphodiesterase inhibitor. In contrast, under no conditions were significant changes in the abundance of the β-MHC mRNA noticed. The changes in mRNA levels were reflected in the amount of myosin isoforms, the relative amount of the V_1 being increased in treated cells [(17) and our unpublished observation].

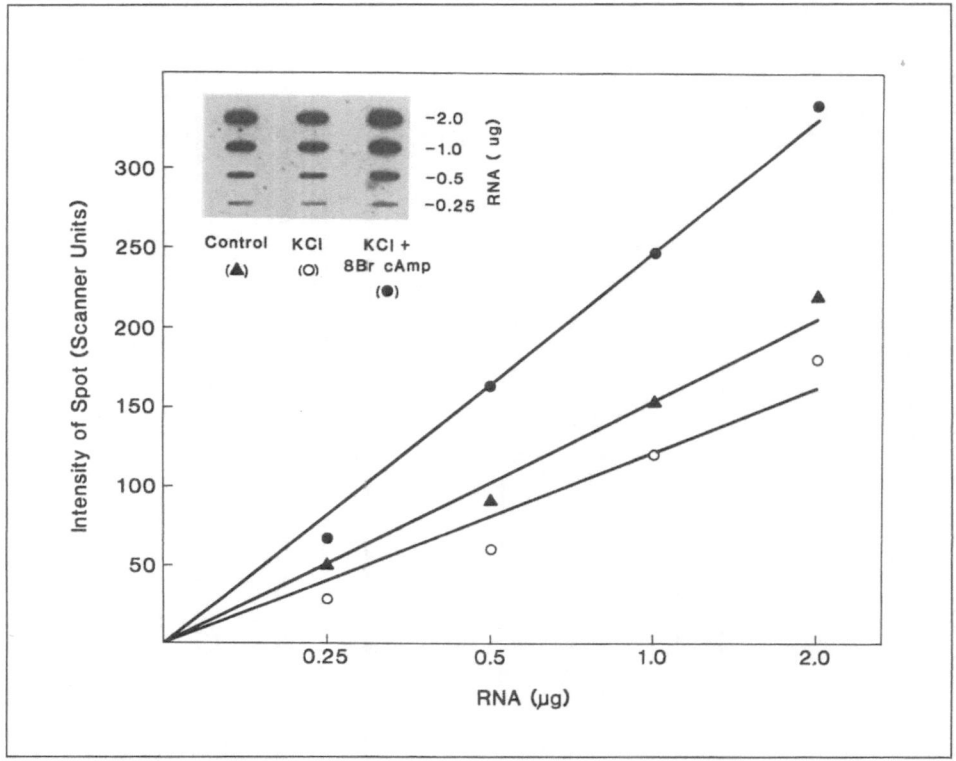

Fig. 2. Expression of α-MHC mRNA in K$^+$-arrested cells following treatment with 8-bromo-cAMP. The culture conditions were as described in legend to Fig. 1. Contractile activity of the cultured cells was arrested by inclusion of 25 mM K$^+$ in the medium. After the contractile activity was abolished the cells were treated with 1 mM 8-bromo-cAMP (8 Br cAMP) for 48 h. Total RNA was isolated and analyzed by slot blot hybridization to α-MHC specific oligonucleotide probe. Quantitation of the extent of hybridization was performed by densitometric scanning of corresponding autoradiograms. Each point represents mean of the data obtained in quadruplicate from three plates. The insert depicts original autograms for four different concentration of RNA obtained from untreated controls, potassium-arrested cells and following treatment of arrested cells with 8-bromo-cAMP

Previous reports have demonstrated that the altered contractile activity of cultured myocytes is reflected in their protein synthetic capacity, as measured by total RNA analysis and assays of protein synthesis (10). In order to determine whether the increased level of α-MHC mRNA is due to increased contractile activity resulting from adrenergic potentiation of the myocytes, we have examined the effect of cAMP in the presence of 25 mM K$^+$ in the medium; this concentration of K$^+$ is known to block contractile activity of the cells (26). As shown in Fig. 2, the effect of 8-bromo-cAMP treatment on the accumulation of α-MHC mRNA in K$^+$-arrested cells was similar to that observed in beating cells. However, the content of α-MHC mRNA is slightly less in K$^+$-arrested cells than in the untreated controls, possibly because of a decreased rate of total protein

Table 1. Effect of the treatment of TPA and A23187 on the expression of β-MHC mRNA

Treatment	Control	Treated
TPA (50 nM)	2.2 ± 0.01	4.6 ± 0.008
TPA (100 nM)	2.6 ± 0.04	5.8 ± 0.03
TPA + A23187	1.8 ± 0.08	10.6 ± 0.11
(50 nM + 2 μM)		

The values are mean of four to five experiments $\pm$ S.E. and represent arbitrary units of densitometrically scanned autoradiographs. The treatment lasted for 48 h and the culture conditions are as those described in lenged to Fig. 1. Phorbol 12-myristate-13-acetate (TPA) was prepared as $4000 \times$ stock solution in dimethylsulfoxide. The calcium inophore (A 23187) was prepared as $1\,000 \times$ stock in absolute ethanol.

synthesis (26). Nevertheless, our results suggest that contraction is not an essential requirement for cAMP-induced MHC switching.

The effect of individual treatments on the level of cAMP was verified by the competitive binding assay with Amersham cAMP kit. After treatment of cells with different agents, the media were removed from the plates and the cells were rinsed three times with 5 ml each of ice-cold phosphate-buffered saline. The cells from each plate were scraped in 1 ml of the above buffer, pelleted by centrifugation, and resuspended in 150 μl of buffer containing 4 mM EDTA and 50 mM Tris buffer pH 7.4. The basal level of cAMP in untreated cells was 2.85 pmol/plate and following treatment with 8-bromo-cAMP without or with phosphodiesterase inhibitor is increased to 30 and 50 pmol/plate, respectively.

We have also examined whether the α-adrenoreceptors play a role in determining the isomyosin composition of the heart. The cultured cells were treated either with phorbol ester (TPA) or calcium ionophore (A 23187) to activate the protein kinase C and inositol triphosphate pathways. As shown in Table 1, both agents have increased the steady state level of β-MHC mRNA, while no change was seen in the abundance of the α-MHC message (data not shown).

Discussion

The mechanism that regulates the growth response of the myocardium to altered hemodynamic load is unknown. Nevertheless, it is clear that the overloaded heart changes its size and phenotype as well. Numerous hypotheses have been proposed to explain the tight coupling between contractile activity and the growth-regulating mechanisms (3), of which the mechanical factors (9), including cell stretch (26), and catecholamines (21) have been recently investigated in some detail. Considering the complexity of the growth process and the multitude of adaptive options of the overloaded heart (7), it is likely that interplay between numerous factors is involved in regulating the gene activities in the myocardium.

The role played by the adrenergic system in the development of cardiac hypertrophy is indicated by numerous reports in which the increased hemodynamic activity has been shown to be accompanied by increased activity of cardiac sympathetic nerves [for review see (12)]. This has been reported in the case of aortic constriction, renal and desoxycorticosterone-induced hypertension, physical exercise, hypoxia and cold exposure. All of these interventions are known to produce cardiac enlargement [for review, see (3)]. Moreover, adrenal medulla denervation has been shown to prevent stress-induced cardiac hypertrophy (25).

That the hemodynamic load is not the sole factor in determining cardiac enlargement was demonstrated by experiments in which pharmacological elimination of pressure overload in spontaneously hypertensive rats does not necessarily eliminate cardiac hypertrophy (20). The interplay of several systems is also evident from the observation that catecholamines and thyroid hormone both have effects on the β-receptors (15).

As far as the effects of heart overload on the expression of specific gene is concerned, the role of more than one factor is also to be anticipated. This is because a given growth stimulus, although resulting in overall acceleration of cardiac growth, frequently upregulates the expression of only one isoform, while it downregulates that of another. For example, in the pressure-overloaded heart, during the early phase of the overload when the level of circulating catecholamine is elevated, the expression of β-MHC is upregulated while that of α-MHC remains unaltered. Later, when the catecholamine content of the heart becomes decreased (2) and down-regulation of β-adrenergic receptors takes place (15), the expression of α-MHC gradually decreases. The complexity of the adrenergic responses of the heart received their full support from in vitro studies in which synergism between α- and β-adrenergic pathways have been found. Thus, the norepinephrine-induced hypertrophy of cultured embryonic myocytes is associated with the potentiation of α-1 receptors and with upregulation of β-MHC gene expression [(21) and this study]. Increasing the level of cAMP that is associated with the β-receptors, on the other hand, leads to increased content of α-MHC (17) and its message [(22) and this study].

The functional consequence of different isoforms present in the heart is not fully understood. It is clear, however, that the shortening velocity of skinned fibers of papillary muscles correlates with myosin isoforms expressed (13). This is most likely because the actin-activated ATPase of individual isoforms differ, the V_1 having about three times higher activity that the V_3 isomyosin (14). It is also known that, in acute experiments, catecholamines increase the rate of rise in tension developed by cardiac muscle (24). Such a high rate is similar to that seen in hearts of small mammals that contain primarily the V_1 isomyosin. Our experiments demonstrate that chronic elevation of intracellular cAMP in cultured cardiac myocytes favors the expression of V_1 isoform of myosin. The β-adrenergic potentiation thus favors the expression of myosin isoform that is compatible with the high rate of rise of tension development. This shift to "faster", less efficient myosin during adrenergic stimulation also explains the observed increase in energy required to develop and maintain tension by such hearts. Matching the pattern of energy utilization to the type of myosin isoform expresses, as shown in this study to be accomplished by cAMP, might determine the nature of adaptive response of the heart. It can be envisioned that such a match or lack of it might lead to generation of other signaling molecule(s) that ensure that the responses of individual components of myocardial cells are in synchrony and appropriate for a given type of functional demand. The broad range of responses seen in adapting hearts (7) might thus have its basis in unequal generation of such signaling molecules. The characterization and isolation of individual molecules or factors will be necessary to find the links between signal transduction pathways that determine the phenotype and, hence, the functional characteristics of the heart.

References

1. Advani SV, Malhotra A, Liang D, Geener DL, Buttrick PM, Scheuer J (1985) Swimming attenuates the shift in myosin isoenzymes in the rat heterotopic cardiac isograft. Circulation 80 (Suppl II):1989

2. Borchard F (1980) Differences between transmitter depletion in human heart hypertrophy and experimental cardiac hypertrophy in Goldblass rats. Basic Res Cardiol 75:118–125
3. Bugaisky LB, Gupta MP, Gupta M, Zak R (1991) Cellular and molecular mechanisms of cardiac hypertrophy. In: Fozzard HA et al. (eds) The Heart and Cardiovascular System, 2nd ed. Raven Press, New York (in press)
4. Buttrick PM, Malhotra A, FActor S, Geener D, Scheuer J (1988) Effects of chronic dobutamine administration on hearts of normal and hypertensive rats. Circ Res 63:173–181
5. Chizzonite RA, Zak R (1984) Regulation of myosin isoenzyme composition in fetal and neonatal rat ventricle by endogeneous thyroid hormones. J Biol Chem 259:12628–12632
6. Hargrove JL, Schmidt FH (1989) The role of mRNA and protein stability in gene expression. FASEB J 3:2360–2370
7. Jacob R (1983) Chronic reactions of myocardium at the myofibrillar level. Reflections on "adaptation" and "disease" based on the biology of long-term cardiac overload. In: Jacob R et al. (eds) Cardiac Adaptation of Hemodynamic Overload, Training and Stress. Steinkopff Verlag, Darmstadt, pp 3–24
8. Kawana M, Ischizuka N, Taira A, Kimata S, Hosoda S (1989) Effects of cardiac sympathetic activity on myosin isozymes of rabbit heart. Circulation 80 (Suppl II):1839
9. Kent RL, Hoober JK, Cooper G (1989) IV. Load responsiveness of protein synthesis in adult mammalian myocardium: role of cardiac deformation linked to sodium influx. Circ Res 64:74–85
10. McDermott P, Morgan HE (1987) Contraction modulates the capacity for protein synthesis during growth of neonatal heart cells in culture. Circ Res 64:542–553
11. Nag AC, Cheng M (1984) Expression of myosin isoenzymes in cardiac-muscle cells in culture. Biochem J 221:21–26
12. Ostman-Smith I (1976) Prevention of exercise-induced cardiac hypertrophy in rats by chemical sympathectomy (Guanethidine treatment). Neurosci 1:497–507
13. Pagani ED, Julian FJ (1984) Rabbit papillary muscle myosin isozymes and the velocity of papillary muscle shortening. Circ Res 54:586–594
14. Pope B, Hoh JFY, Weeds A (1980) The ATPase activities of rat cardiac myosin isoenzymes. FEBS Letters 118:205–208
15. Rupp H, Kissling G, Jacob R (1983) The hormonal and hemodynamic determinants of polymorphic myosin. Perspectives in Cardiovasc Res 7:373–383
16. Rupp H, Wahl R (1990) Influence of thyroid hormones and catecholamines on myosin of swim-exercised rats. J Appl Physiol 68:973–978
17. Rupp H, Berger H-J, Pfeifer A, Werdan K (1991) Effect of positive inotropic agents on myosin isozyme population and mechanical activity of cultured rat heart myocytes. Circ Res (in press)
18. Scarpace P, Abrass IB (1981) Thyroid hormone regulation of rat heart, lymphocyte, and lung-beta-adrenergic receptors. Endocrin 108:1007–1011
19. Shimizu N, Camoretti-Mercado B, Jakovcic S, Zak R (1991) RNA transcription in heart muscle. In: Fozzard HA et al. (eds) The Heart and Cardiovascular System, 2nd ed. Raven Press, New York (in press)
20. Sen S, Tarazi RC, Bumpus FM (1977) Biochemical changes associated with development and reversal and cardiac hypertrophy in spontaneously hypertensive rats. Cardiovasc Res 11:427–433
21. Simpson P (1985) Stimulation of hypertrophy of cultured neonatal rat heart cells through an alpha$_1$ adrenergic receptor and induction of beating through an alpha$_1$ and beta adrenergic receptor interaction. Circ Res 56:884–894
22. Smith WR, Claycomb WC (1989) Expression of alpha and beta myosin heavy chain genes in the rat ventricle cardiac muscle cells. In: Kedes LH, Stockdale FE (eds) Cellular and Molecular Biology of Muscle Development. Liss, New York, pp 359–368
23. Waspe LE, Ordahl CP, Simpson PC (1990) The cardiac beta myosin heavy chain isogene is induced selectively in alphy$_1$ adrenergic receptor stimulated hypertrophy of cultured rat heart myocytes. J Clin Invest 85:1206–1214
24. Winegrad S, McClellan G, Tucker M, Lin L-E (1983) Cyclic AMP regulates myosin isoenzymes in mammalian cardiac muscle. J Gen Physiol 81:749–765

25. Womble JR, Larson DF, Copeland JG, Brown BR, Haddox MK, Russel DH (1980) Adrenal medulla denervation prevents stress-induced epinephrine plasma elevation and cardiac hypertrophy. Life Sci 27:2417–2420
26. Xenophontos XP, Watson PA, Chua BHL, Haneda T, Morgan HE (1989) Increased cyclic AMP content accelerates protein synthesis in rat heart. Circ Res 65:647–656

Authors' address:

Prof. Dr. Radovan Zak
Department of Medicine
Hospital Box 360, 5841 S. Maryland Avenue
The University of Chicago
Chicago, Illinois 60637, USA

The metabolic syndrome and signal transduction of gene expression *

H. Rupp

Physiological Institute II, University of Tübingen, FRG

Summary: Epidemiological studies have clearly shown that the so-called metabolic syndrome which is linked to insulin resistance and a reduced glucose utilization of muscle represents an important risk factor for cardiovascular disease. However, only little is known of the intracellular consequences of insulin resistance. An important feature of an altered substrate utilization is related to signal transduction of gene expression. For the example of myosin heavy chain expression, it is shown that metabolic signals exist which reflect the fuel flux and substrate utilization of the heart muscle cell. The signals were characterized in functional states of the heart associated with altered metabolic influences (fasting, diabetes, sucrose feeding, increased calorie intake, carnitine palmitoyltransferase inhibition). In the pressure-overloaded heart, metabolic interventions which are expected to increase glucose utilization (sucrose feeding, captopril treatment) have a pronounced effect. Although a link with gene expression remains to be established, it should be noted that the sarcoplasmic reticulum Ca^{2+}-pump activity seems to be affected in a functionally comparable manner. It is concluded that metabolic signals alter the protein phenotype of heart muscle and it is expected that a deranged signal transduction affects, not only the heart, but also vascular muscle.

Key words: Metabolic syndrome; myosin; sarcoplasmic reticulum; hypertension; diabetes

Introduction

In recent years increasing evidence was provided for a critical role of metabolic disturbances in the genesis of cardiovascular disease. It appears that a common denominator of the so-called metabolic syndrome with currently unknown genetic defects is an altered response of peripheral organs to insulin. In some tissues insulin resistance occurs, whereas in others, insulin sensitivity is apparently normal. Insulin resistance has been demonstrated so far by epidemiological studies for hypertension, obesity, and non-insulin-dependent diabetes mellitus (NIDDM) (53). In the clinical setting often an overlap is observed and the overall impact on the cardiovascular risk profile is difficult to assess.

Insulin resistance results in basal hyperinsulinemia which represents a compensatory reaction for preserving glucose homeostasis. Hyperinsulinemia was observed in patients with hypertension (15), obesity (63) and NIDDM (63). The glucose tolerance is, however, not perfectly maintained and hyperinsulinemia can give rise to downregulation of insulin receptors (36). One of the deleterious consequences of hyperinsulinemia for the cardiovascular system is related to abnormalities in the profile of blood lipoproteins (67). Although changes in cholesterol are important, only triglycerides and nonesterified free fatty acids (FFA) will be considered in detail in this overview.

---

* The experimental work was supported by the Deutsche Forschungsgemeinschaft and the NATO research grants programme (No. 189/87).

Hypertension

Indications for metabolic disorders came from a number of therapeutic intervention trials showing that treatment of hypertension reduces the all-cause mortality and the risk of stroke and congestive heart failure, but not the risk of coronary heart disease (49). The importance of metabolic disorders is exemplified by the finding that increased serum insulin and triglyceride concentrations have been identified as independent risk factors in prospective epidemiological studies (5). In patients with untreated hypertension, lipid abnormalities are well documented involving higher serum triglyceride, VLDL triglyceride, and FFA concentrations (46, 71).

In adult hypertensive subjects with a considerable degree of insulin resistance, skeletal muscle, but not the liver was identified as a primary site of insulin resistance (15). The cellular mechanisms affected by an altered insulin influence are, however, unclear. Possible insulin-dependent reactions which are impaired involve inhibition of hepatic glucose release and lipolysis, stimulation of transport, oxidation, and nonoxidative disposal of glucose (15). Of the two principal pathways of intracellular glucose metabolism – complete oxidation and non-oxidative disposal (glycogen synthesis and glycolysis) – only the latter was reduced, accounting for virtually all the decrease of total glucose utilization. In contrast to glycolysis, lipolysis responded normally to insulin (15). A positive correlation was observed between the severity of hypertension and the defect in whole-body glucose utilization (15). In this respect, one should take into account also the role of blood FFA. High blood FFA concentrations may cause peripheral hyperinsulinemia by decreasing hepatic insulin degradation (13, 71), and resistance to insulin could be mediated by an increased influence of fatty acids on skeletal muscle (14).

A question which remains unanswered at present is whether a causal relationship exists between insulin resistance and high blood pressure, and it is not known whether secondary hypertension is associated with insulin resistance. A number of mechanisms have been identified which could lead to hypertension in hyperinsulinemic states by mechanisms involving tissues of normal insulin response. Because insulin promotes sodium retention by the distal nephron of the kidney, an increased insulin influence would result in expansion of the extracellular volume and the blood pressure would rise (8). The fact that insulin stimulates sympathetic nervous system activity could also contribute to an increased vascular resistance (84). Insulin seems to play a part also in the well-documented relationship between dietary intake and sympathetic nervous activity (39), and it modulates the activity of various membrane ion transport systems (56). The Na^+-, K^+-ATPase activity is stimulated by insulin (6) and insulin resistance would result in a reduced ATPase activity (26) and thus contribute to smooth muscle hypertrophy and hypertension.

Obesity

Although insulin resistance is a characteristic feature of primary hypertension independent of obesity (71), obesity emerged as an additional risk factor for cardiovascular disease (30). Obesity is present in over half of adult hypertensives, with the consequence that the risk factor profile is further aggravated, as is exemplified by higher insulin, triglyceride, and FFA levels, and a reduced insulin sensitivity (71). In obese subjects, insulin-stimulated glucose utilization and nonoxidative glucose disposal are reduced; in contrast to hypertensives, lipid oxidation is increased (15). Because weight loss was shown to improve insulin sensitivity (19), it is essential to reduce obesity.

Non-insulin-dependent diabetes mellitus (NIDDM)

Hypertension in diabetic patients is more common than in normal subjects and contributes substantially to their increased cardiovascular morbidity and mortality (67). In NIDDM insulin resistance occurs and the insulin-stimulated glucose utilization and non-oxidative glucose disposal are reduced (15, 81). Plasma triglycerides and FFA are increased in patients with NIDDM (38), and persistent abnormalities in lipoprotein composition were observed despite intensive insulin therapy (2). Noteworthy is that in normotensive patients with NIDDM captopril resulted in a rise of skeletal muscle glucose utilization most probably due to increased kinin levels (78, 80).

Strategies for modulating glucose-fatty acid utilization

A reduced insulin sensitivity is expected to result in an altered fuel flux of the muscle cell. This aspect of the metabolic syndrome is currently not taken into account and, thus, evidence will be provided for the possible consequences of an altered cellular substrate utilization. Depending on the degree of insulin resistance and blood FFA concentrations, substrate utilization is expected to change to a various extent. Because there is increasing evidence that cardiac metabolism contributes to signal transduction of gene expression, the regulation of substrate utilization is shown for the heart muscle cell. In Fig. 1, regulatory sites for substrate utilization are depicted schematically, focussing on pharmacological interventions which could shift fuel utilization.

If insulin resistance occurs, the insulin-mediated glucose uptake is expected to be reduced. High levels of FFA impair further glucose uptake (3, 4). The molecular events coupling the insulin-receptor interaction (90, 103) and the glucose transport (3, 4) to regulation of cellular metabolism remain, however, unclear (9, 48, 50, 74). In contrast to glucose, fatty acids are taken up by a diffusion process depending on the plasma FFA concentration (74). In the cytoplasm, fatty acid-binding proteins are responsible for binding and transport of fatty acids and acylcarnitines, and control the transfer of acyl-carnitine to the mitochondrial β-oxidative system (18). Fatty acids are preferentially oxidized rather than being stored as triglycerides because the cytosolic acyl-CoA level is lower than the Km for triglyceride synthesis (35). The "hormone-sensitive" triglyceride lipase was found to be inhibited by long-chain acyl-CoA for matching triglyceride hydrolysis with the supply of extracellular fatty acids and rate of fatty acid oxidation (51). Similar to the fatty acid binding proteins, phospholipid transfer proteins exist which stimulate the transfer of phospholipids between membrane structures (18). Both fatty acid and phospholipid binding proteins could be of potential interest for modulating fatty acid utilization by pharmacological approaches.

Because long-chain fatty acids can cross the inner mitochondrial membrane only as acylcarnitines, the carnitine palmitoyltransferase (CPT) I provides an important target for affecting fatty acid utilization. The activity of CPT I is regulated by malonyl-CoA which reflects intramitochondrial citrate synthesis. Heart muscle of nourished rats contains significant quantities of malonyl-CoA which falls with starvation; malonyl-CoA interacts with CPT I and thereby exerts control over long-chain fatty acid oxidation (52). The malonyl-CoA binding site relevant to CPT I inhibition is situated on the outer side of the outer membrane, whereas the overt CPT I activity resides on the inner side of the outer membrane (58). The CPT II which resides on the inner surface of the inner mitochondrial membrane forms acyl-CoA, and carnitine shuttles back to the mitochondrial inner membrane space (18). Carnitine cannot be synthesized by the heart

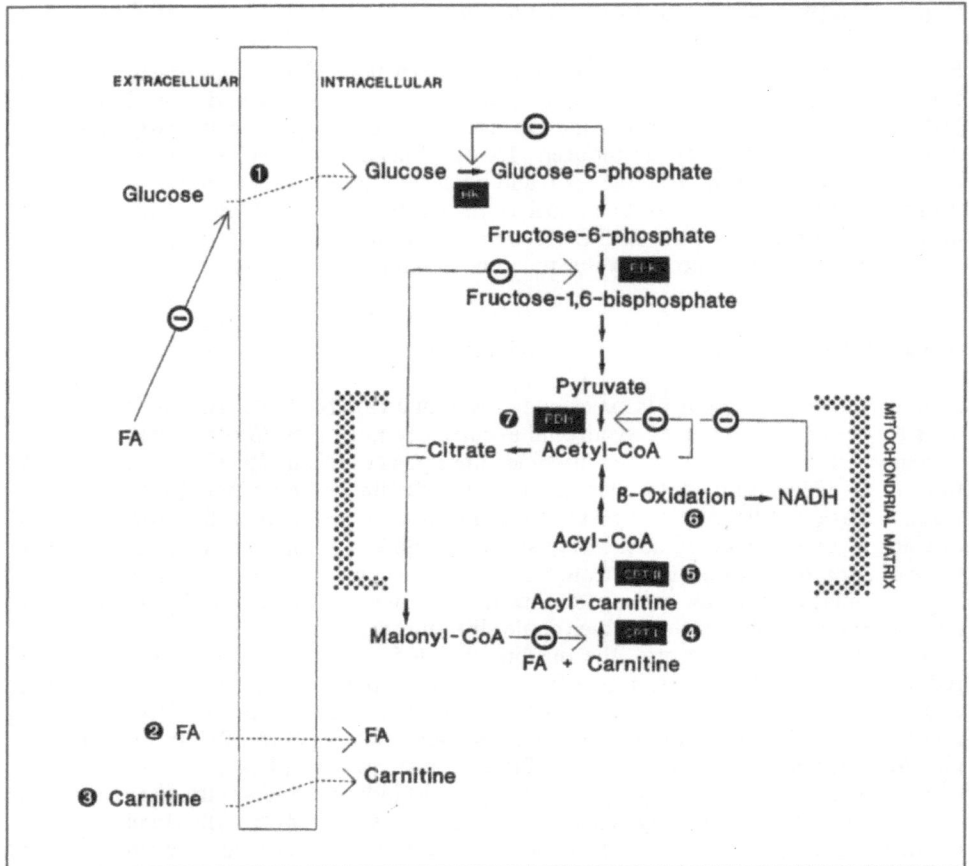

Fig. 1. Strategies for modulating myocardial metabolism. The numbers refer to possible pharmacological intervention sites. Point 1, agents that increase glucose transport: insulin (90, 99, 103); "insulin sensitizer" increasing insulin binding (28, 29), kinins increasing glucose uptake (10, 79); point 2, lipid and fatty acid lowering drugs; point 3, carnitine supplementation; point 4, CPT I inhibitors (methylpalmoxirate, oxfenicine, etomoxir); point 5, CPT II inhibitor (2-(3-methylcinnamylhydrazono)-propionate) (91) and carnitine-acylcarnitine translocase inhibitor (sulfobetaine) (64); point 6, fatty acyl-CoA dehydrogenase and β-ketothiolase inhibitors; point 7, pyruvate dehydrogenase kinase inhibitors, pyruvate dehydrogenase phosphatase activators (103). Abbreviations used are: HK, hexokinase; PFK, phosphofructokinase; PDH, pyruvate dehydrogenase complex; CPT, carnitine palmitoyl transferase; FA, nonesterified free fatty acids. [For details on pharmacological interventions, see (93, 105)]

muscle cell and is taken up against a concentration gradient in an exchange-diffusion process; under physiological conditions, deoxycarnitine is exported in exchange against carnitine (94). The action of carnitine is seen also in its stabilizing action on membrane fluidity, due to its interaction with acylcarnitines which have a detergent effect (34).

Under aerobic conditions, fatty acids are the preferred myocardial substrate and glucose metabolism is downregulated (62). The underlying glucose-fatty acid cycle (74) was shown to operate both in vitro and in vivo (14, 31, 40, 44, 74, 102). Based mostly on in vitro assays, it was demonstrated that metabolism of fatty acids inhibits glucose phosphorylation (hexokinase and phosphofructokinase) and the activity of pyruvate dehydrogenase (Fig. 1). In the intact beating heart, it was shown that the major inhibition occurs at the pyruvate dehydrogenase reaction (102). Pyruvate dehydrogenase kinase (not shown), which inactivates pyruvate dehydrogenase, is stimulated when the ratios of acetyl CoA/CoA and NADH/NAD increase. The ability of dichloroacetate to inhibit pyruvate dehydrogenase kinase, restoring carbon flux through the pyruvate dehydrogenase reaction in the presence of fatty acids is further support for the crucial role of pyruvate dehydrogenase inactivation (102).

Using an inhibitor of CPT I, post-insulin receptor defects could be differentiated. A lipid metabolism-dependent defect caused by metabolites of fatty acid oxidation could be dissociated from a lipid metabolism-independent defect associated with the activation of glucose uptake and glycogen synthesis (82).

States of reduced glucose utilization in animal models

Currently, best documented are changes in substrate utilization in starved rats and rats with insulin-dependent diabetes. Glucose utilization is impaired because of a reduced insulin secretion and high blood fatty acid concentrations (74). In starved rats glycogen, citrate, and the fructose 6-phosphate/fructose 1,6-bisphosphate ratio were increased, and glycogen stores could be raised by increasing the plasma FFA availability in starved rats (108). However, glucose-6-phosphate and citrate accumulated in hearts of ketotic diabetic rats, but not in rats with chronic diabetes (83). Only in ketotic diabetic hearts was glycolysis inhibited, whereas in chronic diabetes, the impaired glucose metabolism primarily reflected a reduced uptake of glucose (83). In genetically diabetic mice, cardiac triglyceride and long-chain acylcarnitine levels were increased; FFA levels were not altered (96). Diabetic rats exhibited lower serum and cardiac carnitine levels (101) which were normalized by an increased carnitine intake (66). A reduced cardiac carnitine level would be deleterious for the diabetic heart, because insulin-stimulated glucose uptake is impaired and the glycolytic flux could not be increased in a compensatory manner. Administration of carnitine normalized, not only cardiac carnitine levels, but also reduced plasma triglyceride and FFA levels (66), also thus relieving, most probably, the inhibitory effect of FFA on glucose uptake; in support of this dual action of carnitine would be the finding that serum glucose levels were reduced in carnitine-treated diabetic rats (66). The lipid lowering effect of carnitine also occurred in normal rats (66). It is noteworthy that plasma triglyceride levels were reduced and cardiac carnitine content was increased also by treadmill exercise of diabetic rats (65).

Less is known of the effects of insulin-resistant states. In obese Zucker rats with diminished insulin responsiveness, the cardiac uptake and conversion of glucose was impaired (82). Whole-body glucose utilization and uptake were, however, increased (37), suggesting that peripheral tissues differ with respect to their insulin sensitivity. In this respect it should be mentioned that dietary interventions involving a continuous high sucrose intake induce insulin resistance, hyperinsulinemia, and hypertriglyceridemia (23).

States of increased glucose utilization in animal models

Cardiac metabolism changes in the rat during development in response to oxygen and substrate availability. The fetus is relatively more dependent on anaerobic glycolysis, using glucose as its major substrate. The mature heart is almost exclusively aerobic, with fatty acids as the major substrate (97). Intriguing is the finding that a shift from fatty acid-to-carbohydrate oxidation was observed in the surviving, non-infarcted tissue of the rat after myocardial infarction (25).

Because in NIDDM with increased serum FFA, glucose utilization is decreased also via the glucose-fatty acid cycle, drugs were designed which improve glucose utilization by reducing fatty acid oxidation. Based on the discovery that 2-bromopalmitate inhibits the carnitine-dependent oxidation of fatty acids, the 2-oxiranecarboxylates methylpalmoxirate (41), clomoxir (104), oxfenicine (21), and etomoxir (11, 105) were developed. These drugs proved effective in inhibiting liver gluconeogenesis by reducing acetyl-CoA, which is required as an allosteric activator of pyruvate carboxylase; ketogenesis is also markedly inhibited (92). In addition, etomoxir reduced fatty acid biosynthesis, most probably by inhibiting acetyl-CoA carboxylase, resulting in reduced serum triglycerides and FFA [(100); Rupp H, Hansen M, unpublished]. It should be mentioned that CPT I is inhibited also by the hypoglycemic sulfonylureas tolbutamide and glyburide (7); the role of this inhibition in the therapy of diabetes remains to be assessed. It should be mentioned that the switch in favor of glucose utilization in normal hearts is associated with an increased cardiac growth. When rats were given methylpalmoxirate and fed a diet containing the medium chain fatty acid octanoate which can diffuse directly into the mitochondrial matrix and thus bypasses the site of CPT I inhibition, the cardiac hypertrophy was prevented (41). For oxfenicine, it was shown that the heart weight was increased in a dose-related manner (21). The hypertrophy was due to uniform myocardial hypertrophy involving all cardiac chambers; a disproportion of mitochondria and myofibrils was not observed. Whether the hypertrophy process was solely due to the decreased energy-forming capacity of heart muscle (21) is not known. Thus, the CPT I inhibitors should be used only for normalizing a reduced glycolytic flux, but not for shifting fuel utilization of the normal heart in the direction of an enhanced glucose oxidation.

States of unclear substrate utilization in animal models

The substrate utilization is not clearly defined in a number of functional states of the heart. In the hypertrophied heart due to pressure overload arising from aortic constriction (32) and in salt-sensitive hypertensive Dahl rats (106), the desoxyglucose uptake was increased, whereas the uptake of a fatty acid analogue was reduced. Although this does not unequivocally indicate a reduced fatty acid utilization (32), the reduced fatty acid ex traction could arise from a decreased coenzyme A and carnitine content of pressure-overloaded heart (76, 77). Cardiomyopathic hamsters were reported to exhibit also depressed cardiac carnitine concentrations and a depressed fatty acid oxidation (107). Also in chronically volume-overloaded heart, carnitine transport was decreased, resulting in a reduced carnitine concentration; myocardial triglyceride accumulation was, however, not observed (12). Intriguing is the finding that in hypertrophied hearts of spontaneously hypertensive rats (SHR) the carnitine levels were elevated; the cardiac carnitine transport system was not reduced, but serum carnitine levels were increased (16). Thus, the consequences of reduced cardiac carnitine levels could be examined by studying rats with overloaded hearts differing in carnitine content. Also in human heart, depressed carnitine levels cannot be considered as a general characteristic of an overload. In patients with dilated cardiomyopathy and congestive heart failure, cardiac total carnitine was reduced, although plasma free and total carnitine levels were elevated (75). However, in patients with end-stage heart failure, the myocardial carnitine was reduced only in a few cases and plasma carnitine was increased (69). Clearly, more work is required to define the carnitine level which is limiting for fatty acid utilization and to examine the functional consequences of cardiac carnitine depletion. When fatty acid utilization is reduced due to carnitine deficiency, the question should be addressed whether the potential of an increased glucose oxidation is impaired due to insulin deficiency, insulin resistance or high blood FFA levels.

Also unclear is the substrate utilization of heart during maturation and aging. In vivo insulin-stimulated glucose utilization was reduced during maturation and the phenomenon was fully developed as early as 4 months of age (61). The marked increase in body weight that occurs during this period was thought to be responsible for the decline in glucose utilization (61). In vivo insulin resistance did not develop when the weight gain was prevented by calorie restriction (61). The reduced whole-body glucose uptake can mainly be attributed to a lower glucose uptake of skeletal muscle for which a nadir was observed also by 4 months, with no change noted with further aging (20). Insulin-induced glucose uptake by skeletal muscle from 12-month-old rats was not depressed, but markedly enhanced in non-obese rats reared in a hypermetabolic state caused by exposure to hypergravity (54).

An increased cardiac metabolism occurs during physical exercise. The present evidence is not in favor of a shift in substrate utilization and it appears that the glucose-fatty acid cycle is not effective (1, 108). It was suggested that the muscle glycogenolysis stimuli induced by exercise are sufficiently strong to overrule the inhibition by increased plasma FFA (1). One has also to take into account that an inhibitory action of NADH is not likely to occur when energy consumption is high; also citrate is expected to leave mitochondria only when citrate production exceeds utilization. In accordance, cardiac citrate concentration was related to plasma FFA in the rest period after physical exercise, demonstrating that the glucose-fatty acid cycle was effective (108). When considering possible changes in metabolism, one has to take into account that muscle has the potential of adapting to exercise (27). Thus, the activity of CPT I (24) and the insulin sensitivity were increased in trained rats (55).

Metabolic influences on cardiac gene expression

The metabolic syndrome represents a recent addition to a list of various metabolic disturbances involving amino acid metabolism disorders, storage diseases, neuromuscular diseases, diseases of metal and pigment metabolism, carnitine deficiency, and connective tissue disorders (17). If the myocardial cell is affected, these metabolic disorders are manifested clinically as cardiomyopathy. In the case of the metabolic syndrome affecting substrate utilization, one has to take into account that signal transduction of gene expression involves also metabolic influences. Best documented currently are these effects for the expression of rat myosin heavy chains (MHC) which are decisive for the mechanical and energetical performance of the contractile apparatus. Although the myosin gene expression responds also to signals such as thyroid hormones (47, 98) and catecholamines (22, 85, 95), there is increasing evidence in favor of additional signals related to cardiac metabolism. When rats were intermittently food-deprived involving fasting every other day for 6 weeks, the proportion of myosin V3 ($\beta\beta$-MHC) was increased and the

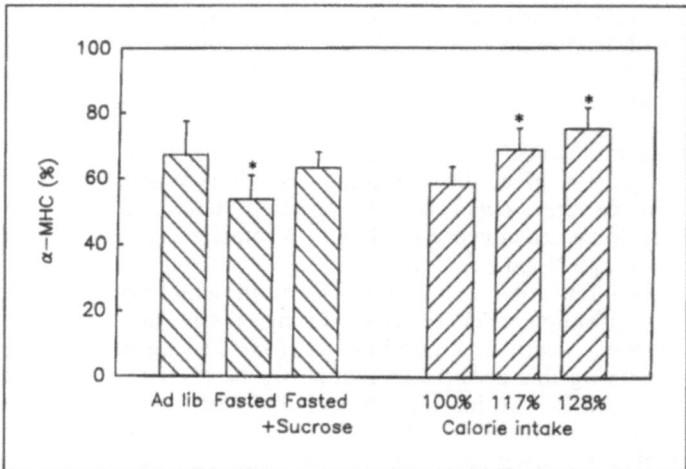

Fig. 2. Effect of a chronically altered calorie intake on α-MHC expression. Rats were intermittently fasted (1 day fasting/1 day ad libitum feeding) and received either tap water or 0.8% sucrose drinking solutions (87). The calorie intake was increased by feeding rats 10% or 20% sunflower oil diets which resulted in a calorie intake of 117% and 128% of rats fed a regular 5% sunflower oil diet (Rupp H, Hansen M, unpublished). Statistical comparisons ($p < 0.05$) were made between experimental rats and rats fed ad libitum the regular diet. Note, the differences in α-MHC expression of control rats arises from different ages

proportion of myosin V1 (αα-MHC) was reduced, corresponding to a switch in gene expression in favor of β-MHC (87) (Fig. 2). When the rats were given drinking solutions containing 0.8% sucrose, the change in MHC expression was prevented (Fig. 2). Because circulating thyroid hormones were not affected by sucrose feeding, it can be concluded that the signal resulting in an increased β-MHC expression was not related to an altered thyroid influence. The sucrose feeding resulted in reduced plasma glucose concentrations particularly after refeeding, which indicates an enhanced peripheral glucose utilization. When the amount of complex carbohydrates in the rat chow was increased from 55% to 75%, the effect of food-restriction could also be prevented (57). When the calorie intake of the rats was increased by providing diets with an increased fat content which does not affect serum FFA concentrations, the MHC expression was changed in an opposite direction. In rats fed 10% or 20% sunflower oil, the proportion of α-MHC increased (Fig. 2), again circulating thyroid hormones could not explain the altered MHC expression. It thus appears that the MHC expression responds to the nutritional status of the organism, indicating a continuum ranging from underfed to normal fed and overfed rats.

At a given calorie intake, the MHC expression depends on the type of substrate utilized. In diabetic rats, β-MHC expression was markedly increased, which can partially be prevented by administration of etomoxir (Fig. 3). It turned out that an increased α-MHC expression does, however, not require inhibition of CPT I because feeding a 5% octanoate/decanoate diet which prevented cardiac hypertrophy did not prevent the increase in α-MHC (Fig. 3) (Rupp H, Elimban V, Dhalla NS, unpublished). Both etomoxir or the octanoate/decanoate diet had no influence on general growth characteristics, plasma insulin, glucose, and thyroid hormones. However, etomoxir markedly reduced plasma triglycerides and led thus, most probably, to an increased glucose uptake. These

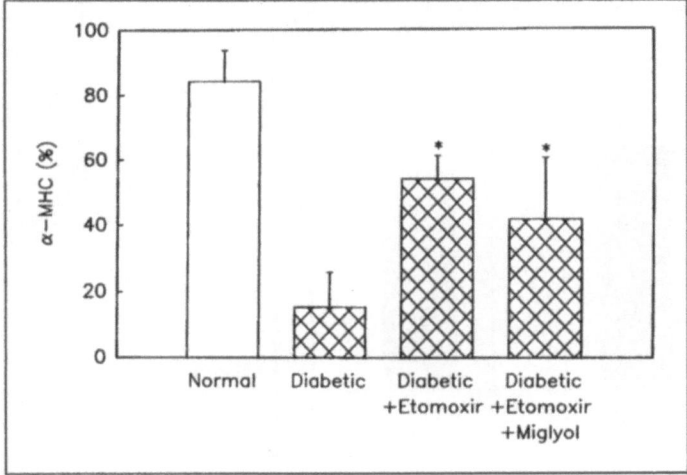

Fig. 3. Effect of chronic diabetes (65 mg/kg streptozotocin) on α-MHC expression. Diabetic rats were treated with 15 mg/kg etomoxir and fed either a regular diet or a 5% octanoate/decanoate ("miglyol") diet. A complete normalization of α-MHC expression was not achieved by etomoxir, most probably because insulin-mediated glucose uptake and plasma triiodothyronine concentrations were reduced (Rupp H, Elimban V, Dhalla NS, unpublished). Statistical comparisons (p < 0.05) were made between etomoxir-treated rats and untreated diabetic rats

data demonstrate that increased plasma triglyceride or FFA concentrations markedly impair the metabolic signals whenever glucose uptake is reduced. In normal rats, etomoxir had a much smaller effect, suggesting that MHC expression responds more sensitively to metabolic signals in states of a reduced glucose utilization.

Further support for a role of metabolic signals was derived from a sucrose treatment of rats with pressure overloaded hearts (86). The increased β-MHC expression of the pressure overloaded heart could be prevented by providing 0.8% sucrose drinking solutions which had, however, no significant effect in normal rats (Fig. 4). Based on the effect of sucrose in intermittently fasted rats, one could deduce that the sucrose feeding improved glucose utilization of the heart; thyroid hormones were not altered.

Evidence in favor of metabolic signals for gene expression of sarcolemmal or sarcoplasmic reticulum ion transport systems or ion channels is currently not available. It is, however, known that the activity of a number of membrane systems is altered in states characterized by metabolic disorders (67). In the studies examining the role of metabolic signals for MHC expression, also the Ca^{2+}-stimulated ATPase activity of the sarcoplasmic reticulum Ca^{2+} pump was determined (86, 87). The sarcoplasmic reticulum Ca^{2+} pump is an important determinant of Ca^{2+} sequestration during diastole of the heart and it is well documented that the rate of Ca^{2+} uptake is depressed in diabetic and overloaded hearts (42, 67). The sucrose and the etomoxir treatments increased, not only α-MHC expression, but also the ATPase activity of the sarcoplasmic reticulum Ca^{2+} pump [(86, 87); Rupp H, Elimban V, Dhalla NS, unpublished]. These interventions improved, therefore, the potential of the heart for fast contraction and relaxation. In this respect, it should be noted that carnitine treatment also normalized the sarcoplasmic reticulum Ca^{2+} transport activity of diabetic rats (45). Carnitine influences blood lipoproteins and

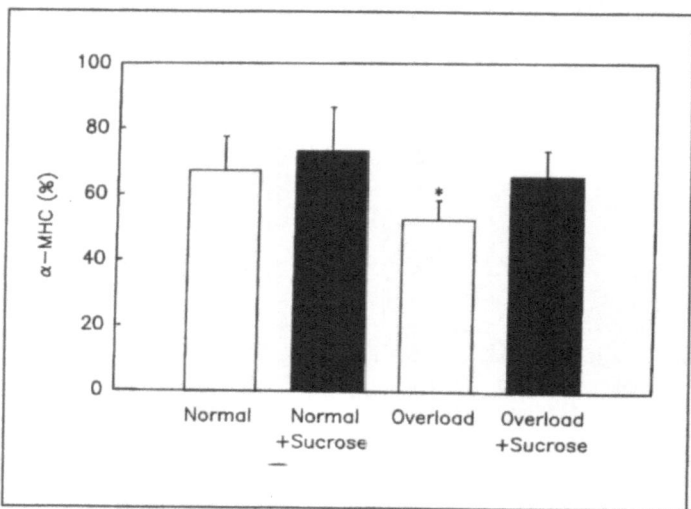

Fig. 4. Effect of a chronic sucrose treatment of rats with pressure-overloaded heart (abdominal aorta constriction) on α-MHC expression. Rats received a regular diet and either tap water or 0.8% sucrose solutions (86). Statistical comparisons (p < 0.05) were made between experimental rats and normal rats

the synthesis of cardiac acylcarnitines, yet the mechanism of the beneficial effect of carnitine remains unclear. It is also not known whether gene expression of the sarcoplasmic reticulum Ca^{2+} pump increased, or whether phospholamban which regulates the Ca^{2+} pump activity (42) was affected either by increasing gene expression or by changing the phosphorylation state. Compared with sarcoplasmic reticulum, much less is currently known of sarcolemmal ion transport systems or channels (67, 68, 89).

In view of the evidence that metabolic signals are important for myocardial subcellular structures, the goal of antihypertensive treatments should be the normalization of metabolic disorders. This is exemplified by the antihypertensive treatment of SHR. Early evidence indicated that blood pressure normalization of SHR with hydralazine was not sufficient for normalizing MHC expression, suggesting that the increased β-MHC of untreated SHR could not be solely attributed to the pressure overload (88). A comparison of various antihypertensive treatments demonstrates that the failure of hydralazine to normalize MHC expression was not unique but was shared by other antihypertensive drugs (Fig. 5). Noteworthy is that the angiotensin-converting-enzyme inhibitor captopril was the drug with the most pronounced effect on MHC expression. Experimental evidence showing that the increased α-MHC expression in the captopril-treated SHR arises from an improved cardiac glucose utilization is, however, still missing. In this respect, the effect of various antihypertensive treatments on insulin sensitivity of hypertensive patients should be considered.

During $β_1$-selective adrenergic blockade with metoprolol or atenolol, insulin sensitivity was decreased by 20% or 13%, respectively; serum insulin, glucose, and triglyceride concentrations were increased by both treatments, but not fatty acid concentrations (73). Also the diuretic agent hydrochlorothiazide decreased insulin sensitivity by approximately 11% and increased serum triglyceride concentrations (70). In contrast, treatment with captopril increased the insulin sensitivity by 11% (70). The increased

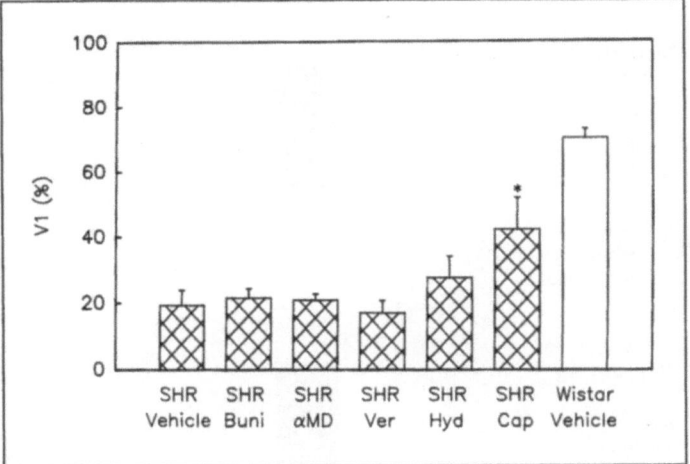

Fig. 5. Treatment of SHR with the β-blocking drug bunitrolol (Buni, 40 mg/kg), α-methyldopa (αMD, 400 mg/kg), verapamil (Ver, 40 mg/kg), hydralazine (Hyd, 80 mg/kg) or captopril (Cap, 50 mg/kg). The blood pressure (mm Hg) was reduced by α-methyldopa (185 $\pm$ 6), verapamil (185 $\pm$ 17), hydralazine (136 $\pm$ 10) and captopril (138 $\pm$ 6) compared with untreated SHR (219 $\pm$ 10); bunitrolol had no significant influence on blood pressure (213 $\pm$ 18). Data from Nagano (60), with exception of the captopril data which are from the MD thesis of Kanemura (33). Statistical comparisons ($p < 0.05$) were made between treated and untreated SHR. In captopril-treated SHR, the proportion of V3 was reduced and the α-MHC expression was thus increased

glucose disposal could arise from local accumulation of bradykinin, which stimulates glucose uptake (78, 80). Captopril had no effect on serum lipoproteins (70). Also, α-adrenergic blockade using prazosin increased insulin sensitivity (72). The calcium-channel-blocker diltiazem did not appear to produce any negative metabolic effects (43). Although rat cardiac MHC expression and in vivo glucose utilization of hypertensive patients are different phenomena, it is nonetheless noteworthy that captopril proved to be an efficient drug for improving α-MHC expression in SHR, as well as for improving metabolic disorders in human subjects.

In conclusion, based on the increasing evidence that metabolic signals play a role for subcellular structures of the heart muscle cell, the pharmacological therapy of diseases associated with metabolic disorders should be aimed at normalizing the underlying metabolic defects. In this respect, it should be pointed out that the metabolic signals are one component of the signal transduction which determines the protein phenotype of the heart muscle cell (Fig. 6). Changes in signal transduction can lead, not only to qualitative changes in gene expression as seen for myosin, but also to quantitative alterations in gene expression as exemplified by sarcoplasmic reticulum (59). Because the protein phenotype of the myocyte is decisive for the mechanical performance, changes in signal transduction should always be considered under the aspect of an altered heart function. One should also take into account that signal transduction mechanisms characterized for heart muscle are expected to be applicable also to smooth muscle. One could thus speculate that metabolic disturbances affect gene expression also of smooth muscle and increase by this mechanism the risk for coronary heart disease.

Acknowledgements. The helpful discussions of M. Hansen are gratefully acknowledged.

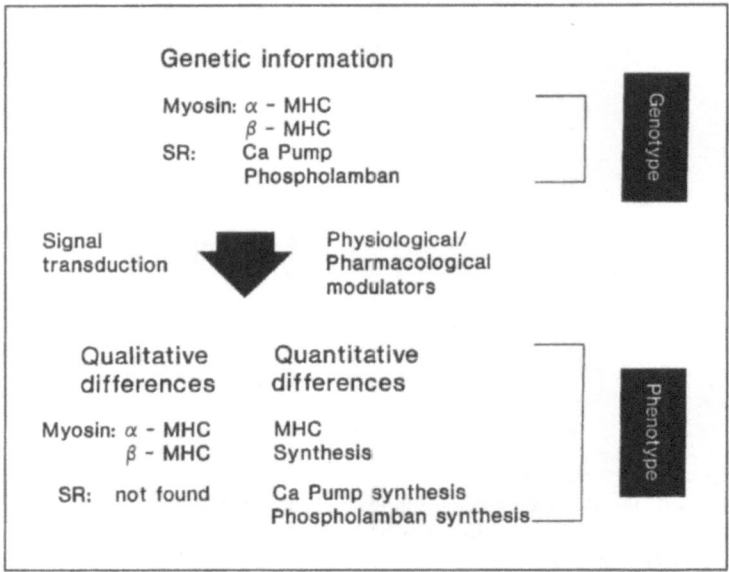

Fig. 6. Physiological and pharmacological modulation of signal transduction of gene expression and consequences for the protein phenotype of the heart muscle cell exemplified for myosin and sarcoplasmic reticulum

References

1. Auclair E, Satabin P, Servan E, Guezennec CY (1988) Metabolic effects of glucose, medium chain triglyceride and long chain triglyceride feeding before prolonged exercise in rats. Eur J Appl Physiol 57:126–131
2. Bagdade JD, Buchanan WE, Kuusi T, Taskinen MR (1990) Persistent abnormalities in lipoprotein composition in noninsulin-dependent diabetes after intensive insulin therapy. Arteriosclerosis 10:232–239
3. Bihler I (1986) The interrelationship between glucose transport and functional activity. In: Rupp H (ed) The Regulation of Heart Function. Thieme Inc, New York Stuttgart, pp 178–185
4. Bihler I (1988) The role of membrane transport in the control of glucose metabolism and its coupling to cellular function. Can J Physiol Pharmacol 66:549–560
5. Castelli WP (1986) The triglyceride issue: a view from Framingham. Am Heart J 112:432–437
6. Clausen T (1986) Regulation of active Na^+-K^+ transport in skeletal muscle. Physiol Rev 66:542–580
7. Cook GA (1987) The hypoglycemic sulfonylureas glyburide and tolbutamide inhibit fatty acid oxidation by inhibiting carnitine palmitoyltransferase. J Biol Chem 262:4968–4972
8. DeFronzo RA (1981) The effect of insulin on renal sodium metabolism. A review with clinical implications. Diabetologia 21:165–171
9. Denton RM, Pogson CI (1976) Metabolic regulation. Chapman and Hall, London
10. Dietze G (1982) Neue Aspekte zur durchblutungssteigernden und insulinähnlichen Wirkung der Muskelarbeit: Mögliche Beteiligung des Kallikrein-Kinin-Prostaglandin Systems. Klin Wochenschr 60:429–444
11. Eistetter K, Wolf HPO (1986) Etomoxir. Drugs of the Future 11:1034–1036
12. El Alaoui Talibi Z, Moravec J (1989) Carnitine transport and exogenous palmitate oxidation in chronically volume-overloaded rat hearts. Biochim Biophys Acta 1003:109–114

13. Evans DJ, Murray R, Kissebah AH (1984) Relationship between skeletal muscle insulin resistance, insulin-mediated glucose disposal, and insulin binding: effects of obesity and body fat topography. J Clin Invest 74:1515–1525
14. Ferrannini E, Barrett EJ, Bevilacqua S, DeFronzo RA (1983) Effect of fatty acids on glucose production and utilization in man. J Clin Invest 72:1737–1747
15. Ferrannini E, Buzzigoli G, Bonadonna R, Giorico MA, Oleggini M, Graziadei L, Pedrinelli R, Brandi L, Bevilacqua S (1987) Insulin resistance in essential hypertension. N Engl J Med 317:350–357
16. Foster KA, O'Rourke B, Reibel DK (1985) Altered carnitine metabolism in spontaneously hypertensive rats. Am J Physiol 249:E183–E186
17. Gilbert EF (1987) The effects of metabolic diseases on the cardiovascular system. Am J Cardiovasc Pathol 1:189–213
18. Glatz JF, van der Vusse GJ (1989) Intracellular transport of lipids. Mol Cell Biochem 88:37–44
19. Golay A, Felber JP, Dusmet M, Gomez F, Curchod B, Jequier E (1985) Effect of weight loss on glucose disposal in obese and obese diabetic patients. Int J Obes 9:181–191
20. Goodman MN, Dluz SM, McElaney MA, Belur E, Ruderman NB (1983) Glucose uptake and insulin sensitivity in rat muscle: changes during 3–96 weeks of age. Am J Physiol 244:E93–E100
21. Greaves P, Martin J, Michel MC, Mompon P (1984) Cardiac hypertrophy in the dog and rat induced by oxfenicine, an agent which modifies muscle metabolism. Arch Toxicol 7 (Suppl):488–493
22. Gupta MP, Gupta M, Stewart A, Zak R (1991) Activation of alpha-myosin heavy chain gene expression by cAMP in cultured fetal rat heart myocytes. Biochem Biophys Res Commun 174:1196–1203
23. Gutman RA, Basilico MZ, Bernal CA, Chicco A, Lombardo YB (1987) Long-term hypertriglyceridemia and glucose intolerance in rats fed chronically an isocaloric sucrose-rich diet. Metabolism 36:1013–1020
24. Guzman M, Castro J (1988) Effects of endurance exercise on carnitine palmitoyltransferase I from rat heart, skeletal muscle and liver mitochondria. Biochim Biophys Acta 963:562–565
25. Hansen CA, Fellenius E, Neely JR (1986) Metabolic rates in normal and infarcted myocardium. Can J Cardiol (Suppl A):1A–8A
26. Hilton PJ (1986) Cellular sodium transport in essential hypertension. N Engl J Med 314:222–229
27. Holloszy JO, Coyle EF (1984) Adaptations of skeletal muscle to endurance exercise and their metabolic consequences. J Appl Physiol 56:831–838
28. Hosokawa T, Ando K, Tamura G (1985) An ascochlorin derivative, AS-6, reduces insulin resistance in the genetically obese diabetic db/db mouse. Diabetes 34:267
29. Hosokawa T, Ando K, Tamura G (1985) Effect of oral treatment with a new hypoglycemic agent, AS-6, on the metabolic activities of adipocytes in db/db mice: a comparative study. Biochem Biophys Res Commun 126:471
30. Hubert HB, Feinleib M, McNamara PM, Castelli WP (1983) Obesity as an independent risk factor for cardiovascular disease: a 26-year follow-up of participants in the Framingham Heart Study. Circulation 67:968–977
31. Jenkins AB, Storlien LH, Chisholm DJ, Kraegen EW (1988) Effects of nonesterified fatty acid availability on tissue-specific glucose utilization in rats in vivo. J Clin Invest 82:293–299
32. Kagaya Y, Kanno Y, Takeyama D, Ishide N, Maruyama Y, Takahashi T, Ido T, Takishima T (1990) Effects of long-term pressure overload on regional myocardial glucose and free fatty acid uptake in rats. A quantitative autoradiographic study. Circulation 81:1353–1361
33. Kanemura M (1987) Regression of cardiac hypertrophy and alteration of left ventricular myosin isoenzyme. Tokyo Jikeikai Medical J 102:1243–1254
34. Kobayashi A, Watanabe H, Fujisawa S, Yamamoto T, Yamazaki N (1989) Effects of L-carnitine and palmitoylcarnitine on membrane fluidity of human erythrocytes. Biochim Biophys Acta 986:83–88
35. Kohn MC, Garfinkel D (1983) Computer simulation of metabolism in palmitate-perfused rat heart. I. Palmitate oxidation. Ann Biomed Eng 11:361–384

36. Kolterman OG, Insel J, Saekow M, Olefsky JM (1980) Mechanisms of insulin resistance in human obesity. Evidence for receptor and postreceptor defects. J Clin Invest 65:1272–1284

37. Krief S, Bazin R, Dupuy F, Lavau M (1988) Increased in vivo glucose utilization in 30-day-old obese Zucker rat: role of white adipose tissue. Am J Physiol 254:E342–E348

38. Laakso M, Sarlund H, Mykkänen L (1990) Insulin resistance is associated with lipid and lipoprotein abnormalities in subjects with varying degrees of glucose tolerance. Arteriosclerosis 10:223–231

39. Landsberg L, Young JB (1985) Insulin-mediated glucose metabolism in the relationship between dietary intake and sympathetic nervous system activity. Int J Obes 9 (Suppl 2):63–68

40. Lassers BW, Wahlqvist ML, Kaijser L, Carlson LA (1971) Relationship in man between plasma free fatty acids and myocardial metabolism of carbohydrate substrates. Lancet 2:448–450

41. Lee SM, Bahl JJ, Bressler R (1985) Prevention of the metabolic effects of 2-tetradecylglycidate by octanoic acid in the genetically diabetic mouse (db/db). Biochem Med 33:104–109

42. Limas C (1986) Calcium transport by the cardiac sarcoplasmic reticulum in different functional states of the heart. In: Rupp H (ed) The Regulation of Heart Function. Thieme Inc, New York Stuttgart, pp 145–158

43. Lithell HO, Pollare T, Berne C (1990) Insulin sensitivity in newly detected hypertensive patients: influence of captopril and other antihypertensive agents on insulin sensitivity and related biological parameters. J Cardiovasc Pharmacol 15 (Suppl 5):S46–S52

44. Löffler G, Petrides PE, Weiss L (1988) Physiologische Chemie. Springer, Berlin Heidelberg New York

45. Lopaschuk GD, Tahiliani AG, Vadlamudi RV, Katz S, McNeill JH (1983) Cardiac sarcoplasmic reticulum function in insulin- or carnitine-treated diabetic rats. Am J Physiol 245:H969–H976

46. MacMahon SW, Macdonald GJ, Blacket RB (1985) Plasma lipoprotein levels in treated and untreated hypertensive men and women. Arteriosclerosis 5:391–396

47. Mahdavi V, Izumo S, Nadal-Ginard B (1987) Developmental and hormonal regulation of sarcomeric myosin heavy chain gene family. Circ Res 60:804–814

48. Martin BR (1987) Metabolic Regulation. A Molecular Approach. Blackwell Scientific Publications, Oxford

49. Maxwell MH (1988) Beyond blood pressure control. Effect of antihypertensive therapy on cardiovascular risk factors. Am J Hypertens 1:366S–371S

50. McCormack JG, Denton RM (1986) Ca^{2+} ions as a link between functional demands and mitochondrial metabolism in the heart. In: Rupp H (ed) The Regulation of Heart Function. Thieme Inc, New York Stuttgart, pp 186–200

51. McDonough KH, Neely JR (1988) Inhibition of myocardial lipase by palmityl CoA. J Mol Cell Cardiol 20 (Suppl 2):31–39

52. McGarry JD, Mills SE, Long CS, Foster DW (1983) Observations on the affinity for carnitine, and malonyl-CoA sensitivity, of carnitine palmitoyltransferase I in animal and human tissues. Demonstration of the presence of malonyl-CoA in non-hepatic tissues of the rat. Biochem J 214:21–28

53. Modan M, Halkin H, Almog S, Lusky A, Eshkol A, Shefi M, Shitrit A, Fuchs Z (1985) Hyperinsulinemia: a link between hypertension, obesity and glucose intolerance. J Clin Invest 75:809–817

54. Mondon CE, Dolkas CB, Oyama J (1981) Enhanced skeletal muscle insulin sensitivity in year-old rats adapted to hypergravity. Am J Physiol 240:E482–E488

55. Mondon CE, Dolkas CB, Reaven GM (1980) Site of enhanced insulin sensitivity in exercise-trained rats at rest. Am J Physiol 239:E169–E177

56. Moore RD (1983) Effects of insulin upon ion transport. Biochim Biophys Acta 737:1–49

57. Morris GS, Herrick RE, Baldwin KM (1989) Dietary carbohydrates modify myosin isoenzyme profiles of semistarved rats. Am J Physiol 256:R976–R981

58. Murthy MS, Pande SV (1987) Malonyl-CoA binding site and the overt carnitine palmitoyltransferase activity reside on the opposite sides of the outer mitochondrial membrane. Proc Natl Acad Sci USA 84:378–382

59. Nagai R, Zarain-Herzberg A, Brandl CJ, Fujii J, Tada M, MacLennan DH, Alpert NR, Periasamy M (1989) Regulation of myocardial Ca^{2+}-ATPase and phospholamban mRNA expression in response to pressure overload and thyroid hormone. Proc Natl Acad Sci USA 68:2966–2970

60. Nagano M (1987) Cardiac regression of spontaneously hypertensive rats treated with hypotensive drugs. In: Papp JGY (ed) Cardiovascular Pharmacology '87. Akademiai Kiado, Budapest, pp 315–322

61. Narimiya M, Azhar S, Dolkas CB, Mondon CE, Sims C, Wright DW, Reaven GM (1984) Insulin resistance in older rats. Am J Physiol 246:E397–E404

62. Neely JR, Morgan HE (1974) Relationship between carbohydrate and lipid metabolism and the energy balance of heart muscle. Ann Rev Physiol 36:413–459

63. Olefsky JM, Kolterman OG, Scarlett JA (1982) Insulin action and resistance in obesity and noninsulin-dependent type II diabetes mellitus. Am J Physiol 243:E15–E30

64. Parvin R, Goswami T, Pande SV (1980) Inhibition of mitochondrial carnitine-acylcarnitine translocase by sulfobetaines. Can J Biochem 58:822–830

65. Paulson DJ, Kopp SJ, Peace DG, Tow JP (1987) Myocardial adaptation to endurance exercise training in diabetic rats. Am J Physiol 252:R1073–R1081

66. Paulson DJ, Schmidt MJ, Traxler JS, Ramacci MT, Shug AL (1984) Improvement of myocardial function in diabetic rats after treatment with L-carnitine. Metabolism 33:358–363

67. Pierce GN, Beamish RE, Dhalla NS (1988) Heart Dysfunction in Diabetes. CRC Press, Boca Raton

68. Pierce GN, Ramjiawan B, Dhalla NS, Ferrari R (1990) Na-H exchange in cardiac sarcolemmal vesicles isolated from diabetic rats. Am J Physiol 258:H255–H261

69. Pierpont ME, Judd D, Goldenberg IF, Ring WS, Olivari MT, Pierpont GL (1989) Myocardial carnitine in end-stage congestive heart failure. Am J Cardiol 64:56–60

70. Pollare T, Lithell H, Berne C (1989) A comparison of the effects of hydrochlorothiazide and captopril on glucose and lipid metabolism in patients with hypertension. N Engl J Med 321:868–873

71. Pollare T, Lithell H, Berne C (1990) Insulin resistance is a characteristic feature of primary hypertension independent of obesity. Metabolism 39:167–174

72. Pollare T, Lithell H, Selinus I, Berne C (1988) Application of prazosin is associated with an increase of insulin sensitivity in obese patients with hypertension. Diabetologia 31:415–420

73. Pollare T, Lithell H, Selinus I, Berne C (1989) Sensitivity to insulin during treatment with atenolol and metoprolol: a randomised, double blind study of effects on carbohydrate and lipoprotein metabolism in hypertensive patients. British Med J 298:1152–1157

74. Randle PJ, Tubbs PK (1979) Carbohydrate and fatty acid metabolism. In: Berne RM, Sperelakis N, Geiger SR (eds) Handbook of Physiology, section 2: the Cardiovascular System, vol 1. The Heart. American Physiological Society, Bethesda, pp 805–844

75. Regitz V, Shug AL, Fleck E (1990) Defective myocardial carnitine metabolism in congestive heart failure secondary to dilated cardiomyopathy and to coronary, hypertensive and valvular heart diseases. Am J Cardiol 65:755–760

76. Reibel DK, O'Rourke B, Foster KA (1987) Mechanisms for altered carnitine content in hypertrophied rat hearts. Am J Physiol 252:H561–H565

77. Reibel DK, Uboh CE, Kent RL (1983) Altered coenzyme A and carnitine metabolism in pressure-overload hypertrophied hearts. Am J Physiol 244:H839–H843

78. Rett K, Lotz N, Wicklmayr M, Fink E, Jauch KW, Günther B, Dietze G (1988) Verbesserte Insulinwirkung durch ACE-Hemmung beim Typ-II-Diabetiker. Dtsch Med Wochenschr 113:243–249

79. Rett K, Wicklmayr M, Dietze G (1990) Metabolic effects of kinins: historical and recent developments. J Cardiovasc Pharmacol 15 (Suppl 6):S57–59

80. Rett K, Wicklmayr M, Dietze G, Mehnert H (1990) Clinical studies with ACE-inhibitors in diabetes. Horm Metab Res Suppl 22:69–74

81. Rizza RA, Mandarino LJ, Gerich JE (1981) Mechanism and significance of insulin resistance in non-insulin-dependent diabetes mellitus. Diabetes 30:990–995

82. Rösen P, Herberg L, Reinauer H (1986) Different types of postinsulin receptor defects contribute to insulin resistance in hearts of obese Zucker rats. Endocrinol 119:1285–1291

83. Rösen P, Windeck P, Zimmer HG, Frenzel H, Burrig KF, Reinauer H (1986) Myocardial performance and metabolism in non-ketotic, diabetic rat hearts: myocardial function and metabolism in vivo and in the isolated perfused heart under the influence of insulin and octanoate. Basic Res Cardiol 81:620–635

84. Rowe JW, Young JB, Minaker KL, Stevens AL, Pallotta J (1981) Effect of insulin and glucose infusions on sympathetic nervous system activity in normal man. Diabetes 30:219–225

85. Rupp H, Berger HJ, Pfeifer A, Werdan K (1991) Effect of positive inotropic agents on myosin isozyme population and mechanical activity of cultured rat heart myocytes. Circ Res 68:1164–1173

86. Rupp H, Elimban V, Dhalla NS (1988) Sucrose feeding prevents changes in myosin isoenzymes and sarcoplasmic reticulum Ca^{2+}-pump ATPase in pressure-loaded rat heart. Biochem Biophys Res Commun 156:917–923

87. Rupp H, Elimban V, Dhalla NS (1989) Diabetes-like action of intermittent fasting on sarcoplasmic reticulum Ca^{2+}-pump ATPase and myosin isoenzymes can be prevented by sucrose. Biochem Biophys Res Commun 164:319–325

88. Rupp H, Jacob R (1983) The interrelationship between normalization of pressure load of heart and hypertrophy and myosin isoenzyme population in the SHR (abstract). J Mol Cell Cardiol 15 (Suppl 2):63

89. Rupp H, Jacob R, Dhalla NS (1990) Coordinated regulation of the subcellular structures of the heart and the consequence for assessing cardiac contractility. In: Jacob R (ed) Evaluation of Cardiac Contractility. Fischer, Stuttgart New York, pp 22–44

90. Saltiel AR, Cuatrecasas P (1988) In search of a second messenger for insulin. Am J Physiol 255:C1–C11

91. Schmidt FH, Deaciuc IV, Kühnle HF (1985) A new inhibitor of the long-chain fatty acid transfer across the mitochondrial membrane: 2-(3-methylcinnamylhydrazono)-propionate (BM42.304). Life Science 36:63–67

92. Selby PL, Sherratt HSA (1989) Substituted 2-oxiranecarboxylic acids: a new group of candidate hypoglycaemic drugs. Trends Pharmacol 10:495–500

93. Sherratt HSA (1981) Inhibition of gluconeogenesis by non-hormonal hypoglycaemic compounds. In: Hue L, Van de Werve G (eds) Short-term Regulation of Liver Metabolism. Elsevier/North-Holland Biomedical Press, Amsterdam, pp 199–227

94. Siliprandi N, Di Lisa F, Pivetta A, Miotto G, Siliprandi D (1987) Transport and function of L-carnitine and L-propionylcarnitine: relevance to some cardiomyopathies and cardiac ischemia. Z Kardiol 76 (Suppl 5):34–40

95. Smith WR, Claycomb WC (1989) Expression of alpha and beta myosin heavy chain genes in the rat ventricular cardiac muscle cell. In: Kedes LH, Stockdale FE (eds) Cellular and Molecular Biology of Muscle Development. Liss Inc, New York, pp 359–368

96. Stearns SB (1983) Carnitine content of skeletal and cardiac muscle from genetically diabetic (db/db) and control mice. Biochem Med 29:57–63

97. Tripp ME (1989) Developmental cardiac metabolism in health and disease. Pediatr Cardiol 10:150–158

98. Umeda PK, Darling DS, Kennedy JM, Jakovcic S, Zak R (1987) Control of myosin heavy chain expression in cardiac hypertrophy. Am J Cardiol 59:49A–55A

99. Urumow T, Wieland OH (1990) A small G-protein involved in phosphatidylinositol-4-phosphate kinase activation. FEBS Lett 263:15–17

100. Vaartjes WJ, De Haas CGM, Haagsman HP (1986) Effects of sodium 2-5-(4-chlorophenyl)pentyl-oxirane-2-carboxylate (POCA) on intermediary metabolism in isolated rat liver cells. Biochem Pharmacol 35:4267–4272

101. Vary TC, Neely JR (1982) A mechanism for reduced myocardial carnitine levels in diabetic animals. Am J Physiol 243:H154–H158

102. Weiss RG, Chacko VP, Gerstenblith G (1989) Fatty acid regulation of glucose metabolism in the intact beating rat heart assessed by carbon-13 NMR spectroscopy: the critical role of pyruvate dehydrogenase. J Mol Cell Cardiol 21:469–478

103. Wieland OH, Urumow T, Drexler P (1989) Insulin, phospholipase, and the activation of the pyruvate dehydrogenase complex: an enigma. Ann NY Acad Sci 573:274–284

104. Wolf HPO, Engel DW (1985) Decrease of fatty acid oxidation, ketogenesis and gluconeogenesis in isolated perfused rat liver by phenylalkyl oxirane carboxylate (B 807-27) due to inhibition of CPT I (EC 2.3.1.21). Eur J Biochem 146:359–363
105. Wolf HPO (1990) Aryl-substituted 2-oxirane carboxylic acids: a new group of antidiabetic drugs. In: Bailey CJ, Flatt PR (eds) New Antidiabetic Drugs. Smith-Gordon, London, pp 217–229
106. Yonekura Y, Brill AB, Som P, Yamamoto K, Srivastava SC, Iwai J, Elmaleh DR, Livni E, Strauss HW, Goodman MM, Knapp FF Jr (1985) Regional myocardial substrate uptake in hypertensive rats: a quantitative autoradiographic measurement. Science 227:1494–1496
107. York CM, Cantrell CR, Borum PR (1983) Cardiac carnitine deficiency and altered carnitine transport in cardiomyopathic hamsters. Arch Biochem Biophys 221:526–533
108. Zorzano A, Balon TW, Brady LJ, Rivera P, Garetto LP, Young JC, Goodman MN, Ruderman NB (1985) Effects of starvation and exercise on concentrations of citrate, hexose phosphates and glycogen in skeletal muscle and heart. Evidence for selective operation of the glucose-fatty acid cycle. Biochem J 232:585–591

Authors' address:

Dr. H. Rupp
Physiologisches Institut II
der Universität Tübingen
Gmelinstraße 5
W-7400 Tübingen, FRG

A new concept for the mechanism of Ca^{++}-regulation of muscle contraction. Implications for physiological and pharmacological approaches to modulate contractile function of myocardium

B. Brenner

Department of General Physiology, University of Ulm, FRG

Summary: Recent development of an experimental protocol to determine kinetics of active cross-bridge turnover in muscle allows analysis of possible Ca^{++}-effects on cross-bridge turnover kinetics. This analysis enabled us to distinguish the two main hypotheses about the mechanism of regulation of muscle contraction. In the first hypothesis, the number of actively turning over cross-bridges is changed, while cross-bridge turnover kinetics are unaffected by Ca^{++} (regulation by "cross-bridge recruitment"). In the other hypotheses, cross-bridge turnover kinetics are controlled by Ca^{++}, while the number of actively turning over cross-bridges is essentially unaffected (regulation by "rate modulation"). It is found that the major mechanism of regulation of muscle contraction is by a change in the rate constant (f_{app}) that determines the transition of a cross-bridge from the weak-binding (non-force generating) configuration to its strong-binding (force generating) configuration. It is demonstrated that the concept of "rate modulation" requires reinterpretation of force-pCa relations and of the mechanisms of physiological and pharmacological modulation of force-pCa relations. On this basis, an additional mechanism for positive inotropic interventions is demonstrated which may have advantages over the previously established mechanisms.

Key words: Cross-bridge recruitment; Ca^{++}-dependent rate constants; cross-bridge turnover kinetics; force-pCa relation; positive inotropic interventions

Introduction

It is generally accepted that muscle contraction is the result of a cyclic interaction of the myosin heads, the cross-bridges, with actin. In recent concepts [for summary, see (9)], cross-bridges are assumed to exist in two main configurations, a high-affinity configuration (configuration of the "strong-binding states") and a low-affinity configuration (the configuration of the "weak-binding states") in which cross-bridges cannot contribute to force generation. During active turnover, cross-bridges are assumed to cycle between these two main configurations as ATP is hydrolyzed. In this concept, force generation or filament sliding are the result of a structural change associated with the transition of an attached cross-bridge from the low affinity configuration to its high affinity (force-generating) configuration (Fig. 1).

Regulation of muscle contraction was previously thought to occur by control of the number of actin sites to which cross-bridges can attach and complete their active turnover. Thus, in this concept, the change in active force (or in ATPase) with increasing Ca^{++}-concentration results from an increase in the number of cross-bridges involved in active turnover while the turnover kinetics of active cross-bridges are independent of Ca^{++} [cross-bridge "recruitment"; (20)]. This concept was based on the finding that in demembranated ("skinned") frog fibers an increase in free Ca^{++} did not significantly af-

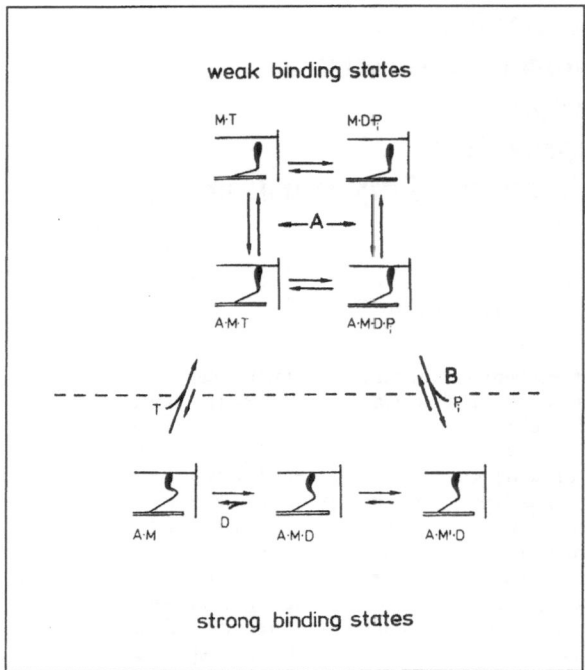

Fig. 1. Simplified diagram of cross-bridge action in muscle derived from recent biochemical kinetic schemes (12, 21, 23). In the weak-binding states, cross-bridges reversibly bind to actin (detach/reattach rapidly). In the strong-binding states equilibrium for reversible actin interaction is far on the side of attachment. Thus, for simplicity, detached states are omitted. Relative magnitude of arrows indicates qualitatively the change in free energy across the corresponding reaction step. A = actin, M = myosin, T = ATP, D = ADP, P_i = inorganic phosphate. "A" and "B" indicate the steps which were previously assumed to be blocked/unblocked to provide regulation by cross-bridge recruitment. "A": steric blocking of cross-bridge attachment (11, 14, 18). "B": on/off-control of the P_i-release reaction (7, 8)

fect the maximum unloaded shortening velocity (v_{max}). Furthermore, Ca^{++} appeared to have no effect on the shape of the force-velocity relation (20). X-ray diffraction studies of the second actin layer line were interpreted to indicate that tropomyosin moves on the surface of the actin filament upon binding of Ca^{++} to troponin C. Based on this interpretation, it was suggested that the postulated cross-bridge recruitment is mediated by blocking/unblocking of cross-bridge attachment to actin in states prior to force generation [steric-blocking hypothesis of regulation (11, 14, 18); "A" in Fig. 1].

As an alternative, it was proposed (15) that regulation of muscle contraction, in principle, could occur by Ca^{++}-dependent modulation of cross-bridge turnover kinetics, e.g., by modulation of the rate constant "f" which in the two-state cross-bridge model of Huxley (13) describes the transitions from the nonforce- to the force-generating state. In the more complex recent cross-bridge cycles with two groups of states of different actin affinity (e.g., Fig. 1) this rate constant (now termed f_{app}) describes the probability for the transition of a cross-bridge from the weak-binding (non-force generating) configuration to its strong-binding (force generating) configuration (3).[1]

Although from biochemical, mechanical, and structural studies it became clear that regulation cannot occur via blocking/unblocking of cross-bridge *attachment* in the low affinity states ("A" in Fig. 1), and although the idea was proposed that regulation acts on a subsequent reaction step, e.g., release of inorganic phosphate from the attached low-affinity cross-bridge [(7, 8); "B" in Fig. 1], the concept was still retained that regulation occurs via cross-bridge recruitment. That is, it remained unchallenged that an increase in activation is mediated by recruitment of new actively turning over cross-bridges, and not by altering turnover kinetics of already active ones.

Experimental protocol to probe for Ca^{++}-effects on cross-bridge turnover kinetics

Conclusive distinction between the two general hypotheses, i.e., recruitment vs change in turnover kinetics, remained impossible until recently, because measurements of force, fiber stiffness, and fiber ATPase under isometric conditions, or of the maximum speed of shortening (v_{max}) do not allow to distinguish between the two alternative hypotheses. The ratio of isometric ATPase over isometric force [e.g., (16)] is proportional to g_{app} under isometric conditions (i.e., when cross-bridges are positively strained and generate active force) where g_{app} describes the probability for a cross-bridge to change from the strong-binding configuration back to its weak-binding configuration (3). Measurements of v_{max} only provide information about g_{app} after a cross-bridge has released its strain due to filament sliding during fiber shortening ["g_2" in the notation of (13)]. Consequently, although both v_{max} and ATPase/force were found Ca^{++}-independent, these findings only ruled out Ca^{++}-effects on g_{app} of the strained or unstrained cross-bridge in the strong-binding configuration. No approach, however, was available which could provide unambiguous evidence about possible Ca^{++}-effects on f_{app}. Recently, however, we developed an experimental approach (1) which provides direct information about the magnitude of cross-bridge turnover kinetics, specifically about f_{app} (Fig. 2). In this approach, a period of unloaded (or lightly loaded) shortening is used to shift the distribution of cross-bridges between force- and nonforce-generating states toward the non-force-generating states (Fig. 2; note the much lower fiber stiffness during isotonic shortening which is about 15% of the isometric value). After a restretch to establish original filament overlap, force and stiffness redevelop. The time-course of the redevelopment of force and stiffness reflects the reincrease in occupancy of the strong-binding (force-generating) cross-bridge states. It was demonstrated (2, 3) that the rate constant of force redevelopment (k_{redev}) essentially reflects the sum of the rate constant characterizing the transition from the non-force to the force-generating states (f_{app}), plus the rate constant(s) for the return to the non-force-generating states (mainly g_{apr}).

Evidence for Ca^{++}-effects on cross-bridge turnover kinetics

Based on the above interpretation, measurements of k_{redev} at different Ca^{++}-concentrations allow to distinguish between the two hypotheses about regulation of mus-

---

[1] The apparent rate constant "f_{app}" cannot be assigned to any single reaction step within the cross-bridge cycle, but depends on the rate constant of P_i-release and all rate constants/equilibrium constants defined within the group of weak-binding states. Note that the magnitude of f_{app}, however, is mainly determined by a slow reaction step within the weak-binding states (5). This step is either the hydrolysis step [(21); scheme of Fig. 1], or a slow isomerization of the states $M \cdot D \cdot P_i / AM \cdot D \cdot P_i$ (23).

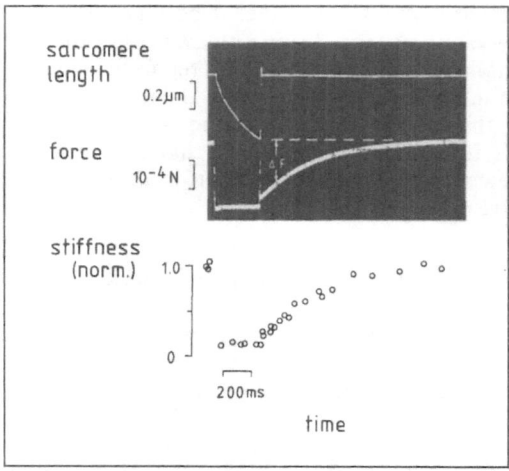

Fig. 2. Experimental protocol for recording time-course of force redevelopment after a period of isotonic shortening. Top trace: sarcomere length recorded by laser light diffraction. Middle trace: force. Bottom trace: apparent fiber stiffness measured during ramp-shaped stretches. Speed of stretches was set to about 1000 (nm/half-sarcomere)/s such that fiber stiffness reflects occupancy of force-generating states. Initially, the fiber is contracting under isometric conditions. Then the fiber is allowed to shorten under very low load (<3% of isometric force). After restretch to the original overlap, redevelopment of force is observed again under isometric conditions. To provide precise isometric conditions, sarcomere length was recorded by laser light diffraction and servo controlled during the period of force redevelopment (5). Skinned rabbit psoas fiber. [Reproduced by permission from (1).]

cle contraction. For cross-bridge recruitment, k_{redev} should be unaffected by Ca^{++} and only the steady state level of force should change (Fig. 3a, solid lines). For modulation of f_{app} by Ca^{++}, k_{redev} should increase with Ca^{++}-activation (Fig. 3a, dashed lines compared to uppermost solid line). The experiment reveals that the time-course of force redevelopment becomes faster when Ca^{++} is raised (Fig. 3b). This directly indicates that Ca^{++} affects cross-bridge turnover kinetics.

Since the ratio of isometric ATPase over isometric force is essentially Ca^{++}-independent (3, 16) the faster force redevelopment at higher Ca^{++}-concentrations is the result of an increase in f_{app}, while g_{app} (proportional to ATPase/force) is unaffected or only very little affected. This suggested that Ca^{++}-regulation exerts its effect by control of f_{app}. However, the question remained whether Ca^{++}-dependence of force, stiffness, and ATPase is fully accounted for by the Ca^{++} effect upon f_{app} or whether, in addition, some cross-bridge recruitment (Ca^{++}-dependent change in the number of actively turning over cross-bridges) has to be considered. Detailed analysis of Ca^{++}-dependence of force redevelopment, together with measurements of isometric force, isometric stiffness, and fiber ATPase at different levels of Ca^{++}-activation revealed [see (3) for details] that, at least for force levels above 25% of maximum tension, the Ca^{++}-mediated changes in isometric force, fiber stiffness, and fiber ATPase are essentially the result of the changes in f_{app} with Ca^{++} (Fig. 4). If cross-bridge recruitment occurs at all, it must be restricted to activation levels below 25% of full activation.

The concept of regulation via modulation of f_{app} by Ca^{++} ("rate modulation") found additional support by reinvestigation of force-velocity relations (4). In skinned rabbit

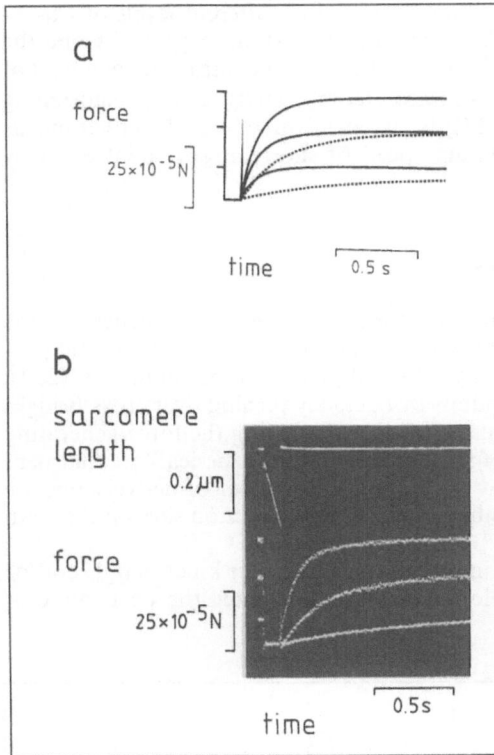

Fig. 3. Force redevelopment at different levels of Ca^{++}-activation. *a* Solid lines: expected behavior for regulation by cross-bridge recruitment (either via steric blocking of cross-bridge attachment, "A" in Fig. 1, or via blocking/unblocking of the P_i-release reaction "B" in Fig. 1). Dashed lines and uppermost solid line: expected behavior for regulation via modulation of cross-bridge turnover kinetics (f_{app}). Dashed lines for $^1/_3$ and $^2/_3$ of full activation, uppermost solid line for full activation. *b* Experimentally observed behavior: traces of three different levels of Ca^{++}-activation are shown (full activation, about two-third and somewhat less than one-third of full activation). Activation level is defined by the observed active force normalized with respect to maximum force at saturating Ca^{++}-concentrations. Skinned rabbit psoas fiber. [Reproduced by permission from (3).]

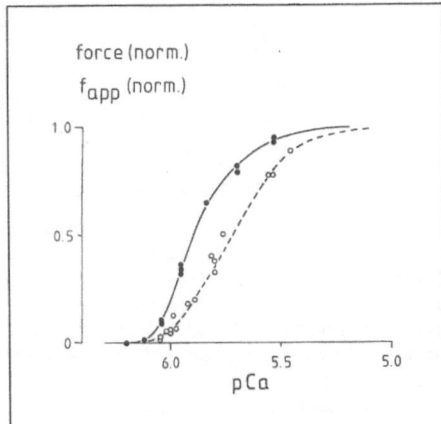

Fig. 4. Effect of sarcoplasmic Ca^{++}-concentration on force and f_{app}. Skinned rabbit psoas fiber. Experimental temperature 5° C. Note that Ca^{++}-sensitivity (pCa for half-maximum values) and slope of the two curves are different. [Reproduced by permission (3).]

psoas fibers the shape of force-velocity relations recorded at different levels of Ca^{++}-activation was found to change with Ca^{++}-activation, just as expected from the dependence of f_{app} on sarcoplasmic free Ca^{++}-concentration. In contrast, detachment of cross-bridges which became negatively strained (compressed) during shortening [determined by "g_2" in the notation of (13)] is independent of Ca^{++}-activation, as evidenced by the fact that v_{max} (the maximum speed of shortening) is unaffected by Ca^{++}.

Implications of regulation via turnover kinetics

The most significant implication of regulation via turnover kinetics (f_{app}) instead of the previously assumed recruitment concerns interpretation of force-pCa relations and possible mechanisms for their modulation by physiological/pharmacological means [(2, 3); Fig. 5]. Active force is proportional to the number of actively turning over cross-bridges times the fraction of actively turning over cross-bridges occupying the force-generating states [equal to $f_{app}/(f_{app}+g_{app})$, see (3) for details]. In the "classical" recruitment hypothesis, $f_{app}/(f_{app}+g_{app})$ is unaffected by Ca^{++} and the number of actively turning over cross-bridges is determined by the number of activated interaction sites on the actin filaments. This, in turn, is determined by Ca^{++}-binding to troponin C.

For the recruitment hypothesis, changes in cross-bridge turnover kinetics (f_{app} and/or g_{app}) by some physiological or pharmacological intervention alter the occupancy of

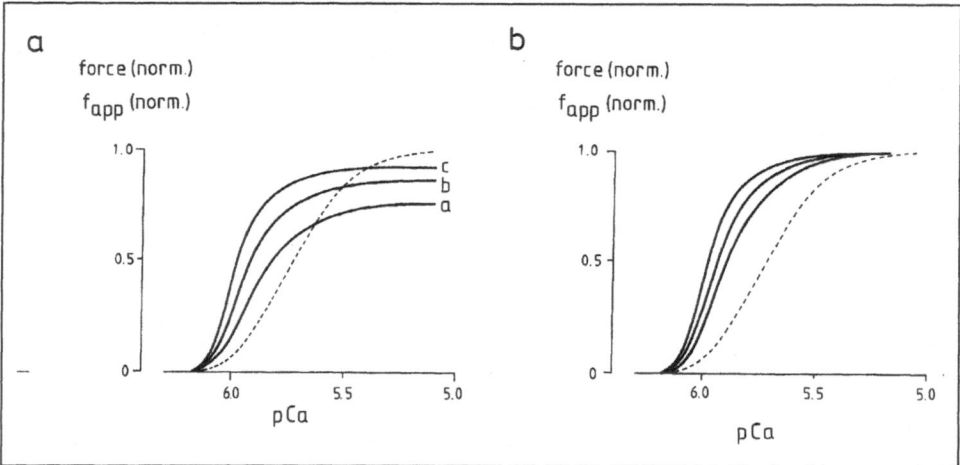

Fig. 5. Expected effects of changes in cross-bridge turnover kinetics (f_{app} and g_{app}) on force-pCa relations for regulation via Ca^{++}-dependent modulation of f_{app} ("rate modulation"). *a* Force-pCa relations as calculated. For calculation of force-pCa relations the experimentally determined f_{app}-pCa relation shown in Fig. 4 was used. Three different ratios of f_{app}/g_{app} at maximum activation were assumed. For curve "a" the assumed ratio is 3/1, for curves "b" and "c" 6/1 and 12/1, respectively. Force is proportional to number of turning over cross-bridges times $f_{app}/(f_{app}+g_{app})$ [for details, see (3)]. The number of turning over cross-bridges and g_{app} are essentially Ca^{++}-independent. Proportionality factor and number of turning over cross-bridges set to 1. *b* All calculated force-pCa relations normalized to their force level at saturating Ca^{++}-concentrations

force-generating states $[f_{app}/(f_{app}+g_{app})]$, however, to the same extent for all Ca^{++}-concentrations. Thus, only the vertical scaling of force-pCa-relations is expected to change, and the resulting force pCa-relations should be identical if normalized to maximum force at saturating Ca^{++}-concentrations.

This is very different for the hypothesis of Ca^{++}-regulation via "rate modulation" [(2, 3); Fig. 5]. Assuming unchanged Ca^{++}-binding to the regulatory proteins (f_{app}-pCa relation of Fig. 4 remains unaffected), changes in cross-bridge turnover kinetics (f_{app} or g_{app}) by any physiological or pharmacological intervention do not simply scale the calculated force level at each Ca^{++}-concentration, as for the recruitment concept, but also affect apparent Ca^{++}-sensitivity (pCa for 50% activation) and slope of the force-pCa relation (Fig. 5a). This is more clearly illustrated by normalizing force-pCa relations with respect to active force at saturating Ca^{++}-concentration (Fig. 5b). This results from the fact that at low levels of activation (magnitude of f_{app} is comparable to magnitude of g_{app}), changes in f_{app} or g_{app} have a larger effect on the ratio $f_{app}/(f_{app}+g_{app})$ than at high activation levels ($f_{app}>>g_{app}$). Note that apparent Ca^{++}-sensitivity and the slope of the force-pCa relations depend on cross-bridge turnover kinetics (Fig. 5) and are very different from these parameters for the f_{app}-pCa relation (Fig. 4). This implies that force-pCa relations neither directly reflect Ca^{++}-sensitivity nor cooperativity of Ca^{++}-binding to the regulatory proteins.

Implications for physiological modulation of contractile function

Based on the recruitment concept, effects of myosin P-light chain phosphorylation on the force-pCa relation were found difficult to be accounted for (19). At low activation levels, phosphorylation increased active force much more than at high activation levels. On the basis of the recruitment concept, neither increased Ca^{++}-binding to troponin C (maximum force should not change) nor changes in turnover kinetics (should affect force at all activation levels by same factor) could account for these observations. Following the proposal of our "rate modulation" concept for regulation of muscle contraction and its implications for interpretation of force-pCa relations [(2, 3); Fig. 5] it was demonstrated that the observed effects of myosin P-light chain phosphorylation on force-pCa relations apparently are the result of an increase in f_{app} with myosin P-light chain phosphorylation (6, 17, 24).

Implications for possible mechanisms of inotropic interventions

Possible mechanisms for inotropic interventions are schematically illustrated in Fig. 6. The two previously described mechanisms for inotropic interventions are illustrated in Fig. 6a, b. By these interventions either the intracellular Ca^{++}-transients are increased ["amplitude modulation"; (22); Fig. 6a], or Ca^{++}-binding to troponin C is enhanced ["sensitivity modulation", e.g., by "Ca^{++}-sensitizers"; (22); Fig. 6b]. On the basis of Ca^{++}-regulation via "rate modulation" (change in f_{app} with Ca^{++}), we have to consider an additional third mechanism for positive inotropic interventions. Changes in cross-bridge turnover kinetics can cause changes in the force-pCa relation (Fig. 5) which result in enhanced active force for a given Ca^{++}-transient (Fig. 6c). Since, again, the pCa for 50% activation is affected, this again is sensitivity modulation, and drugs acting by this mechanism also represent "Ca^{++}-sensitizers". However, in addition to Ca^{++}-sensitivity, the slope of force-pCa relations is also affected to some extent. Since this sensitivity modulation results from a different mechanism and results in different side effects (see

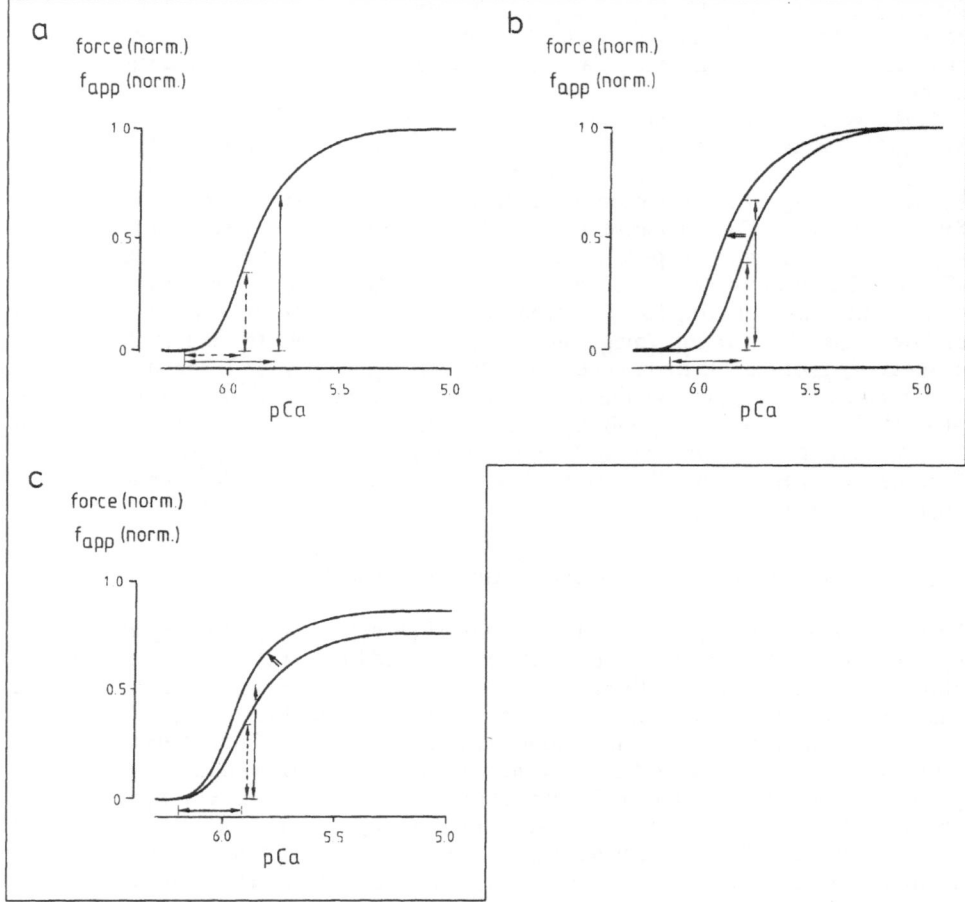

Fig. 6. Schematic diagrams for possible mechanisms of positive inotropic drugs. Horizontal arrows qualitatively illustrate the assumed intracellular Ca^{++}-transients. *a* "Amplitude modulation" [cf. (22)]. Increase in isometric force by increased Ca^{++}-transient. Dashed arrows: Ca^{++}-transient and resulting force without positive inotropic intervention. Solid arrows: with positive inotropic intervention. *b* "Sensitivity modulation" [cf. (22)]. Increased Ca^{++}-responsiveness by Ca^{++}-sensitizer which increases Ca^{++}-affinity to troponin C ("class I" Ca^{++}-sensitizer), resulting in leftward shift of force-pCa relation. At submaximal Ca^{++}-concentrations the same Ca^{++}-transient results in a larger isometric force. Note that in the presence of this type of Ca^{++}-sensitizer for full relaxation a lower Ca^{++}-concentration is required than under control conditions. Dashed arrow: force under control conditions. *c* Increased Ca^{++}-responsiveness by Ca^{++}-sensitizer which affects f_{app} or g_{app} (class IIa or class IIb Ca^{++}-sensitizer), resulting in leftward shift and steeper force-pCa relation. Two curves from Fig. 5a. Dashed arrow, force under control conditions. Note that full relaxation in the presence of a class II Ca^{++}-sensitizer does not require as low Ca^{++}-concentrations as relaxation in the presence of a class I Ca^{++}-sensitizer. For effect on economy see text

next paragraph), this class of Ca^{++}-sensitizers ("class II") should not be mixed up with the other class of Ca^{++}-sensitizers which acts through improved Ca^{++}-binding to troponin C ("class I" sensitizers).

Drugs which shift the force-pCa relation to lower free Ca^{++}-concentrations (to the left in Figs. 5, 6), i.e., any Ca^{++}-sensitizer, will require lower free Ca^{++}-concentrations for full relaxation. Thus, all Ca^{++}-sensitizers may lead to the problem of incomplete relaxation. However, for Ca^{++}-sensitizers of class II (acting via turnover kinetics) this effect is much reduced (Fig. 6c). Enhancement of Ca^{++}-binding to troponin C by force-generating cross-bridges at low activation levels [e.g., (10)], however, may cause some additional leftward shift of the low end of the force-pCa relation expected (from calculation) for "class II" Ca^{++}-sensitizers (Fig. 6c) or for increased myosin P-light chain phosphorylation [(6, 17, 24); Fig. 5]. Thus, the advantage of class II Ca^{++}-sensitizers over class I Ca^{++}-sensitizers concerning incomplete relaxation may be reduced somewhat by this effect.

A second difference in "side effects" concerns effects of Ca^{++}-sensitizers upon the economy of force (or pressure) development. As judged by "tension cost", defined as isometric ATPase/isometric force and which is proportional to g_{app}, Ca^{++}-sensitizers of class I (increase in Ca^{++}-binding to TnC) have no effect. For Ca^{++}-sensitizers of class II, one has to distinguish sensitizers which act via a) increased f_{app}, from those which act via b) a decrease in g_{app}. In the former case tension cost is unaffected (or only very little affected), in the latter example tension cost decreases as Ca^{++}-responsiveness is increased. Consequently, with a Ca^{++}-sensitizer of class II(b), the same transient in sarcoplasmic Ca^{++}-concentration will not only lead to larger active force (increased Ca^{++}-responsiveness), but also to improved economy of force generation (reduced tension cost). However, due to the apparent coupling between the magnitude of g_{app} for isometric conditions with g_{app} for unstrained cross-bridges during shortening [g_2 in the notation of (13)] the improved economy is expected to lead to reduced maximum speed of shortening which was shown to be determined by g_2 (13). Thus, reduction of maximum speed of shortening may put a limit to the extent to which g_{app} can be reduced by a class II(b) Ca^{++}-sensitizer before pump function of myocardium becomes significantly impaired.

Conclusions

Our finding that Ca^{++}-regulation is mediated by "rate modulation" (Ca^{++}-dependent change in f_{app}) and not by cross-bridge recruitment requires reinterpretation of force-pCa relations and their changes upon physiological and pharmacological interventions. Regulation by rate modulation opens up an additional mechanism for inotropic interventions (class IIa and class IIb Ca^{++}-sensitizers). The "class II" of Ca^{++}-sensitizers may be associated with less severe problems of incomplete relaxation, and some of these Ca^{++}-sensitizers (class IIb) are expected to even improve economy of pressure development.

References

1. Brenner B (1985) Correlation between the cross-bridge cycle in muscle and the actomyosin ATPase cycle in solution. J Muscle Res Cell Motil 6:659–664
2. Brenner B (1986) The cross-bridge cycle in muscle. Mechanical, biochemical, and structural studies on single skinned rabbit psoas fibers to characterize cross-bridge kinetics in muscle for correlation with the actomyosin-ATPase in solution. Basic Res Cardiol 81, 1:1–15

3. Brenner B (1988) Effect of Ca^{2+} on cross-bridge turnover kinetics in skinned single rabbit psoas fibers: implications for regulation of muscle contraction. Proc Natl Acad Sci USA 85:3265–3269
4. Brenner B (1989) Effect of Ca^{++}-activation upon force-velocity-relation. Further evidence for Ca^{++}-regulation affecting cross-bridge turnover kinetics. Biophys J 55:407a
5. Brenner B, Eisenberg E (1986) The rate of force generation in muscle: correlation with actomyosin ATPase in solution. Proc Natl Acad Sci USA 83:3542–3546
6. Brenner B, Morano I (1990) Effects of myosin light chain phosphorylation on isometric force and cross-bridge turnover kinetics. Pflüg Arch 415:R73
7. Brenner B, Schoenberg M, Chalovich JM, Greene LE, Eisenberg E (1982) Evidence for cross-bridge attachment in relaxed muscle at low ionic strength. Proc Natl Acad Sci USA 79:7288–7291
8. Chalovich JM, Chock PB, Eisenberg E (1981) Mechanism of action of troponin-tropomyosin. J Biol Chem 256:575–578
9. Eisenberg E, Hill TL (1985) Muscular contraction and free energy transduction in biological systems. Science 227:999–1006
10. Güth K, Potter JD (1987) Effect of rigor and cycling cross-bridges on the structure of troponin C and on the Ca^{2+}-specific regulatory sites in skinned rabbit psoas fibers. J Biol Chem 262:13627–13635
11. Haselgrove JC (1973) X-ray evidence for the conformational change in the actin-containing filaments of vertebrate striated muscle. Cold Spring Harb Symp Quant Biol 37:341–352
12. Hibberd MG, Trentham DR (1986) Relationships between chemical and mechanical events during muscular contraction. Ann Rev Biophys Chem 15:119–161
13. Huxley AF (1957) Muscle structure and theories of contraction. Prog Biophys 7:255–318
14. Huxley HE (1973) Structural changes in the actin- and myosin-containing filaments during contraction. Cold Spring Harb Symp Quant Biol 37:361–376
15. Julian FJ (1969) Activation in a skeletal muscle contraction model with modification for insect fibrillar muscle. Biophys J 9:547–570
16. Kushmerick MJ, Krasner B (1982) Force and ATPase rate in skinned skeletal muscle fibers. Fed Proc 41:2232–2237
17. Metzger JM, Moss RL, Giulian GG, Greaser ML (1988) Increased rate of tension redevelopment at submaximal (Ca^{++}) in fast-twitch skeletal muscle following myosin light chain phosphorylation. Biophys J 53:23a
18. Parry DAD, Squire JM (1973) Structural role of tropomyosin in muscle regulation. Analysis of the x-ray diffraction patterns from relaxed and contracting muscles. J Mol Biol 75:33–55
19. Persechini A, Stull JT, Cooke R (1985) The effect of myosin phosphorylation on the contractile properties of skinned rabbit skeletal muscle fibers. J Biol Chem 260:7951–7954
20. Podolsky RJ, Teichholz LE (1970) The relation between calcium and contraction kinetics in skinned muscle fibers. J Physiol 211:19–35
21. Rosenfeld SS, Taylor EW (1984) The ATPase mechanism of skeletal and smooth muscle actosubfragment 1. J Biol Chem 259:11908–11919
22. Rüegg JC (1986) Calcium in muscle activation. A comparative approach. Springer, Berlin Heidelberg New York
23. Stein LA, Schwarz RP, Chock PB, Eisenberg E (1979) Mechanism of actomyosin adenosine triphosphatase. Evidence that adenosine 5′-triphosphate hydrolysis can occur without dissociation of the actomyosin complex. Biochemistry 18:3895–3909
24. Sweeney HL, Stull JT (1990) Alteration of cross-bridge kinetics by myosin light chain phosphorylation in rabbit skeletal muscle: implications for regulation of actin-myosin interactions. Proc Natl Acad Sci USA 87:414–418

Authors' address:

Prof. Dr. B. Brenner
Allgemeine Physiologie
Universität Ulm
Albert-Einstein-Allee 11
W-7900 Ulm, FRG

Large and rapid changes of myofibrillar total calcium during the cardiac cycle. Electron probe microanalysis of voltage-clamped guinea-pig ventricular myocytes *

M. F. Wendt-Gallitelli [1], G. Isenberg [2], T. Voigt [1], and C. Ross [1]

[1] Physiologisches Institut II, University of Tübingen
[2] Institut für Angewandte Physiologie, Köln, FRG

Summary: At 36° C and 2 mM $[Ca^{2+}]_0$, single guinea-pig ventricular myocytes were voltage clamped with patch electrodes. When paired pulsing had potentiated the contraction to the maximum, the cells were shock-frozen for electron probe microanalysis (EPMA). Shock-freezing was timed at the end of diastole (-80 mV) or at different times during systole ($+5$ mV).

The same paired-pulse protocol was applied to another group of myocytes from which contraction was recorded and $[Ca^{2+}]_i$ was estimated by microfluospectroscopy (50 µM Na-Indo-1). In potentiated cells, during the first pulse, contraction peaked within 128 ± 25 ms after start of depolarization. $[Ca^{2+}]_i$ peaked within 25 ms to 890 ± 220 nM (mean $\pm$ SEM) and fell within 100 ms to about 450 nM.

ΣCa_{myo}, the total calcium concentration in the overlapping myofilaments (A-band), was measured by EPMA in 17 potentiated myocytes. During diastole, ΣCa_{myo} was 2.6 ± 0.4 mmol/kg dry weight (dw), which can be converted to 0.65 mM (mmoles per liter myofibrillar space). Since $[Ca^{2+}]_i$ was 180 nM, we estimate that 99.97% of total calcium is bound.

A time-course for systolic ΣCa_{myo} was determined by shock-freezing 13 cells at different times after start of depolarization to $+5$ mV. ΣCa_{myo} was 5.5 ± 0.3 mmol/kg dw (1.4 mM) after 15–25 ms, 4.6 ± 0.5 mmol/kg dw (1.1 mM) after 30–45 ms, and 3.1 mmol/kg dw (0.8 mM) after 60–120 ms. The fast time-course of ΣCa_{myo} suggests that calcium binds to and unbinds from troponin C at a fast rate. Hence, it is the slow kinetics of the cross-bridges that determines the 130-ms time-to-peak shortening.

Key words: Ventricular heart cell; voltage clamp; free calcium; total calcium; activation of contraction

Introduction

It is the calcium binding to troponin C which activates contraction in cardiac muscle. Total calcium minus free myoplasmic calcium is the Ca^{2+} bound to ligands. If the time-course of the changes in free- and total myoplasmic Ca-concentration can be measured during the contraction cycle, one can obtain quantitative information concerning the regulatory-role Ca^{2+}-ligands play at any time of the contraction style.

Electron probe microanalysis is a method which can measure total calcium, i.e., the sum of free and bound calcium exactly in the region of the overlapping filaments.

With electron probe microanalysis, we have measured (time scale: in milliseconds) the changes of total myofibrillar calcium during contraction in ultrathin cryosections of isolated guinea-pig ventricular myocytes. In voltage-clamp experiments the contraction of the myocytes was potentiated to an optimum via a paired-pulse protocol, and the membrane currents were measured. Afterwards, the myocytes were shock-frozen for cryosectioning and x-ray microanalysis. The same paired-pulse protocol was applied to another group of myocytes from which contraction and free cytosolic Ca^{2+} was estimated by microfluospectrometry.

* Supported by the Deutsche Forschungsgemeinschaft We 879/3-2 and Is 24/7-2

We have chosen this difficult and time-demanding combination of voltage-clamp technique, cryosectioning, and electron probe microanalysis on single myocytes, because we are convinced that measurements of changes in total myofibrillar calcium during activation and relaxation give complementary information to that obtained by measurements of free calcium with microfluospectrometry: for the first time, we can give evidence that the total calcium in the myofibrillar region increases to millimolar concentrations within a few milliseconds after depolarization and, more surprisingly, large amounts of this calcium are removed rapidly from the filaments when the cell is still contracting.

The single-cell preparations avoid the problem of cell-to-cell heterogenicity that is inherent in multicellular preparations. Due to limited cooling rate, acceptable cryopreservation is achieved only in the outermost cells of multicellular preparations. These cells may not be representative for the multicellular preparation. Furthermore, the method of timed freezing of a single myocyte under voltage-clamp conditions is the only one at this time which makes it possible to document electrical events of the cell membrane up till the very moment of freezing and on the same cell from which the elemental distribution will be analyzed by electron probe microanalysis.

Methods

Myocyte isolation: The methods for preparing single isolated Ca^{2+}-tolerant ventricular myocytes of guinea-pig have been described in detail in (1). Briefly, the heart was retrogradely perfused (36° C) with a Ca-free cell-medium. This was followed by perfusion with the same medium supplemented with 50 mg/l protease and 250 μM $CaCl_2$. The ventricle was chopped and the pieces stirred in the same medium for three periods of 10 min each. The released myocytes were resuspended in a medium containing 0.5 mM $CaCl_2$, and then stored until used. For the experiments, the physiological saline solution contained 150 mM NaCl, 5.4 mM KCl, 2 mM $CaCl_2$, 1.2 mM $MgCl_2$, 5 mM glucose, and 5 mM HEPES/NaOH, pH 7.4.

Voltage-clamp experiments were performed according to the whole-cell configuration of the patch-clamp technique, as described in (10).

Contractile force of the single isolated myocytes was measured as described recently (6).

Rapid transients of free [Ca^{2+}]$_i$ (myoplasmic free calcium) was estimated with the ratio technique of indo-1 fluorescence (5), as described recently (4).

Shock-freezing of the myocyte. The isolated quiescent myocyte with clear cross-striation, superfused at 36° C with a solution containing 2 mM $CaCl_2$, is sucked up with a patch-pipette which serves for both the transfer of the cell from the chamber to a special silver holder, as well as for electrophysiological measurements [for details, see (10)].

The computer generating the voltage-clamp pulses also controls the horizontal movement of chamber and microscope away from the holder, and the vertical movement of the coolant (Fig. 1). Thereafter, at a defined time in the contraction cycle, the myocyte is shock-frozen.

Figure 2 shows the membrane currents of an isolated myocyte as recorded before and during shock-freezing in systole, 40 ms after start of depolarization. Starting from a holding potential of -80 mV, a prepulse of 20 ms activates and deactivates the sodium current. A pulse of 180 ms at $+5$ mV activates the Ca^{2+}-current. After 20 ms repolarization to -45 mV, a 160 ms long pulse to $+50$ mV activates Ca^{2+}-influx via Na^{+}-Ca^{2+}-exchange mechanism. Repolarization to -80 mV induces a large tail current which is thought to represent Ca^{2+}-efflux via the Na^{+}-Ca^{2+}-exchange.

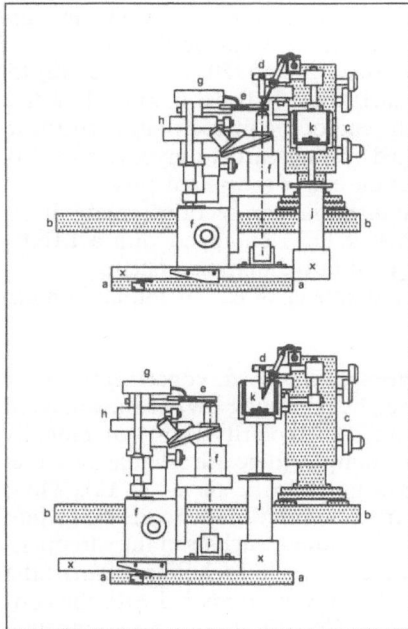

Fig. 1. Device for shock-freezing of voltage-clamped ventricular myocytes, shown before (top) and after (bottom) shock-freezing. The two plates (a) and (b) are fixed independently to prevent transfer of vibrations from the moving parts to the electrode. Plate b supports a Leitz micromanipulator (c) that bears the silver holder (d), and a hydraulic Narashige micromanipulator for the electrode and the head stage of the amplifier. Parts b, c, and d are kept still during the shock-freezing. The sliding stage x supports a simple microscope (f) adapted through a prism (i) to a TV camera (not shown). x also supports, via the manipulator (h), the experimental chamber (e) into which solution flows from the heat exchanger (g). During shock-freezing, the sliding stage (x) is moved backwards by means of pneumatic pistons. When the sliding stage x has positioned the silver holder, cell, and electrode into the air above the beaker with the coolant (k), the beaker is pushed upwards with the piston (j). (With permission from Journal of Physiology 1991, in press)

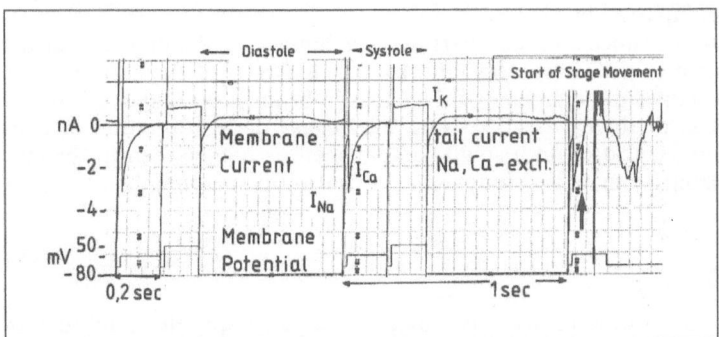

Fig. 2. The membrane current can be used as a protocol to monitor the events during shock-freezing. Shock-freezing during systole, 40 ms after start of depolarization to $+5$ mV. The panel shows the membrane current in response to the voltage clamp protocol (lower trace). During diastole the holding potential is -80 mV. At a rate of 1 Hz, paired voltage clamp pulses are applied. The first pulse starts with a short 20 ms depolarization to -45 mV that activates and inactivates an inward sodium current I_{Na}. A 180 ms pulse to $+5$ mV activates and inactivates an inward calcium current I_{Ca}. After a short 20 ms repolarization to -45 mV, the second pulse depolarizes the membrane to $+50$ mV for 160 ms and induces an outward current carried mostly by K^+ ions. The final repolarization to -80 mV induces a large inward tail current due to electrogenic Na^+-Ca^{2+} exchange. When the cell in the holder is moved out of the experimental chamber no change in the membrane current is seen. Contact with the $-196°$ C coolant (large arrow) is indicated by a large capacitive artifact followed by a large outward current

The currents records before and during freezing are superimposable, and thus disturbances in the membrane function due to vibrations can be excluded. For analysis of myofibrillar calcium during systole, myocytes were frozen 10, 15, 20, 25, 30, 35, 40, 45, 60, 90, 120, 125, 160, 170, 560 ms after start of depolarization. In order to know how fast the myoplasmic total calcium concentration after the end of the paired pulses returns to the low values previously measured in unstimulated resting cardiac myocytes (8–10), myocytes were also shock frozen 1.8 s and 3 min after the end of the paired pulses.

After freezing, the frozen myocytes were cut into ultrathin cryosections, freeze-dried, and analyzed in a Philips electron microscope CM12/STEM equipped with a LINK-energy dispersive Pentafet-detector, and with a full quantitative analysis-system.

For analysis, the electron beam was focused to a diameter of ca. 16 nm, and an appropriate area was scanned.

Concentration units: Since the cryosections have been freeze-dried, concentrations are measured in millimoles of an element per kg dry weight (mmol/kg dw) of the analyzed compartment. These values can be converted to units of molarity (mM) or molality (mmol/kg water) of the analyzed compartment: for example, there are reliable measurements of the water content of mitochondria, showing it to be 66% (7, 12). Thus, 1 mmol/kg dw ΣCa_{mito} can be converted into 0.33 mM (mmol/l mitochondria), or into 0.5 mmol/kg mitochondrial water. Unknown hydration values, such as in the sarcoplasmic reticulum (SR), can be estimated on the basis of the known mitochondrial water: the x-ray continuum, measured, e.g., in SR, or in the A-band, was compared with the continuum in adjacent mitochondria using the same dose of electrons (i.e., same count-time and same beam intensity) [for details, see (11)]. In order to reduce the statistical error of the single measurement of low Ca-concentrations, the analysis-time was prolonged to 600–1000 s. In this way, minimal concentrations of calcium in the range of 0.5 mmol/kg dw or 0.16 mmol/liter compartment can be detected.

The spatial resolution of subcellular compartments is limited by the diameter of the electron beam obtainable in the microscope and by the thickness of the cryosections. Since in modern microscopes the diameter of the electron beam is no longer a limiting factor, it is the thickness of the cryosections that may cause underestimation of concentrations when the concentration in a small compartment is higher than in the surroundings, as the analyzing beam may include some portion of the surroundings.

Results and discussion

Potentiation of contraction: In the ventricle myocyte of the guinea-pig the amplitude of contraction increases with stimulation frequency (positive staircase). In vivo, the heart is beating at a rate of about 3 Hz. For technical reasons the computer-controlled experiments were done at 1 Hz basic frequency and the contraction was potentiated with a paired pulse protocol. Paired pulses increase the peak-force in a beat-to-beat fashion; potentiation become steady after 5 beats (11). The "systole" refers exclusively to the first contraction which was evoked by the clamp-step to +5 mV. In the unloaded myocytes, after a latency of ca. 15 ms, contraction peaked within 110 ms and relaxed within 200 ms to 80%. In four myocytes we observed the effect of paired pulsing on unloaded shortening (Fig. 4).

In Fig. 3, the height of the columns represent the total myofibrillar calcium concentrations measured in diastole and systole.

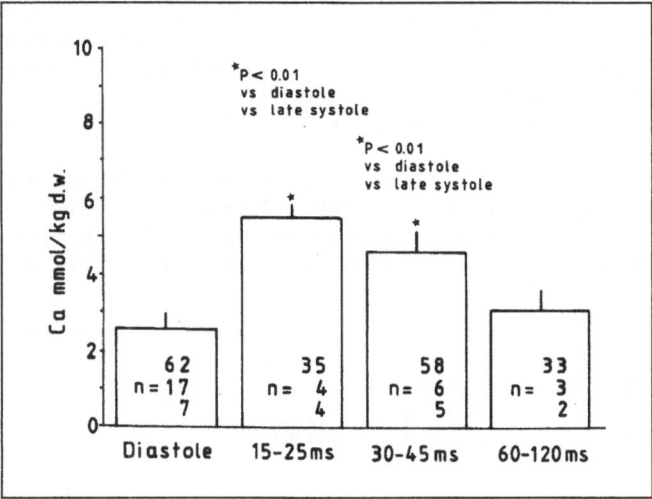

Fig. 3. Total myoplasmic calcium (ΣCa_{myo}) in ventricular myocytes shock-frozen at the end of diastole and during early (15–25 ms), middle (30–45 ms), and late systole (60–120 ms) after contraction was potentiated to a optimum by paired-pulse protocol. n=number of spectra, of cells, of animals. Bars indicate means $\pm$ SEM

1. At the end of the diastole, the total calcium concentration measured in the region of overlapping filaments was 2.6 ± 0.4 (mean $\pm$ SEM) mmol/kg dw (number of spectra $= 62$), which corresponds, in terms of molarity, to 0.65 mM (mmol/liter myofibrillar space). 1.8 s after the end of paired pulsing, ΣCa_{myo} decreased to 1.8 ± 0.4 mmol/kg dw or 0.45 mM (n $= 13$). Three min later, ΣCa_{myo} was 1 ± 0.2 mmol/kg dw or 0.25 mM (n $= 10$). This time-dependent decrease of ΣCa_{myo} after the end of stimulation agrees with the finding that, in unstimulated myocytes, ΣCa_{myo} was not significantly different from zero (10). This reversibility of the potentiation-induced increase in ΣCa_{myo} suggests that it is not an artefact, but rather a phenomenon linked to contractile potentiation.

The diastolic total myofibrillar calcium concentration is eight times higher than that expected on the basis of the known Ca^{2+}-ligands (3). We can exclude that this is an artefact, as values in the range of 2 mmol/kg dw are far above the minimal detectable concentrations and statistically significantly differ from zero. High diastolic Ca-concentrations have already been published by our laboratory: in earlier investigations similar high diastolic concentrations were measured in multicellular preparations of guinea-pig ventricle, the contraction of which had been potentiated with positive inotropic interventions, although diastolic tension was not increased (8).

During diastole, the concentration of myoplasmic free calcium in the myocytes was in the range of 0.2 μM. This means that 0.03% of the total calcium is ionized, and 99.97% is bound. As possible Ca^{2+}-ligands, calmodulin, troponin C, and myosin have been described for the myofibrillar space (3). The concentrations of these ligands are insufficient to explain the present data, hence, we postulate that the myofibrillar space of the ventricular cell contains about 600 μM additional "slow" Ca^{2+} binding sites, i.e., sites with on- and off-rates similar to that of the Ca^{2+},Mg^{2+}-sites of troponin C. With those additional calcium ligands we can adequately model the potentiation-mediated increase in $[Ca^{2+}]_i$ and ΣCa_{myo} and its decay upon rest.

The Ca^{2+},Mg^{2+}-sites of myosin are occupied by Mg^{2+}; their affinities for Ca^{2+} and Mg^{2+} differs only by a factor of 100, and the $[Mg^{2+}]_i$ is four orders of magnitude higher than $[Ca^{2+}]_i$. The Ca^{2+},Mg^{2+}-sites of troponin C would have properties suitable for the potentiation-induced increase in diastolic ΣCa_{myo} and $[Ca^{2+}]_i$. However, the Ca^{2+}-specific site of troponin C can, at best, bind only 100 μM Ca^{2+}, which is a concentration much lower than 650 μM.

2. *During systole,* 15–25 ms after start of depolarization, the total myofibrillar Ca reaches a maximum of 5.5 mmol/kg dw, which corresponds to 1.8 mM. Nested analysis of variance shows that the concentration is significantly higher than the diastolic value. 30–45 ms after start of depolarization the myofibrillar Ca concentration is not sig-

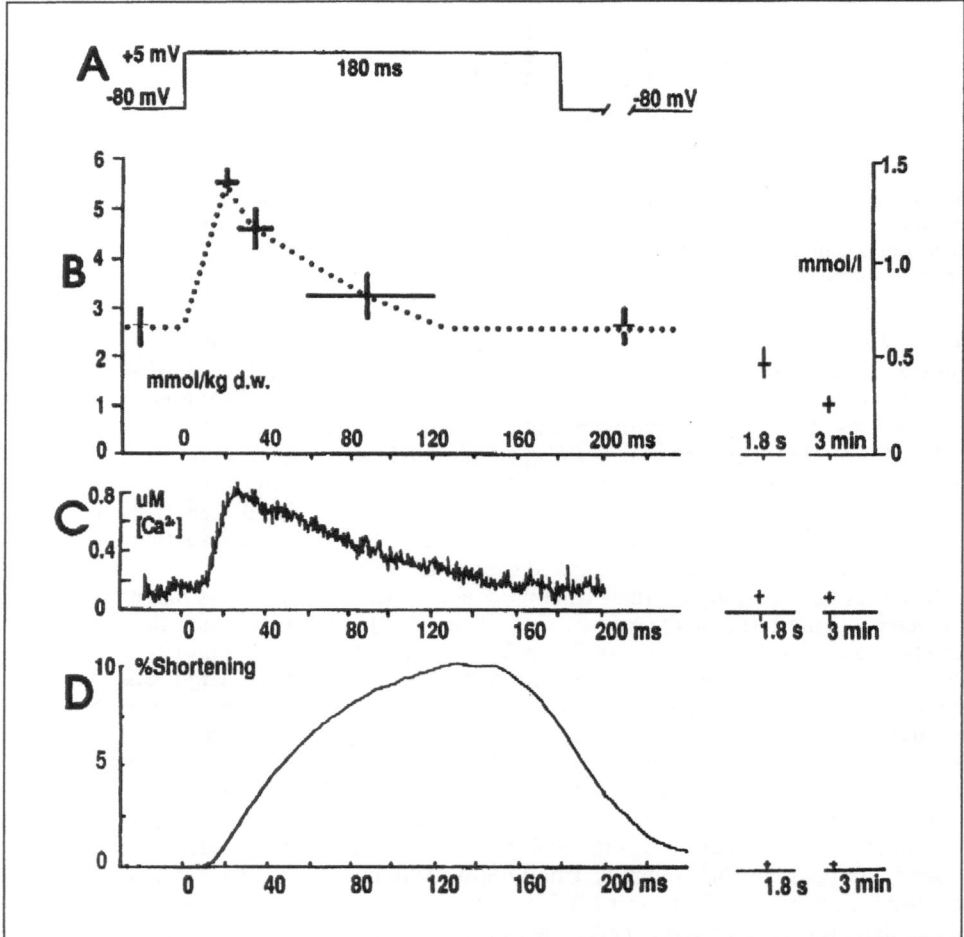

Fig. 4. Time-course of ΣCa_{myo} (B) in comparison with $[Ca^{2+}]$ (C) and isotonic shortening (D). *A* shows the voltage clamp procotol. In *B* the vertical bars indicate $\pm$ SEM of the mean, horizontal bars are the period of time in which measurements were grouped together. *C* and *D* are averages from 10 sweeps. For $[Ca^{2+}]_i$ data were transformed into a linear scale by computer

nificantly lower than in early systole, and is still significantly higher than in diastole. At a time, however, at which contraction has not yet reached its maximum, i.e., 60–120 ms after start of depolarization, the total myoplasmic calcium is decreased to 3.1 mmol/kg dw. This systolic value is no longer significantly different from the diastolic value.

This is shown more clearly in Fig. 4: the time courses of total and free calcium as well as isotonic contraction are plotted in the same time scale. The vertical bars represent the statistical error of the means, the horizontal bars the period of time in which the measurements of single myocytes were grouped together.

The result that the concentration of free calcium peaks at an early time is well known from Ca^{2+} measurements with aequorin (2), but these measurements did not answer the question of whether the rapid decrease is due to a shift of calcium from the aequorin to troponin C, or due to accumulation of calium in the SR. We think that the present results answer this question unequivocally. Figure 4 shows that, not only the free, but also the total calcium decreases to diastolic values a long time before relaxation starts. Thus, the notion that calcium has bound to the low affinity sites of troponin C can be rejected.

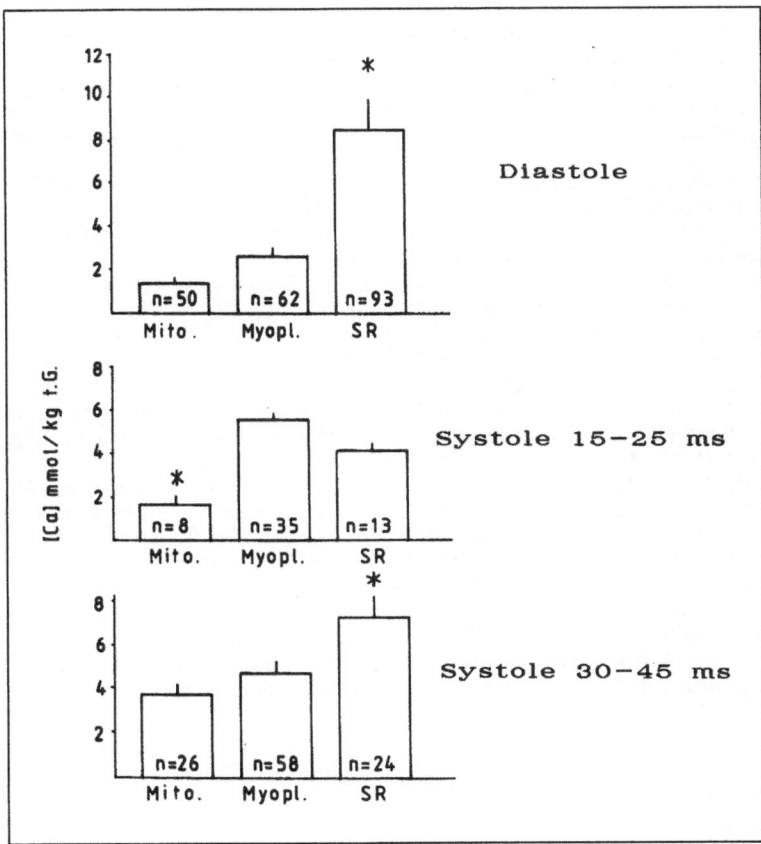

Fig. 5. Total calcium concentration in myoplasma (ΣCa_{myo}), mitochondria (ΣCa_{mi}), and SR (ΣCa_{SR}) at the end of diastole after paired pulses, as well as during early and middle systole. n = number of spectra. Bars indicate means $\pm$ SEM

Further, Fig. 5 shows the total calcium concentration in the SR (ΣCa_{SR}). During diastole, ΣCa_{SR} is significantly higher than ΣCa_{myo}. During early systole the concentration-gradient between myoplasm and SR disappears. Both properties are expected from a Ca^{2+}-release compartment. As soon as 30–45 ms after start of depolarization, ΣCa_{SR} increased again; the values were significantly higher than in myoplasm. This indicates that, at this time, at least part of the myoplasmic Ca^{2+} has been taken up from the SR.

The results about systolic ΣCa_{myo} also show that it is not the myoplasmic calcium concentration which determines the time-to-peak of contraction, but rather the slow kinetic of the cross-bridges. We think that Ca^{2+} binding to troponin C initiates the force-generating process. After this initial activation, the further time-course of contraction and the time-to-peak dissociate from the Ca-concentration, i.e., ΣCa_{myo} can fall while force or shortening can still increase.

References

1. Bendukidze Z, Isenberg G, Klöckner U (1985) Ca-tolerant guinea-pig ventricular myocytes as isolated in the presence of 250 μM free Ca. Basic Res Cardiol 80:13–18
2. Blinks JR, Endo M (1986) Modification of myofibrillar responsiveness to Ca^{2+} as inotropic mechanism. Circulation 73 SIII:85–98
3. Fabiato A (1983) Calcium-induced release of calcium from the cardiac sarcoplasmic reticulum. Am J Physiol 245:C1–C14
4. Ganitkevich VY, Isenberg G (1991) Depolarization-mediated intracellular Ca^{2+} transients in isolated smooth muscle cells of the guinea pig urinary bladder. J Physiol (in press)
5. Grynkiewicz G, Poenie M, Tsien RW (1985) A new generation of Ca^{2+} indicators with greatly improved fluorescence properties. J Biol Chem 260:3440–3450
6. Shepherd N, Vornanen M, Isenberg G (1990) Force measurements from voltage-clamped guinea-pig ventricular myocytes. Am J Physiol 258:H542–549
7. Somlyo AV, Gonzales-Serratos H, Shuman H, McClennan G, Somlyo AP (1981) Calcium release and ionic changes in the sarcoplasmic reticulum of tetanized muscle. An electron probe study. J Cell Biol 90:577–594
8. Wendt-Gallitelli MF (1986) Ca pools involved in the regulation of cardiac contraction under positive inotropy. X-ray microanalysis of rapid frozen ventricular muscles of the guinea pig. Basic Res Cardiol 81:S1, 25–31
9. Wendt-Gallitelli MF, Jacob R, Wolburg H (1982) Intracellular membranes as boundaries for ionic distribution. In situ elemental distribution in guina-pig heart muscle in different defined electromechanical coupling states. Z Naturforsch 37c:712–720
10. Wendt-Gallitelli MF, Isenberg G (1989) X-ray microanalysis of single myocytes frozen under voltage-clamp conditions. Am J Physiol 256:H574–H583
11. Wendt-Gallitelli MF, Isenberg G (1991) Total and free myoplasmic calcium during a contraction cycle: x-ray microanalysis in guinea-pig ventricular myocytes. J Physiol (in press)
12. Werkheiser WC, Bartley W (1957) The study of steady-state concentrations of internal solutes of mitochondria by rapid centrifugal transfer to a fixation medium. Biochem J 66:79–91

Authors' address:

Priv.-Doz. Dr. M. F. Wendt-Gallitelli
Physiologisches Institut II
Gmelinstraße 5
W-7400 Tübingen 1, FRG

Are antisarcolemmal (ASAs) and antimyolemmal antibodies (AMLAs) "natural" antibodies?

B. Maisch [1], L. Drude [1], C. Hengstenberg [1], M. Herzum [1], G. Hufnagel [1], K. Kochsiek [3],
A. Schmaltz [2], U. Schönian [1], and M. D. Schwab [3]

[1] Department of Internal Medicine – Cardiology, Philipps-University Marburg
   (Prof. Dr. B. Maisch),
[2] Department of Pediatric Cardiology, University of Essen (Prof. Dr. A. Schmaltz),
[3] University Hospital of Internal Medicine, Würzburg (Prof. Dr. K. Kochsiek), FRG

Summary: Antisarcolemmal (ASAs) and in particular antimyolemmal antibodies (AMLAs) are a serologic hallmark of inflammatory heart muscle disease and its sequelae. Since they may also occur to a much lesser incidence with increasing age, it was examined whether they also possess properties of "natural antibodies". As natural antibodies, AMLAs and ASAs have specificity for conserved structures on the membrane. They possess cross-reactivity and increase with age. In contrast to natural antibodies, however, they occur most frequently after viral stimulation, and are more often of the IgG- and IgA- than of the IgM-isotype and fix complement in the acute stage of the disease. They also exhibit cytolytic and cytotoxic properties when incubated in vitro with isolated heart muscle cells. In addition, antigenic mimicry has been demonstrated to be operative, since they are cross-reactive to viral proteins.

Key words: Myocarditis; perimyocarditis; dilated cardiomyopathy; antisarcolemmal antibodies; antimyolemmal antibodies; cytolytic serum activity; natural antibodies

Introduction

Our retrospective knowledge of immune reactions has, until the late 1970s, been largely influenced by the opinion that autoantibodies are unwanted and highly pathological phenomena. Nils Jerne has called B-cells and plasma cells producing autoantibodies "forbidden clones" in the framework of his network theory (8). Even earlier, Paul Ehrlich's scenario of immune response described them as "horror autotoxicus". Meanwhile, in systemic autoimmune disorders, as well as in normal healthy individuals, autoantibodies to different constituents of normal cells have been demonstrated. This also applies to autoantibodies to the cardiac myocyte, the cytoskeleton, the connective tissue, the extracellular matrix, the endothelial cells and fibroblasts in different heart muscle diseases and in postcardiac injury syndromes (1, 4–7, 9, 10–31, 33, 34). In fact, the entire cardiac tissue can be a target of cellular and humoral immune reactions (16).

Our knowledge about autoreactive processes has expanded continuously: Autoantibodies and/or natural antibodies (3) and autoreactive T-cells play a part in the immunological "network" that regulates the interaction of lymphocytes, immune regulation, T-cell traffic, "homing" of cells, and the effector mechanisms. In any one of the conditions the cardiac myocyte, the endothelial cells and the fibroblasts, but also the extracellular matrix is exposed to immunocompetent cells. Myocytes, fibroblasts, and vascular endothelium may be partially altered in inflammatory heart muscle diseases (myocarditis, endocarditis, and rejection after heart transplantation, in ischemic heart disease, and in the cardiomyopathies).

Disease-induced changes from viral or bacterial assaults, from ischemia or during a rejection episode predispose the heart to be an excellent target for the recognition by antigen presenting or other immuncompetent cells, or to the response by humoral immunological effector organs. These may be monitored in the myocardium itself by endomyocardial biopsy (14–16, 20, 25). Its fingerprints can be detected even years later in the peripheral blood as circulating autoantibodies (1, 4–7, 9–34). Their incidence in different forms of heart disease has been recently reviewed extensively (16).

From these data the question arises if the anticardiac antibodies in general, or antisarcolemmal or antimyolemmal antibodies in particular are just "natural antibodies", or what is their true pathogenetic relevance?

From recent work in animal models certain characteristics of natural antibodies have become clear:

1) They have specifity for highly conserved structures, e.g., for xanthinoxidase, myelin basic protein, collagen, DNA, cytoplasmatic filaments, the cytoskeleton, thyreoglobulin, myoglobin, sperm proteins, albumin, neural tissue or the FC fragment of IgG.

2) They increase with age.

3) They possess extensive cross-reactivity because their respective autoantigens are ubiquitous. Their immune reaction is polyclonal and polyspecific.

4) In experimental animals they are found in germ-free mice. It is therefore unlikely that they occur primarily as a result of stimulation by bacterial antigens.

It is the purpose of the present investigation to examine, in inflammatory heart disease and dilated cardiomyopathy, the role of antisarcolemmal (ASAs) and antimyolemmal antibodies (AMLAs) with respect to these main characteristics of natural antibodies.

Patients

Ten adult patients with Coxsackie virus B3 and B4 myocarditis [eight male, two female; mean age 33.8 ± 12.4 years; histologically validated as active myocarditis according to the Dallas criteria (2)], 10 patients with biopsy-proven active myocarditis of unknown origin (seven male, three female; mean age 43 ± 14.2 years), 50 adult patients with perimyocarditis [31 male, 29 female; mean age 44.2 ± 8.7 years with pericardial effusion and segmental wall motion abnormality or cardiomegaly in levocardiography or two-dimensional (2D) echocardiography] were selected out of 2100 patients who had undergone endomyocardial biopsy in a 10-year period in Marburg and Würzburg, FRG. With respect to immunohistochemical data, they were also compared to patients with status post myocarditis (n = 22) and status post perimyocarditis (n = 15) without cardiomegaly, and 28 patients with postmyocarditic heart muscle disease or 50 patients with idiopathic dilated cardiomyopathy.

In addition, six children were included with definite myocarditis or perimyocarditis (mean age 2.74 ± 4.96; four male, two female), six children with probable perimyocarditis (two male, four female; mean age 7.17 ± 5.15), 31 children with possible inflammatory heart disease (14 male, 17 female; mean age 8.45 ± 3.82). Controls included 150 healthy adult blood donors (mean age 48.2 ± 12.3 years, 85 male, 65 female), and 48 children from 1 month to 17 years of age). The study with children under the suspicion of myocarditis was conducted in close collaboration with the departments of pediatric cardiology in Würzburg (Prof. Sandhage) and in Tübingen (Prof. Apitz) and Essen (Prof. Schmaltz).

Diagnostic criteria

Histological diagnosis of biopsy-proven myocarditis was based on the Dallas criteria (2). The essential criteria for definite perimyocarditis diagnosed on clinical grounds, included pericardial rubs or effusion with segmental wall motion abnormality by levocardiography and/or 2D echocardiography after exclusion of coronary artery disease by cineangiography. Probable perimyocarditis (this diagnosis was applied in children only due to limited biopsies available) was diagnosed either when pericarditis was associated with rhythm disturbances alone, or when a reversible segmental wall motion abnormality was observed in the context of a viral illness. The diagnosis of possible myocarditis in children was based on the present of reversible rhythm disturbances associated with a viral illness.

Light microscopy

Light microscopical investigations, including routine hematoxylin-eosin staining, were carried out at the pathological-anatomical institutes of the respective contributing centers (Prof. Müller-Hermelink, Würzburg; Prof. Hort, Düsseldorf; Prof. Thomas, Marburg) and our own laboratory.

Immunological methods

Immunohistochemistry: For immunohistochemistry of endomyocardial biopsies the direct technique [as described in (15)] was used. In addition, a double-sandwich technique was used for the demonstration of circulating anti-heart antibodies to bind on the same cryostat section at the same antibody binding site, using TRITC- and FITC-labeled antibodies [F(ab)$_2$ fragments, dilution 1:100; Medac] (15). Furthermore, binding of the monoclonal antibody directed against the membrane attack complex (C_{5b9}) was analyzed (dilution 1:40) by a peroxidase-coupled second antibody (rabbit antimouse IgG) (kindly provided by S. Bhakdi, Institute of Bacteriology, University of Gießen).

Immunoserology

Circulating antiheart and non-organ-specific antibodies were determined on cryostat sections of human, rat, and bovine heart, skeletal muscle, thyroid gland, stomach, kidney, and liver (14, 15, 19–22). Circulating heterologous antimyolemmal antibodies were determined on intact rat cardiocytes isolated by Percoll gradient centrifugation after perfusion with a collagenase (Worthington)-Ringer perfusate (14). Circulating homologous antimyolemmal antibodies were assessed on intact myocytes from human atrial appendages removed during open-heart surgery, minced, and incubated in a calcium-free Ringer collagenase solution [composition according to medium 2 in (22)] at 37° C, sedimented by centrifugation (80 g) after addition of EDTA. Fixation was accomplished by acetone added to the Ringer solution in the same volume centrifugation (22).

Cytolytic serum activity

The pathogenetic relevance of antimyolemmal (AMLAs) and antisarcolemmal (AEAs) antibodies, as well as antiendothelial antibodies (AEAs) was measured in a microcytotoxicity assay using vital cardiocytes as target cells. Antibody mediated cytolysis in the presence of complement was assessed by an index comparing the half-lives of cardiocytes in the presence of the patient's serum and with control sera (pool). Indices < 0.75 indicated significant cardiocytolysis.

Biochemical and Western blot studies

Isolation of membrane proteins of the heart: The sarcolemmal vesicles of the heart of Sprague-Dawley rats (150–200 g) immersed in iced TSE medium (sucrose 0.25 M, Tris/HCl 20 mM. EGTA 1 mM, at pH 7.5) and frozen at $-76°$ C, and of the heart of a histopathologically investigated 17-year-old patient (blood group 0) who died after a spinal operation, were isolated according to (32). Electron microscopic evaluation of the final pellet demonstrated highly enriched membrane vesicles with less than 5% contaminants. Endoplasmatic reticulum and mitochondria were ruled out enzymatically.

SDS polyacrylamide gel electrophoresis and Western blot: SDS polyacrylamide gel (12.5%) electrophoresis of cardiac membrane proteins and of Coxsackie B virus were performed according to standard procedures. The proteins were transferred quantitatively from the polyacrylamide gel to a nitrocellulose sheet (6, 13). The unstained electrophoretic blots were soaked in 5% bovine serum albumin in PBS buffer (10.15 mM NaCl, 10 mM Na_2HPO_4, 2.5 mM KCl, 1.5 mM KH_2PO_4, 0.3% Tween 20, pH 7.4) for 16 h at $0°$ C to saturate non-specific binding sites, and then were rinsed twice in PBS buffer. Each sheet was incubated for 2 h with 100 ml of the patient's serum diluted 1:50 in 5 ml PBS containing 1% bovine serum albumin. Alternatively, peroxidase-labelled lectins, HLA and DR antibodies, and the previously described monoclonal and monospecific antibodies were tested. The sheets were then washed five times in PBS and incubated with goat antihuman $F(ab)_2$-peroxidase conjugate (Medac), ratio 1:500 in PBS, containing 1% bovine serum albumin. The sheets were rinsed 10 times with PBS buffer. For color reaction, the blots were soaked in a freshly prepared, filtered solution of 6 mg 3-amino-9-ethyl-carbazol (Sigma), 7.5 ml DMF (Merck), 0.1 ml HCl 1 M, and 0.15 ml 30% H_2O_2 in 150 ml distilled water at pH 5.5–6.0. The reaction was terminated after 5–10 min by washing with water. The blots were dried and stored protected from light.

To account for minor background staining by the human sera, standard control sera were used in each analysis. Positive antibody binding to one of the bands was accepted only when, compared to the control sera, new bands appeared, or at least a twofold intensity of immunoglobulin binding was observed.

Results and discussion of the characteristics
of natural antibodies with respect to features from ASAs and AMLAs

Antisarcolemmal and antimyolemmal antibodies have specificity
for highly conserved structures

It can be demonstrated that the cardiac sarcolemma and myolemma are highly conserved structures. The sarcolemma and myolemma are first line autoantigens (Fig. 1) in various heart diseases:

AMLAs are characterized by a linear membrane fluorescence with isolated human myocytes (Fig. 2). They can be associated or mimick antilaminin antibodies. The sarcolemmal structure is less easily identified on biopsies, since antibodies against collagen, interstitial tissue, the extracellular matrix may show similar immunofluorescence patterns both when bound ASAs are analyzed (Table 1) or circulating AMLAs and ASAs are evaluated (Table 2).

It becomes clear from the data in Tables 1 and 2 that bound ASAs of the IgM, IgA and IgG class are markers of a secondary immunopathogenesis. Additional complement fixa-

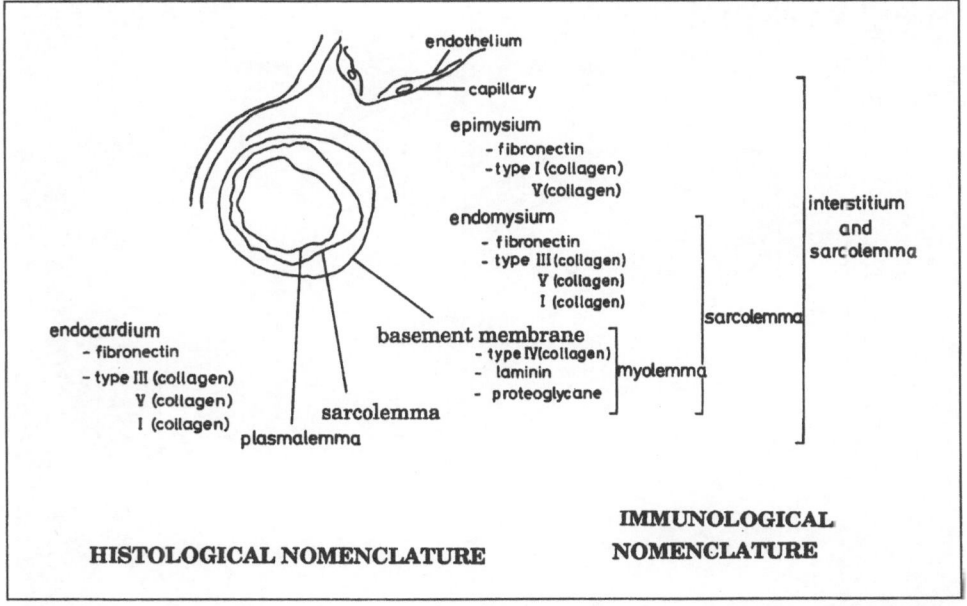

Fig. 1. Cardiac autoantigens. The cardiac sarcolemma and myolemma are highly conserved structures, but constitute only one of the possible cardiac autoantigens

Table 1. Immunohistochemistry in endomyocardial biopsies

Clinical diagnosis	N	Trivalent	IgG	IgM	IgA	C3	C3 or IgM
Myocarditis (active/acute)	20	100[a, b]	90[a, b]	55[a, b]	70[a, b]	70[a, b]	85[a, b]
Perimyocarditis (active/acute)	50	90	90	75	85	80	90
Status post myocarditis (no cardiomegaly)	22	100	95	32	32	36	45
Status post perimyocarditis (no cardiomegaly)	15	73[a]	60[a]	13	7	33[a]	40[a]
Postmyocarditic HMD[c] (cardiomegaly)	28	79[a]	75[a]	18	36[a]	61[a, b]	75[a]
Dilated cardiomyopathy (idiopathic)	50	60[a]	56[a]	48[a, b]	8	12	48[a]
Non-cardiac controls		12	12	0	0	0	0
Coronary artery disease	100	43[a]	41[a]	11	20	3	14

[a] $p > 0.05$ by $\hat{\chi}^2$ analysis when compared to non-cardiac controls.
[b] $p > 0.05$ by $\hat{\chi}^2$ analysis when compared to coronary artery disease.
[c] HMD; Heart muscle disease.

tion is indicative of a secondary immunopathogenesis operating in the individual patients.

As can be derived from Table 2, not only do individuals with inflammatory heart disease or dilated cardiomyopathy possess this antibody in the myocardial tissue and in the peripheral blood, but also do so to a much lesser extent than do healthy controls (Fig. 3).

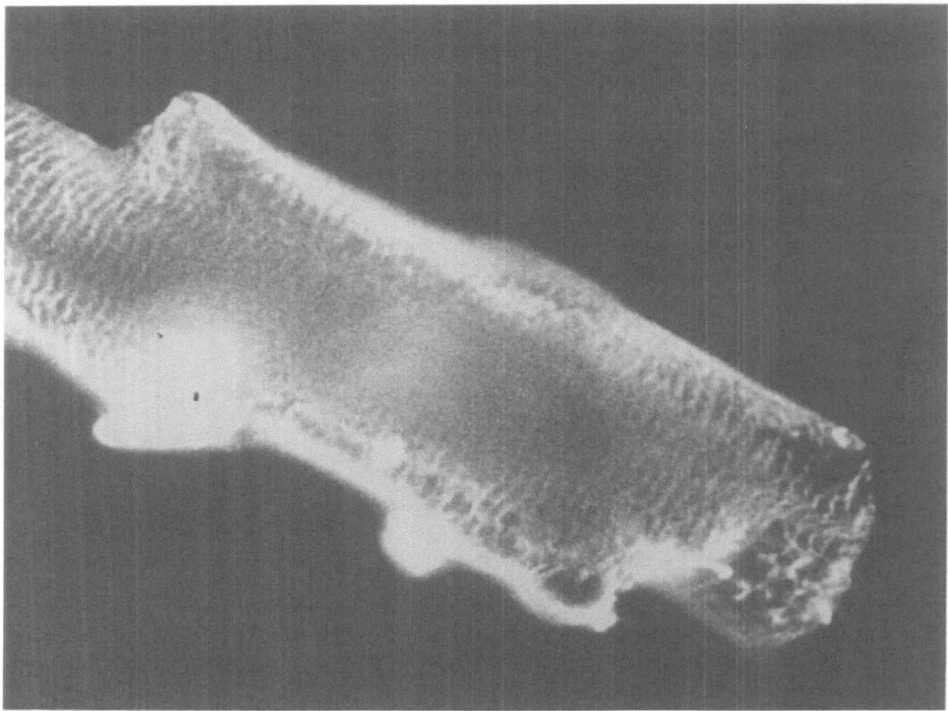

Fig. 2. Circulating antimyolemmal antibodies in a 27-year-old patient with active myocarditis using a human adult myocyte as antigen (titer 1:160). Antilaminin antibodies were demonstrated as concomittant after staining of sarcolemma and Z-bands of isolated rat cardiocytes. The ALA-ELISA was positive as well.

When comparing the disease-associated incidence of circulating ASAs and AMLAs in myocarditis in children and adults, one can derive that in all age groups the antimyolemmal antibodies are a good disease marker (Table 2).

When analyzing possible subgroups of antimembrane antibodies such as antilaminin antibodies, one can derive that the latter may be part of the microheterogeneity of ASAs or AMLAs, but are – at least in our patients – found less frequently than positive ASAs or AMLAs were recorded.

Natural antibodies increase with age

In healthy adults controls (n = 150) 31% of them have low titer AMLAs and 35% of them demonstrate ASAs in the peripheral blood. Incidence of bound ASAs is around 20% of the IgG isotype in healthy controls (post mortem, non cardiac death, n = 20).

Analysis in healthy children demonstrates clearly that in healthy newborns neither ASAs nor AMLAs can be detected; they appear after the first 6 months of age. Their in-

Table 2. Circulating antibodies to the sarcolemma, the extracellular matrix and intermediate filaments (% positive)

	n	AMLAs (homol)	ASAs	ALAs	Z-bands	A-Actin	A-Myosin	A-Tubulin	AIDAs	A-Desmin	A-Vimentin	A-M7	AEAs
Adults:													
Myocarditis	50	90	90	70	15	10	30	0	0	0	0	35	80
Perimyocarditis	50	60	50	60	10	0	20	10	1	0	0	nd	40
Children:													
Perimyocarditis	12	100	100	100	10	0	5	0	0	0	0	nd	70
Healthy controls (adults)	150	31	35	20	5	5	5	0	0	5	0	0	17
Pericarditis	10	80	50	nd	0	0	0	0	0	0	0	0	30
Postpericardiotomy-syndrome	40	90	90	33	12	5	12	0	2	0	0	nd	78
CAD*	96	38	36	nd	5	4	4	0	0	0	0	nd	19

* Coronary artery disease

AMLAs = antimyolemmal antibodies
ASAs = antisarcolemmal antibodies
ALAs = antilaminin antibodies
AIDAs = antintercalated disk antibodies
A-M7 = antimitochondrial antigen M7 antibodies
AEA = antiendothelial antibodies

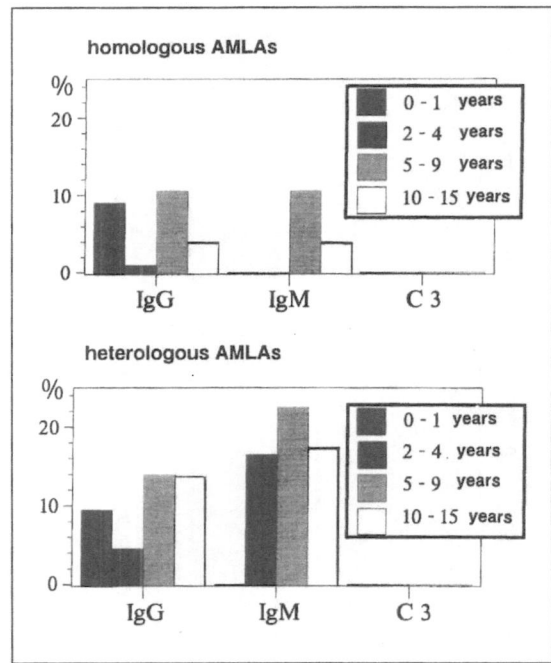

Fig. 3. Age-related incidence of ASAs and AMLAs in children without heart disease

cidence increases gradually (Fig. 3). This property of antimembrane antibodies fits well to the characteristics of natural autoantibodies.

Natural antibodies possess extensive cross-reactivity

Cross-reactivity is a key marker of ASAs and AMLAs. In Coxsackie-B-virus-induced myocarditis this can be clearly stated for several bands of sarcolemmal proteins to which the patients' sera bind. As can be derived from Fig. 4, which sums up Western blot data from 10 patients with Coxsackie-virus-induced myocarditis, antigenic mimicry appear to be a pathogenetic principle of Coxsackie-B-virus-induced active myocarditis.

In a quantitative analysis of 10 patients with CBV myocarditis cross-reactive antibodies fixed on the 220, 110, 48, 35, 31, and 26 Kda bands. Virus-specific epitopes could be detected as 33 and 34 Kda bands, whereas cardioselective epitopes were 90, 78, 72, 67, and 45 Kda bands (29).

Cross-reactivity to other membrane constituents is also possible. In the indirect test with human skeletal muscle tissue about one-third of the sera that bind to the cardiac sarcolemma also fix to the skeletal muscle sarcolemma.

In streptococcal disease, e.g., rheumatic fever cross-reactivity between epitopes of the sarcolemma and the streptococcal membrane has become clear since Kaplan's initial work (9), and has been further clarified by Cunningham et al. (4, 5).

In infective endocarditis induced by streptococci Thometzek et al. (35) have similarily demonstrated cross-reactivity to a number of epitopes of the sarcolemma.

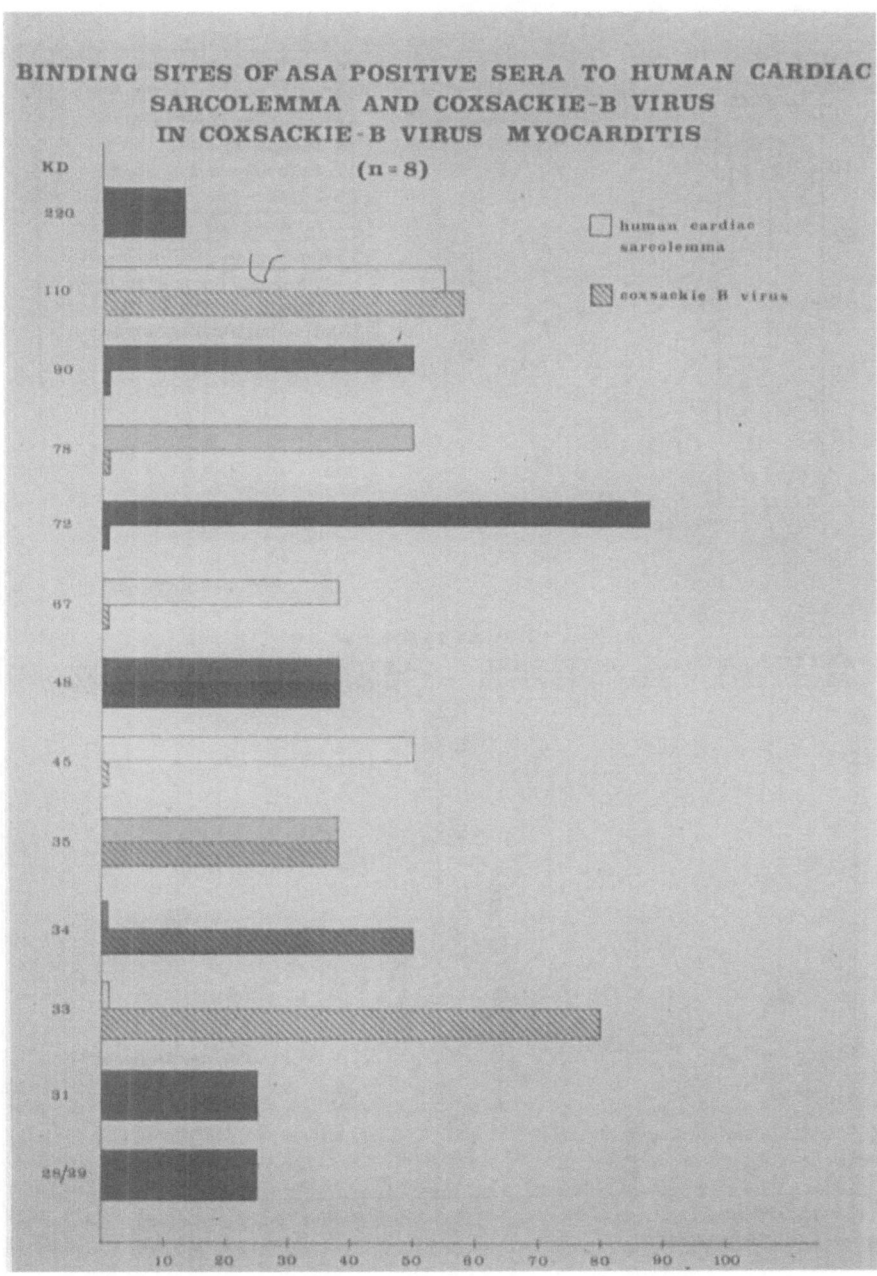

Fig. 4. Cross-reactivity of ASAs to both sarcolemma and Coxsackie-virus-derived proteins can be analyzed from Western blots of patients with biopsy-proven active Coxsackie B virus myocarditis (see text for further explanation)

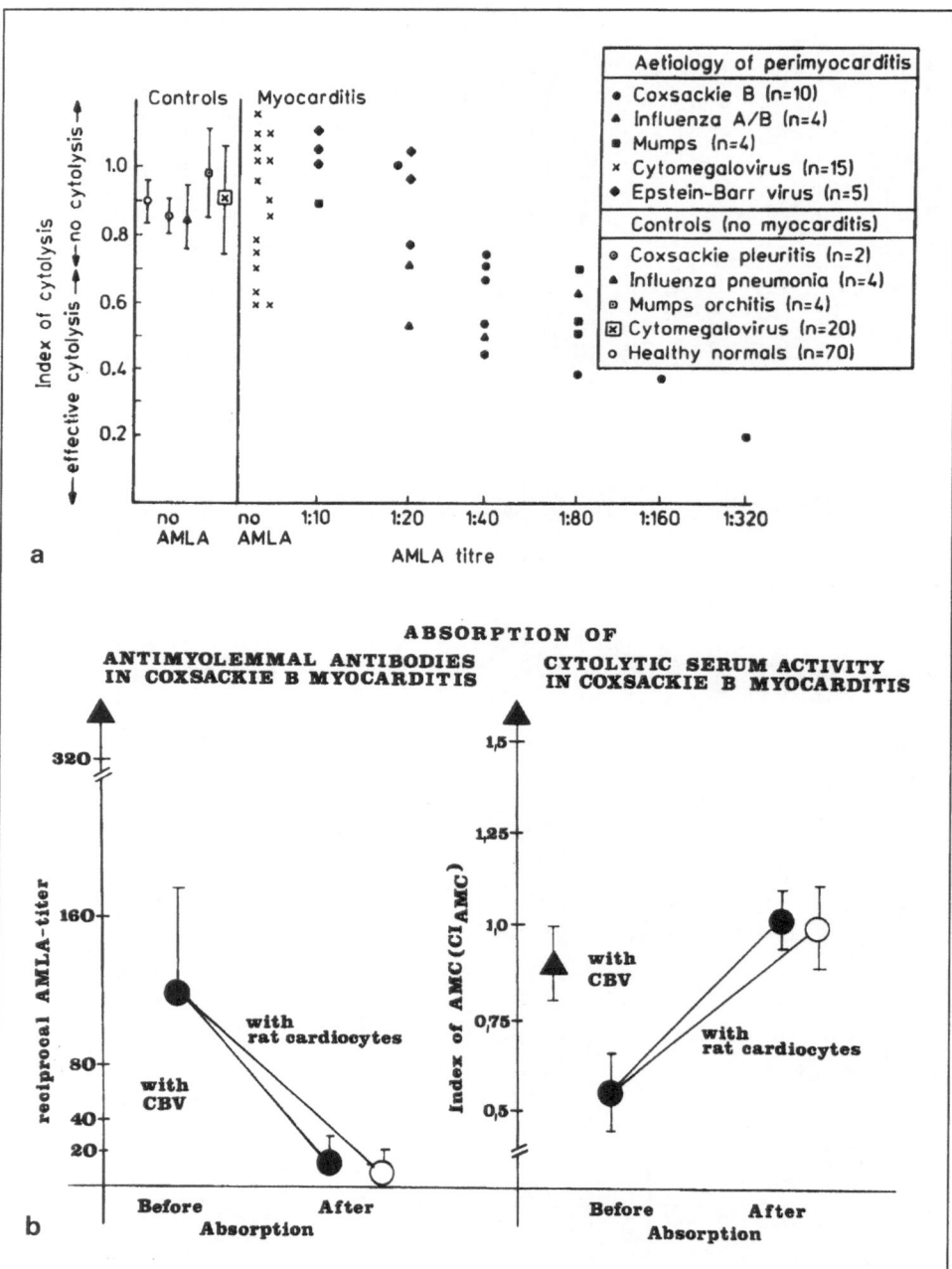

Fig. 5 a. Cytolytic serum activity in viral myocarditis. The antimyolemmal antibody titer correlates well with the cytolytic serum activity in the presence of complement [from (22) with permission]. **b** Cytolytic serum activity can be absorbed out by either virus proteins or cardiac sarcolemma

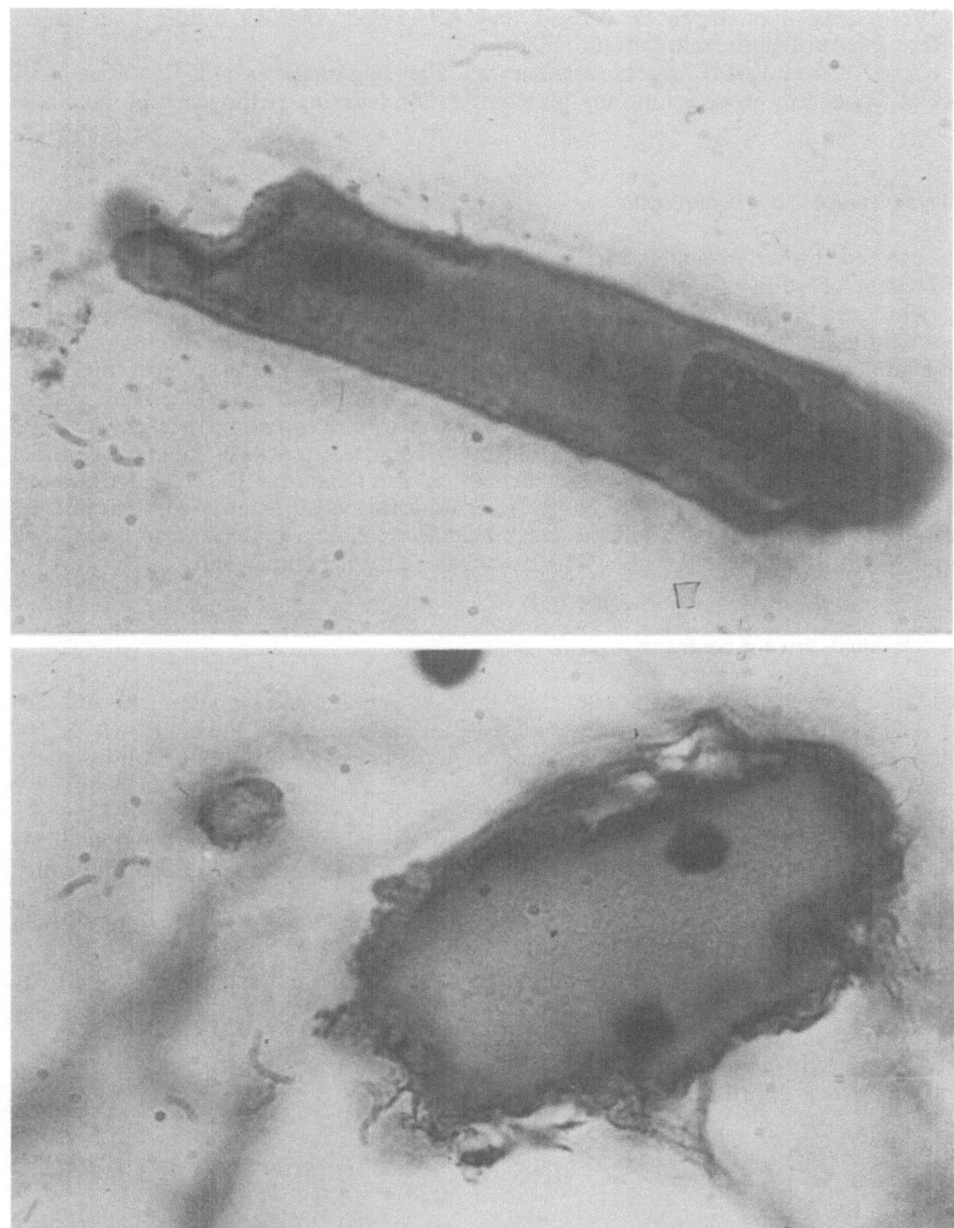

Fig. 6. Fixation of the C_{5b9} "membrane attack complex" in vitro to an intact myocyte after addition of the patients' serum and a complement source at the beginning of the incubation period (a) and 3 h later (b), when the myocyte has undergone spherical contraction

From these data it can be derived that ASAs and AMLAs belong to a micro-heterogeneity of antimembrane antibodies.

Some ASAs and AMLAs are cross-reactive, others are cardiospecific. Cross-reactivity being a common observation may also be the dominanting pathogenetic principle in vivo.

Further evidence and counterevidence

It has been further elucidated by the pathogenetic properties of ASAs and AMLAs in vitro in myocarditis of viral origin (14, 22; Fig. 5) that the cytolytic serum activity of the patients' sera in the presence of complement is associated with high titer of AMLAs. This cytolytic serum activity can be absorbed out by either the Coxsackie B virus or a sar-colemmal preparation, thus clearly indicating that cytolytic AMLAs are operative in ac-tive Coxsackie B and influenza myocarditis. Fixation of complement C_3 and C_4 and of the C_{5b9} complex has been repeatedly demonstrated both in endomyocardial biopsies and with isolated cardiocytes before (Fig. 6a) and immediately after spherical contrac-tions and cell death (Fig. 6b) following incubation with the serum. Recently, Drude et al. (37) could demonstrate with the same sera that even isolated heterologous cardiocytes stimulated in vitro in a specially designed incubator chamber undergoes an accelerated process of cell death when incubated with cytolytic sera and complement.

Conclusions – pro and contra

It can be derived from these studies that AMLAs and ASAs have specificity for con-served structures, and that they possess extensive cross-reactivity, and increase with age. These three characteristics argue for the role of AMLAs and ASAs as natural antibodies.

ASAs and AMLAs may occur, however, as a result of bacterial (e.g., in infective endocarditis and rheumatic fever) and viral stimulation in Coxsackie and influenza myocarditis. They are more often of the IgG- or IgA- than of the IgM-isotype and fix complement. They exert a cytolytic and cytotoxic response less in vitro than that which may be operative in vivo.

All the latter characteristics indicate this from the ASAs and AMLAs induced by a polyclonal stimulation after infection or postcardiac injury.

Subtypes must exist that are not only diagnostic markers but also are pathologically relevant autoantibodies.

Antigenic mimicry is then the governing immunological principle; secondary im-munopathogenesis is the disease process operating in protracted forms of inflammatory and postmyocarditic forms of heart disease.

References

1. Acosta AM, Sadigursky M, Santos-Bush CA (1983) Anti-striated muscle antibody activity produced by Trypanosoma cruzi. Proc Soc Exp Med 172:364
2. Aretz HT, Billingham ME, Edwards WD, Fallon JT, Fenoglio JJ Jr, Olsen EGJ, Schoen FJ (1987) Myocarditis – a pathologic definition and classification. Am J Cardiovasc Pathol 1:3
3. Boyden sV (1963) Natural antibodies and the immune response. Adv Immunol 5:1
4. Cunningham MW, Swerlick RA (1986) Polyspecificity of antistreptococcal murine monoclonal antibodies and their implications in autoimmunity. J Exp Med 164:998

5. Cunningham MW, Hall NK, Krisher KK, Spanier AM (1986) A study of anti-group a streptococcal monoclonal antibodies cross-reactive with myosin. J Immunol 136:293
6. De Scheerder I, Buyzere M de, Algoed L, Lange M de, Delanghe J, Bogaert AM, Clement DL (1987) Characteristic anti-heart antibody patterns in postcardiac injury syndrome, endocarditis and acute myocarditis. Eur Heart J (Suppl J) 8:237
7. Hufnagel G, Pfeifer U, Maisch B (1987) Immunohistological investigations in suspected cardiac sarcoidosis. Eur Heart J (Suppl J) 8:59
8. Jerne NK (1955) The natural selection theory of antibody formation. Proc Nat Acad Sci USA 41:849
9. Kaplan MH (1967) Multiple nature of the cross-reactive relationships between antigens group A streptococci and mammalian tissue. In: Trentin JJ (ed) Cross-reacting antigens and natural antigens. Williams & Wilkins, Baltimore, pp 48–55
10. Maisch B (1985) Rickettsial perimyocarditis – a follow up study. Heart Vessels 2:55
11. Maisch B (1985) Surface antigens of adult heart cells and their use in diagnosis. Basic Res Cardiol (Suppl 1) 80:47
12. Maisch B (1986) Immunologic regulator and effector functions in perimyocarditis, postmyocarditic heart muscle disease and dilated cardiomyopathy. Basic Res Cardiol (Suppl 1) 81:217
13. Maisch B (1987) Immunological mechanisms in human cardiac injury. In: Spry JE (ed) Immunology and molecular biology of cardiovascular disease. In: Shillingfort JP (ed) Current status of clinical cardiology. MTP Press, London, pp 225–252
14. Maisch B (1987) The sarcolemma as antigen in the secondary immunopathogenesis of myopericarditis. Eur Heart J (Suppl J) 8:155
15. Maisch B (1988) The use of myocardial biopsy in heart failure. Eur Heart J (Suppl H) 9:59
16. Maisch B (1989) Autoreactivity of the cardiac myocyte, connective tissue and the extracellular matrix in heart disease and postcardiac injury. Springer Seminar Immunopathol 11:369–395
17. Maisch B, Berg PA, Kochsiek K (1979) Clinical significance of immunopathological findings in patients with postpericardiotomy syndrome. I. Relevance of antibody pattern. Clin Exp Immunol 38:189
18. Maisch B, Berg PA, Schuff-Werner P, Kochsiek K (1979) Clinical significance of immunpathological findings in patients with postpericardiotomy syndrome. II. The significance of serum inhibitors and rosette inhibitory factors. Clin Exp Immunol 38:198
19. Maisch B, Berg PA, Kochsiek K (1980) Autoantibodies and serum inhibition factors (SIF) in patients with myocarditis. Klin Wochenschr 58:219
20. Maisch B, Berg PA, Kochsiek K (1980) Immunological parameters in patients with congestive cardiomyopathy. Basic Res Cardiol 75:219
21. Maisch B, Maisch S, Kochsiek K (1982) Immune reactions in tuberculous and chronic constrictive pericarditis. Am J Cardiol 50:1007
22. Maisch B, Trostel-Soeder R, Stechemesser E, Berg PA, Kochsiek K (1982) Diagnostic relevance of humoral and cell-mediated immune reactions in patients with acute viral myocarditis. Clin Exp Immunol 48:533
23. Maisch B, Deeg P, Liebau G, Kochsiek K (1983) Diagnostic relevance of humoral and cytotoxic immune reactions in primary and secondary dilated cardiomyopathy. Am J Cardiol 52:1071
24. Maisch B, Eichstädt H, Kochsiek K (1983) Immune reactions in infective endocarditis. Part I: Clinical data and diagnostic relevance of antimyocardial antibodies. Am Heart J 106:329
25. Maisch B, Kochsiek K (1983) Humoral immune reactions in uremic pericarditis. Am J Nephrol 3:264
26. Maisch B, Büschel G, Izumi T, Eigel P, Regitz V, Deeg P, Pfeifer U, Schmaltz A, Herzum M, Liebau G, Kochsiek K (1985) Four years of experience in endomyocardial biopsy – an immunohistologic approach. Heart Vessels (Suppl) 1:59
27. Maisch B, Lotze U, Schneider J, Kochsiek K (1985) Antibodies to human sinus node in sick sinus syndrome. N Trend Arrhythmias 1:417
28. Maisch B, Lotze U, Schneider J, Kochsiek K (1986) Antibodies to human sinus node in sick sinus syndrome. PACE 9:1101
29. Maisch B, Bauer E, Thometzek P, Herzum M, Kochsiek K (1987) Autoreactive immune mechanisms in infective endocarditis. Eur Heart J (Suppl J) 8:311

30. Maisch B, Bauer E, Cirsi M, Thometzek P (1990) Cytolytic cross-reactive antibodies directed against the cardiac membrane of adult human myocytes in Coxsackie B myocarditis – analysis by Western blot, immunofluorescence test and antibody-mediated cytolysis of cardiocytes (in press)
31. Neu N, Beisel K, Traystman M, Rose N, Craig SW (1987) Autoantibodies specific for the cardiac myosin isoform are found in mice susceptible to coxsackie virue B3-induced myocarditis. J Immunol 138:2488
32. Obermayer U, Scheidler J, Maisch B (1987) Antibodies against micro- and intermediate filaments in carditis and dilated cardiomyopathy – are they a diagnostic marker? Eur Heart J (Suppl J) 8:181
33. Paris S, Fosset M, Samuel D, Ailhand G (1977) Chick embryo plasma membrane from cardiac muscle cells having respiratory control and tolerance to calcium. Biochem Biophys Res Comm 72:327–333
34. Schultheiss (1987) The mitochondrium as antigen in inflammatory heart disease. Eur Heart J (Suppl J) 8:203
35. Schultheiss H-P, Bolte HD (1985) Immunological analysis of autoantibodies against the adenine nucleotide translocator in dilated cardiomyopathy. J Mol Cell Cardiol 17:601
36. Thometzek P, Maisch B (1987) Antibodies cross-reactive to streptococci in infective endocarditis. Eur Heart J (Suppl J) 8:319
37. Drude L, Wiemers F, Maisch B (1991) Impaired myocyte function in vitro incubated with sera from patients with myocarditis. Eur Heart J 12 (Suppl B) (in press)

Authors' address:

Prof. Dr. Bernhard Maisch
Department of Internal Medicine – Cardiology
Philipps-University Marburg
W-3550 Marburg, FRG

Chemiluminescence as a marker of myocardial ischemia

B. Török

Institute of Experimental Surgery, University School of Medicine Pécs, Hungary

Summary: Dog experiments were performed using the measurement of tissue chemiluminescence to clarify the peculiar role of reactive oxygen species in ischemic heart damage. Following left thoracotomy and pericardiotomy, the left anterior descending coronary artery (LAD) was ligated for 2 h and 24 h. Epicardial and endocardial muscle specimens were excised, homogenized, and centrifuged to detect chemiluminescent difference in the supernatants after t-butyl hydroperoxide induction at each time interval. Characteristic alterations were found between the infarcted region, border zone, and intact area. The induced photoemission differs in an altered kinetic as well as in intensity values. It is assumed that interrelations exist between the observed light burst and the actual scavenger state. Antioxidant application advantageously modifies the chemiluminescence effect, especially at the border zone. Induced chemiluminescence is a good method to characterize ischemically altered myocardial cellular metabolism.

Key words: Myocardial ischemia; free oxygen radicals; singlet oxygen; chemiluminescence

Introduction

In myocardial ischemic state the normal oxidative metabolism is inhibited and pathologic intermediates accumulate. The mechanisms of inhibition and accumulation are integral with the oxygen-derived free radical action of destroying, for example, the polyunsaturated fatty acids in the membrane bilayer (11, 13, 15, 16, 19, 24).

The peroxidative process in which the reactive oxygen species: O_2^-, H_2O_2, $OH^{\cdot}$ participate is well-outlined and can conventionally be measured by the accumulation of TBA reactive materials and the loss of endogenous scavenging molecules (glutathione level, SOD activity, etc.). The factors above give, however, only indirect signals for the events.

EPR spectroscopy can directly characterize the ischemic insult, signaling the changes in myocardial tissue lipids (29), but the method is complicated and very expensive. On the other hand, low-level chemiluminescence is a promising, quick, and easily performed method (2, 20, 23, 25). The present report demonstrates chemiluminescence in myocardial tissue, analyzing the photoemission kinetics in normal and ischemic conditions.

Materials and methods

Experimental protocol

Adult mongrel dogs were intramuscularly premedicated with droperidol (1.5 mg/kg), fentanyl (0.03 mg/kg), atropine (0.05 mg/kg), then anesthetized intravenously with hexobarbital-Na (50 mg/kg), and after endotracheal intubation, artificially ventilated

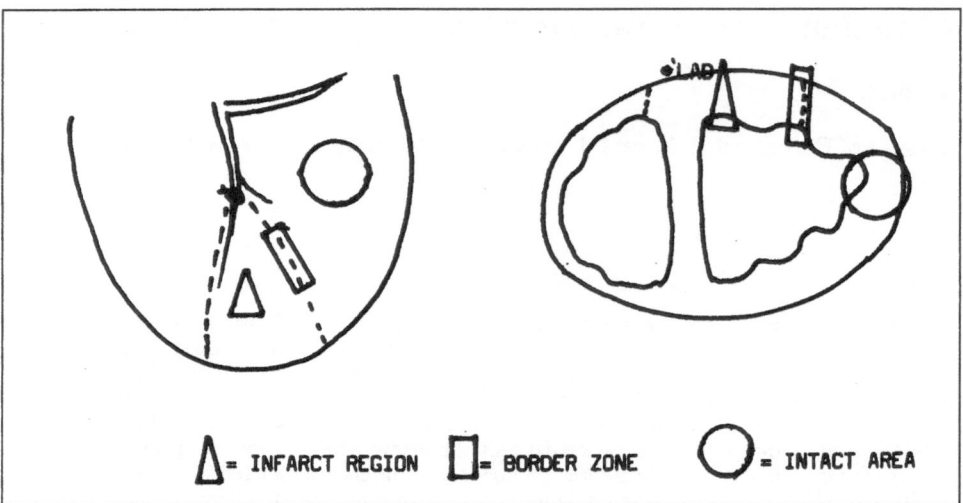

Fig. 1. Scheme of experiments. Left anterior descending (LAD) coronary artery was ligated for 2 h and 24 h. Muscle specimens were taken by excision from the infarcted region, border zone, and intact area: $\triangle$, $\square$, and $\bigcirc$, respectively. The transmural myocardial samples were divided into epicardial and endocardial segments

with O_2-N_2O gas mixture in a ratio of 1:4. Following left thoracotomy and pericardiotomy, the left anterior descending coronary artery (LAD) was dissected free and ligated under the first major diagonal branch (Fig. 1). Two h and 24 h after ligature the hearts were excised and myocardial muscle samples were taken from three different regions: the central infarcted region, border zone and non-infarcted musculature with intact blood supply.

Preparation of muscle samples

The quickly excised heart specimens were homogenized with ice-cold physiologic saline solution in a ratio of 1:9. Homogenates were centrifuged for 10 min with 16000 rpm and the supernatant was kept at 0° C until measurement.

Photon counting

Supernatant chemiluminescence signal detection was performed by photon-counting technique with a six-channel B 9505 Luminometer (Berthold, Wildbad, FRG) at 37° C. 500 µl supernatant was then mixed with 150 µl of 0.1 per cent t-butyl hydroperoxide and the luminescence was continuously monitored using the automatic time scale mode.

Results

The spontaneous photoemission of supernatants gained from myocardial tissue samples was very low; its intensites reaching only twice the "background" level of the applied photomultiplyers. Nonetheless, with this method it was not possible to discriminate between normal and ischemic heart tissue, although the ischemic supernatants show a little (but not significantly) higher light emission.

The t-butyl hydroperoxide induces effective changes in the chemiluminescence events. The light emission of samples shows an exponential alteration. After an initial lag phase an emission burst appeared quickly, rising to a plateau followed by a slow decay toward the background state. Very characteristic differences between ischemic and normal tissue manifest themselves at the upslope of increased photoemission, peak duration and the rate of light exhaustion. Isolated mathematical analysis of the peak values, time differences in the burst phase or integration values for a strict time period may be misleading. According to our initial observations the whole shape of photoemission kinetic has to be evaluated; only in such a manner is it possible to demonstrate the essence of changes.

Figure 2a demonstrates the photoemission curves of ischemic, border, and intact region from a 2-h infarcted heart. The changes are evident: discriminative alterations are present in the upslope, peak and integration photon values of the samples. Figure 2b shows the light emission in a 24-h ischemic heart; the differences are again obvious. A comparison to detect direct proportionality between the 2-h and 24-h infarction is not given. Nevertheless, the velocity of light emission and peak values are higher after long-term ischemia.

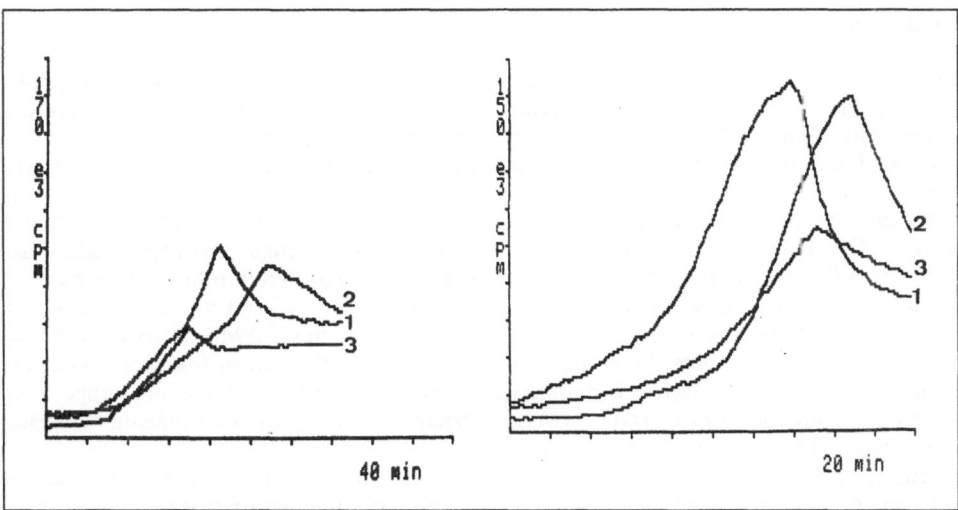

Fig. 2a. Dynamics of light emission in a 2-h infarct case. Ordinate: photon numbers $\times 10^3$; abscissa: time in min. Measuring time: 28 min. Channel 1: infarct region. Peak (P): 87; Integral value (I): 1281; Channel 2: border zone. P: 77; I: 1200; Channel 3: intact area. P: 50; I: 906. **b** Chemiluminescence affects in a 24-h infarct case. Measuring time: 20 min. Channel 1: infarct region. P: 140; I: 1290; Channel 2: border zone. P: 134; I: 981; Channel 3: intact area. P: 82; I: 809

Table 1. Range of chemiluminescence markers in regional ischemic heart (values in percentage of the control with extremes)

LAD ligature	Total photon count		Photon peak value		Apperarance of peak
	Infarct	Border	Infarct	Border	
2 Hour	+15 (0–41)	+ 1 (0–25)	+21 (0–72)	+ 8 (0–59)	Fast
24 Hour	+33 (17–83)	+25 (2–59)	+48 (19–137)	+38 (10–101)	Rapid

Remarks: The percentual alterations of chemiluminescence markers characterize the trend of changes after infarction. At any rate, the data requires further investigations to clear the role of intact and of reversibly or already irreversibly damaged cells in the events.

Table 1 contains the range of chemiluminescence markers of all measured cases (eight and 11 animals, respectively) in percentage values. According to observations, the cause of great differences may be partly due to the manual excision, partly due to the actual collateral circulation of excised samples, producing different mixtures of intact and irreversibly damaged cells.

It is obvious from the data that addition of t-butyl-hydroperoxide to the supernatant effectively catalyzes a process yielding a diverse and intense light emission pattern differing, not only in an altered kinetics, but also in intensity values.

Discussion

The present study demonstrates that the measurement of t-butyl hydroperoxide-induced chemiluminescence provides a good indicator for differentiation of myocardial tissue injuries. Although similar chemiluminescence has been observed in intact and perfused organs, tissue homogenates and subcellular fractions (2–7, 12, 20, 26), data from heart tissue is almost lacking.

Kinetic analysis of the chemiluminescence emission by Barsacchi et al. (1) established a relationship between the oxidative stress caused by cumene hydroperoxide and prostaglandin release from the heart. Kuzuya et al. (18) reported luminol-enhanced chemiluminescence differences between viable and irreversibly injured myocardium in the fifth minute of measurement. Our data indicates that t-butyl hydroperoxide-induced photoemission may reflect the actual scavenger state in the myocardium. Namely, the pathognomonic cellular ischemic damage must be viewed as a metabolic imbalance. The toxic overproduction of free radicals and the decreased ability to neutralize them causes a progressive lipid peroxidation chain reaction.

Our chemiluminescence measurements are correlated to these events. Differences between ischemic and nonischemic tissues in yielding photoemission can be explained by the altered catalytic reaction upon addition of t-butyl hydroperoxide. In samples from the infarcted region, we observed a steeper rise and higher light emission plateau than in samples of intact areas. Not only the peak values, but also the duration and exhaustion of the induced light emission are well outlined differences between the infarcted and intact myocardial areas.

According to Cadenas et al. (8–10) the light emission from the free radical decomposition requires the homolytic scission of the hydroperoxide in order to generate the chemiluminescent species. It can be assumed that this mechanism can be applied to our methods. In consequence of ischemia the capability for catalytic reaction is increased with accumulation of released cytochromes which are likely the most important compounds to trigger an increased photoemission. Concomitantly, the decreased ability of endogenous trapping produced by the gradual loss of scavenging effect on supplemental t-butyl hydroperoxide causes a subsequent perturbation in glutathione status (14, 23). Ischemia produces discriminative changes in samples which remain temporarily "hidden", though induction with organic hydroperoxide is already able to demonstrate the altered kinetic of tissue deterioration. By analogy, t-butyl hydroperoxide-induced chemiluminescence is similar to a photographic negative; the visible picture does not appear at exposure, but only subsequent to the photo-development process.

It must be remarked that the chemiluminescence of the border zone may be intermediate to the infarcted and intact areas. Quantitative problems may stem from the variability of manual excision, i.e., on the quantity of already irreversibly injured and accidentally excised still viable cells. However, following 24-h ischemia, the border zone does show an increased photoemission signalling an active metabolic process in this region.

Additional luminometric investigations are needed to clarify changes following ischemia of variable intervals, not only in the acute phase, but also during the chronic healing process. Correlations must include interpretation of other characteristics of lipid peroxidation, e.g., changes in TBA reactive materials, glutathione status, defending enzymes, etc. At any rate, according to our earlier dog experiments (21, 22, 27, 28) the MDA accumulation and simultaneous decrease in GSH level, SOD activity, and more importantly, the changes of some endoperoxide derivatives (6-keto $PGF_{1\alpha}$ and TXB_2) give distinct alterations that can be brought into connection with the observed changes of chemiluminescence.

In conclusion, myocardial ischemic damage is two-fold: oxy-radicals contribute to the worsening toxic insult of ischemic injury and the gradual breakdown of ubiquituous endogenous scavenger compounds (glutathiones, SOD, vitamins, etc.), and exert less cellular protection. Oxygen-derived free radicals (primarily the dangerous $OH^{\cdot}$ radicals) evidently participate in the lipid peroxidation process. There is strong evidence that peroxy radicals are also produced which later generate singlet oxygen and/or excited carbonyl groups. Photoemission of the singlet-triplet transition of excited carbonyl groups and dimol emission of singlet oxygen are the basis of the measured luminometric differences. In this context, two important notes should be made: i) light burst is always present in cell-deteriorating processes, and ii) the light emission depends on the availability of "breakdown materials" from which compounds with higher luminescence capacity are produced. So, the t-butyl hydroperoxide-induced chemiluminescence may provide crucial diagnostic information about the state of myocardial cellular metabolism and the extension of hypoxic tissue injuries.

Acknowledgements. The helpful suggestions of Prof. K. Jobst and Dr. T. Köszegi (Department of Clinical Chemistry), and the excellent technical assistance of Mrs. Ildikó Hepp are acknowledged.

References

1. Barsacchi R, Camici P, Pelosi G, Nanni N, Benassi A, Giannessi D, Ursini F (1986) Chemiluminescence: a tool to investigate oxidative stress in the heart. In: Novelli GP, Ursini F (eds)
   Oxygen free radicals in shock. Karger, Basel New York, pp 175–179
2. Boveris A, Cadenas E, Reiter R, Filipkowski M, Nakase Y, Chance B (1980) Organ chemiluminescence: noninvasive assay for oxidative free radical reactions. Proc Natl Acad Sci USA
   77:347–351
3. Cadenas E, Boveris A, Chance B (1980) Chemiluminescence of lipid vesicles supplemented with
   cytochrome c and hydroperoxide. Biochem J 188:577–583
4. Cadenas E, Müller A, Brigelius R, Esterbauer H, Sies H (1983) Effects of 4-hydroxynonenal on
   isolated hepatocytes. Biochem J 214:479–487
5. Cadenas E (1984) Biological chemiluminescence. Photochemistry and Photobiology 40:823–830
6. Cadenas E, Sies H (1984) Low-level chemiluminescence as indicator of singlet molecular oxygen
   in biological systems. Methods in Enzymol 105:221–231
7. Cadenas E, Sies H (1982) Low-level chemiluminescence of liver microsomal fractions initiated
   by t-butyl hydroperoxide. Relation to microsomal hemoprotein, oxygen dependence, and lipid
   peroxidation. Eur J Biochem 124:349–356
8. Cadenas E, Varsavsky AI, Boveris A, Chance B (1980) Low-level chemiluminescence of
   cytochrome c-catalyzed decomposition of hydrogen peroxide. FEBS Lett 113:141–144
9. Cadenas E, Varsavsky AI, Boveris A, Chance B (1981) Ultraweak chemiluminescence of brain
   and liver homogenates induced by oxygen organic hydroperoxide. Biochem J 198:645–654
10. Cadenas E, Boveris A, Chance B (1980) Low-level chemiluminescence of hydroperoxide supple-
    mented cytochrome c. Biochem J 187:131–140
11. De Groot H, Littauer A (1989) Hypoxia, reactive oxygen, and cell injury. Free Rad Biol
    6:541–551
12. DiLuzio NR, Stege TE (1977) The role of ethanol metabolites in hepatic lipid peroxidation. In:
    Fischer MM, Ranking IG (eds) Alochol and the liver. Plenum Press, New York, pp 45–62
13. Farber JL, Chien KR, Mittnach S (1981) The pathogenesis of irreversible cell injury in
    ischemia. Am J Pathol 102:271–281
14. Guarnieri C, Flamigni F, Rizzuto S, Vaona I, Caldarera CM (1987) Altered thiol group status
    in the heart ornithine decarboxylase inactivated following perfusion with t-butyl
    hydroperoxide. Int J Biochem 19:931–935
15. Hearse DJ, Humphrey IM, Bullock GR (1978) The oxygen paradox and the calcium paradox:
    two facets of the same problem? J Mol Cell Cardiol 10:641–668
16. Hess ML, Manson NH (1984) Molecular friend and foe. The role of the oxygen free radical
    system in the calcium paradox, the oxygen paradox and ischaemia/reperfusion injury. J Mol
    Cell Cardiol 16:969–985
17. Hoves RM, Steele RH (1971) Microsomal chemiluminescence induced by NADPH and its rela-
    tion to lipid peroxidation. Res Commun Chem Pathol Pharmacol 2:619–625
18. Kuzuya T, Hoshida S, Nishida M, Kim Y, Fuji H, Kitabakate A, Kamada T, Tada M (1989)
    Role of free radicals and neutrophils in canine myocardial reperfusion injury: myocardial sal-
    vage by a novel free radical scavenger, 2-octadecyl-ascorbic acid. Cardiovasc Res 23:323–330
19. McCord JM (1985) Oxygen-derived free radicals in postischemic tissue injury. N Engl J Med
    312:159–163
20. Ohkohchi N, Kanno M, Terashima T, Taguchi Y, Mori S, Saeki R, Usa T, Inaba H, Miyayawa
    T (1989) Assessment of the viability of liver allografts by chemiluminescence. Transpl Proc
    21:1332–1334
21. Röth E, Kelemen D, Török B, Nagy A, Pollak S (1989) Dynamics of prostacyclin and throm-
    boxane during myocardial ischemia. Prog Clin Biol Res 308:907–911
22. Röth E, Török B, Kelemen D, Pollák S (1989) Free radical mediated injuries after coronary
    artery occlusion. Basic Res Cardiol 84:388–395
23. Schulte-Herbrüggen T, Cadenas E (1985) Electronically excited state generation during the
    lipoxygenase-catalyzed aerobic oxidation of arachidonate. The effect of reduced glutathione.
    Photobiochem Photobiophys 10:35–52

24. Shlafer M, Kane PF, Wiggins VY, Kirsh MM (1982) Possible role for cytotoxic oxygen metabolites in the pathogenesis of cardiac ischemic injury. Circulation 66:185–192
25. Sies H (1986) Biochemistry of oxidative stress. Angew Chem Int Ed Eng 25:1058–1071
26. Sugioka K, Nakano M (1976) A possible mechanism of the generation of singlet molecular oxygen in NADPH-dependent microsomal lipid peroxidation. Biochim Biophys Acta 423:203–216
27. Török B, Röth E, Bar V, Pollák Z (1986) Effects of antioxidant therapy in experimentally induced heart infarcts. Basic Res Cardiol 83:223–228
28. Török B, Röth E, Trombitás K (1988) Concordance of structural and functional alterations in myocardial ischemic states. Basic Res Cardiol 83:223–228
29. Zweier JL, Kuppusamy P, Lutty GA (1988) Measurement of endothelial cell free radical generation: evidence for a central mechanism of free radical injury in postischemic tissues. Proc Natl Acad Sci USA 85:4046–4050

Authors' address:

Prof. Dr. B. Török
Dept. of Experimental Surgery
University of Medicine Pécs
Kodály Zoltan u. 20
H-7643 Pécs
Hungary

Part III: Significance of Neuroendocrine
Mechanisms for the Development of Heart Failure

Role of neuroendocrine mechanisms in the pathogenesis of heart failure *

A. J. G. Riegger

Medizinische Universitätsklinik Würzburg, FRG

Summary: In chronic heart failure, neurohumoral mechanisms play an important role in the regulation of cardiac performance by direct influences on systolic and diastolic function of the myocardium, and indirectly, by modulation of pre- and afterload. Important vasoconstrictor, fluid- and sodium-retaining factors are the renin-angiotensin-aldosterone system, sympathetic nerve activity and vasopressin; vasodilator, volume, and sodium-eliminating factors are atrial natriuretic peptide, vasodilator prostaglandins like prostacyclin and prostaglandin E_2, dopamine, bradykinin, and possibly, endothelial derived relaxing factor (EDRF).

There is evidence from experimental and clinical studies that the sympathetic nerve activity is stimulated in the early phase of the disease, as well as is the secretion of atrial natriuretic peptide which increases in relation to a rise in preload. In early or mild heart failure, atrial natriuretic peptide suppresses the activity of the renin-angiotensin-aldosterone system, which may prevent an increase in peripheral vascular resistance and preserve renal blood flow. In more severe heart failure, the renin-angiotensin-aldosterone system is activated, leading to an increase of peripheral and renal vascular resistance and fluid and sodium retention. This is associated with an increased production of vasodilator prostaglandins. In severe heart failure, mostly in connection with hyponatremia, a nonosmolar, inappropriately high secretion of vasopressin can be demonstrated.

These findings suggest that early interventions in order to suppress unfavorable neurohumoral mechanisms or to support protective factors like atrial natriuretic peptide may be of particular importance in the treatment of congestive heart failure with the aim of a retardation of the progression of the disease, which would result in an improvement of survival.

Key words: Heart failure; renin; atrial natriuretic peptide; sympathetic activity; circulation; kidney function

Introduction

Vasoconstrictor and vasodilator neurohumoral factors are both activated in severe congestive heart failure. It has been demonstrated that pharmacological intervention in the late stage of the disease by blockade of one of the major vasoconstrictor sodium- and fluid-retaining mechanisms of the renin-angiotensin-aldosterone system, by converting enzyme inhibition, results in an improvement of survival and symptomatology (2).

As congestive heart failure has an extremely bad prognosis once severe symptoms have developed, early intervention into the pathophysiological process of the disease may be an important goal in order to achieve a prevention or retardation of the deterioration of cardiac function. To develop appropriate therapeutic principles, it is of particular importance to understand the complicated concert of neurohumoral mechanisms in the regulation of cardiac performance during the development of congestive heart failure.

---

* The study was supported by the Deutsche Forschungsgemeinschaft.

Therefore, we have studied hemodynamic, neurohumoral, and renal changes in an animal model of experimental chronic congestive heart failure, induced by rapid right ventricular pacing (11).

Mild experimental heart failure

We recently studied hemodynamic, neurohumoral, and renal changes during the development of congestive heart failure in an animal model of low cardiac output due to rapid right ventricular pacing (12) in an early stage of the disease that resembled relatively mild heart failure. The experimental setting allows to modify the severity of heart failure by adjusting the pacemaker to different heart rates. In this experiment mild heart failure was induced by chronic rapid right-ventricular pacing using a heart rate of 240 beats/min.

Figure 1 demonstrates hemodynamic changes following right-ventricular pacing in six conscious, chronically instrumented dogs. Rapid right-ventricular pacing resulted in a significant decrease of cardiac output, mixed venous oxygen saturation measured in blood from the pulmonary artery, a considerable fall in mean arterial pressure, and a continuous increase of mean right atrial pressure. Systemic vascular resistance increased only transiently during the first day of pacing, and then returned rapidly to basal values.

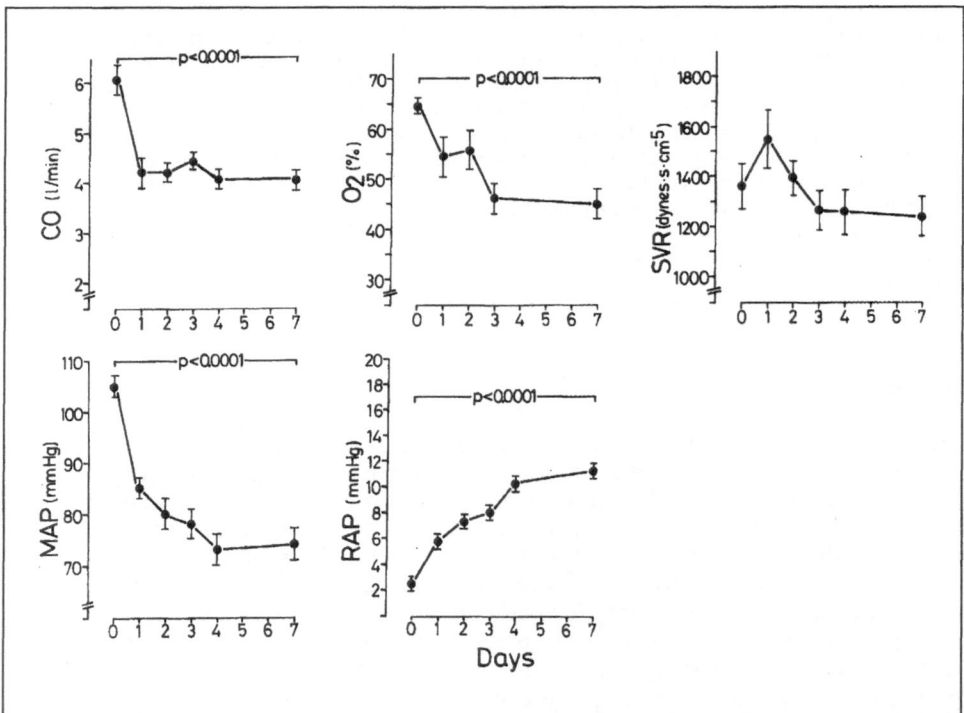

Fig. 1. Cardiac output (CO), mixed venous oxygen saturation (02), systemic vascular resistance (SVR), mean arterial pressure (MAP), and mean right atrial pressure (RAP) during the induction of congestive heart failure due to rapid right ventricular pacing [adapted from (12)]

Neurohumoral changes are shown in Fig. 2. In parallel to the increase of right atrial pressure, we found a significant stimulation of the secretion of atrial natriuretic peptide with a linear correlation coefficient of $r = 0.66$ ($p < 0.001$). According to the deterioration of cardiac function, we observed a stimulation of sympathetic nerve activity indicated by increased plasma levels of norepinephrine.

Surprisingly, we found a significant suppression of renin secretion, indicated by a significant decrease of plasma renin concentration in the aorta, renal vein, and pulmonary artery. This inhibitory effect on renin was maintained throughout the 7 days of pacing. In parallel to the decrease of plasma renin concentration, we observed a tendency to a reduction of plasma aldosterone levels. This confirms data previously published (7) in the same experimental setting where we found a significant suppression of plasma renin concentration and aldosterone during the first 4 days of pacing. The inhibition of the renin-angiotensin-aldosterone system in the early phase of the development of congestive

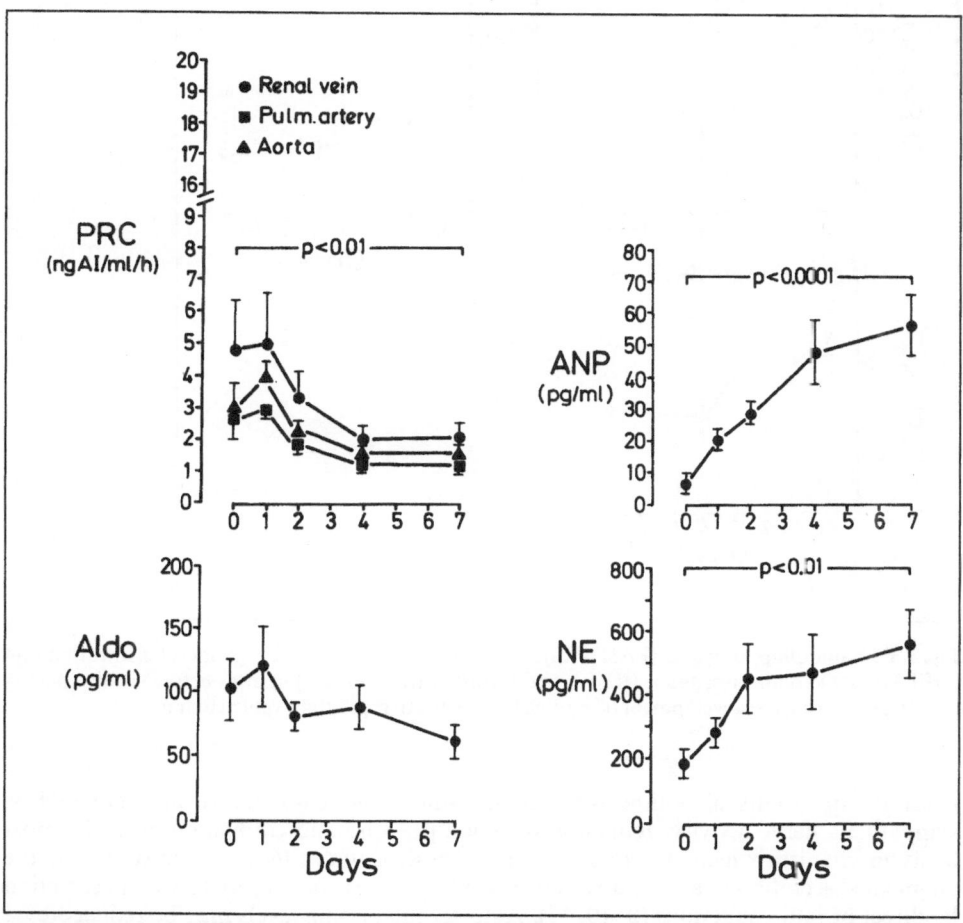

Fig. 2. Plasma renin concentration (PRC), atrial natriuretic peptide (ANP), plasma aldosterone (Aldo), and plasma norepinephrine (NE) during rapid right ventricular pacing [adapted from (12)]

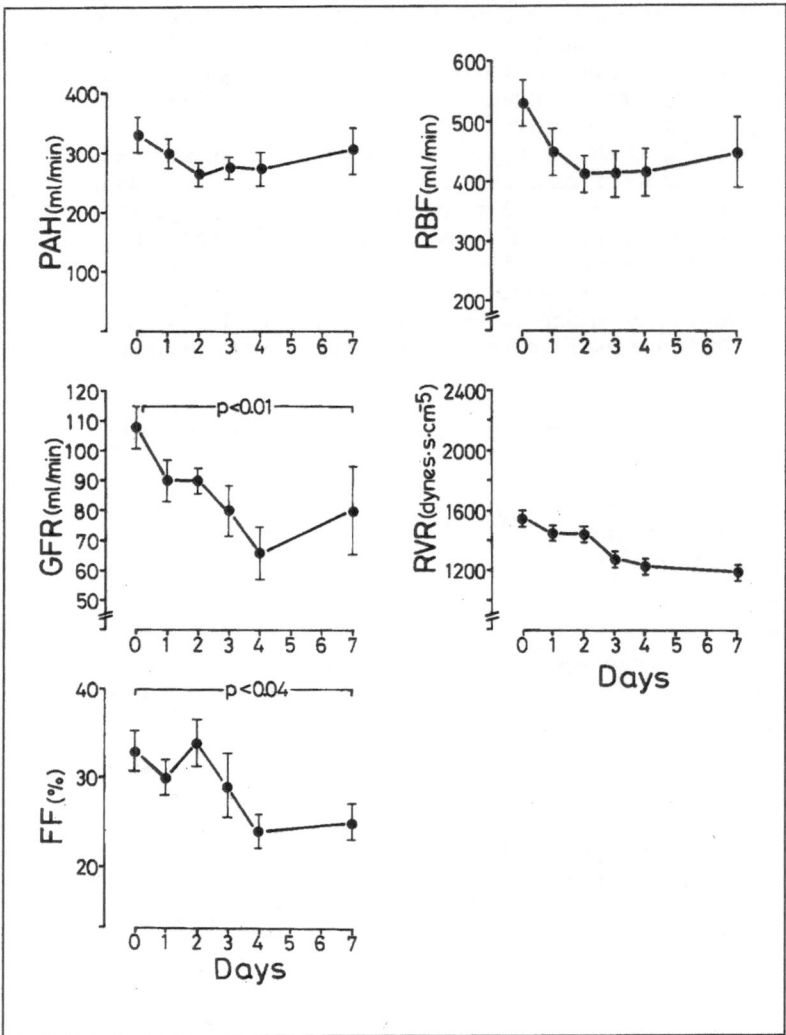

Fig. 3. Paraaminohippuric acid (PAH) clearance, renal blood flow (RBF), glomerular filtration rate (GFR), renal vascular resistance (RVR), and filtration fraction (FF) in dogs before cardiac pacing (day 0) and during the development of cardiac failure due to rapid right ventricular pacing

heart failure occurs at a time when major stimuli of renin release are activated as sympathetic nerve activity, reduction of blood pressure and cardiac output. The most likely mechanism which suppresses the renin system under these circumstances is the augmented secretion of atrial natriuretic peptide which is able to suppress renin secretion by direct or indirect actions (8, 10, 15). Aldosterone plasma levels may be reduced by a direct inhibitory effect of atrial natriuretic peptide on the zona glomerulosa of the adrenal gland and by a reduction of the angiotensin II plasma levels (5).

Changes of renal excretory parameters are shown in Fig. 3. Despite a significant reduction of cardiac output, we observed no significant changes of effective renal plasma flow (PAH-clearance), renal blood flow, or renal vascular resistance. We found, however, a significant reduction of glomerular filtration rate and filtration fraction. This can be explained by a lack of constriction of the vas efferens of the glomerulum due to the reduced formation of angiotensin II, a mechanism which normally would maintain glomerular filtration rate by increasing filtration pressure when blood pressure and/or cardiac output are reduced. During the first 7 days of pacing, we observed no significant changes of urine flow and of the plasma concentrations of creatinine and blood urea nitrogen.

Thus, the experimental data in an animal model of mild heart failure suggest that in an early stage of the disease atrial natriuretic peptide may play an important role in the pathogenic process of heart failure by suppressing the renin-angiotensin-aldosterone system, preventing an increase of peripheral vascular resistance and maintaining renal blood flow.

The mechanisms leading to activation of the sympathetic nervous system and the renin-angiotensin system, as well as to the nonosmolar stimulation of vasopressin in heart failure are not fully understood, but it is thought that one principal contributing factor is baroreceptor dysfunction.

Under physiologic conditions, vagal afferents exert a tonic inhibitory influence on the vasomotor center regulating sympathetic nerve activity (3) and, thereby, via renal nerve activity, renin secretion (9), as well as by the release of vasopressin (14). In experimental heart failure, a decreased electrical activity of vagal afferents from left atrial receptors and attenuated reflex effects on diuresis of left atrial distension have been demonstrated (1, 6, 16, 17).

It has been hypothesized that a decreased activity of vagal afferents might contribute to the activation of neurohumoral systems in congestive heart failure. Therefore, we studied the effects of vagal nerve blockade (4) by local anesthesia on neurohormones in six conscious dogs before and after induction of heart failure by rapid right ventricular pacing (250 beats/min, 10 days). In healthy dogs vagal blockade significantly increased plasma vasopressin levels (from 1.5 ± 0.6 to 13.7 ± 10.5 pg/ml, $p < 0.02$), without significantly affecting plasma catecholamines and renin. After 10 days of pacing, mean arterial pressure and cardiac output were decreased, right atrial and pulmonary arterial pressures and plasma levels of norepinephrine, dopamine, and atrial natriuretic peptide were increased. In this state, vagal blockade significantly increased plasma renin activity (from 1.52 ± 0.43 to 3.18 ± 0.54 ng AI/ml/h, $p < 0.02$) and led to an excessive increase of plasma vasopressin (from 4.2 ± 3.3 to 89.1 ± 54.9 pg/ml, $p < 0.02$), this increase being significantly higher than in healthy dogs. We conclude that in these dogs with low cardiac output state, which resembles early heart failure, vagal afferent activity is increased and effectively suppresses renin and vasopressin. This does not exclude the possibility that in later stages of heart failure vagal afferent dysfunction may develop, resulting in neurohumoral disinhibition.

Severe experimental heart failure

In a previous experiment (13), we induced more severe heart failure by increasing the rate of right ventricular pacing up to 260 beats/min. This resulted in more profound reduction of cardiac output, reduced mean arterial pressure, increase in mean pulmonary arterial and right atrial pressure, and in a significant increase of atrial natriuretic peptide. Under these conditions the pattern of hemodynamic, neurohumoral, and renal regula-

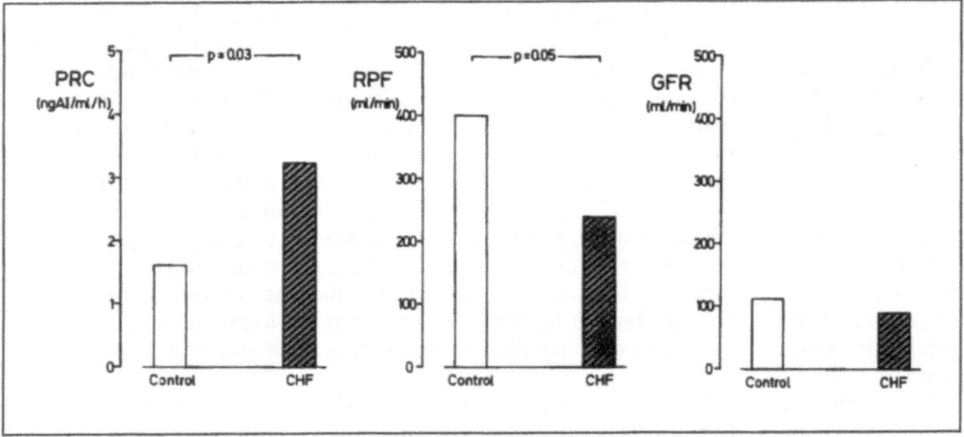

Fig. 4. Plasma renin concentration (PRC), renal plasma flow (RPF), and glomerular filtration rate (GFR) in dogs before (control) and after the induction of severe congestive heart failure (CHF)

tion was substantially different compared to early or mild heart failure. In this situation of more severe circulatory impairment the beneficial effects of atrial natriuretic peptide were overridden by vasoconstrictor mechanisms, resulting in a significant increase of renin secretion and peripheral vascular resistance (Fig. 4). In severe heart failure, we found a reduction of renal blood flow, whereas glomerular filtration rate was well preserved (Fig. 4), resulting in an increase of filtration fraction. These changes of renal functional parameters can be partly explained by an increase of vascular resistance of the vas efferens of the glomerulum due to the increased stimulation of the renin-angiotensin system.

Conclusions

There is evidence from experimental studies in congestive heart failure that neurohumoral and renal changes differ considerably in the early phase of the pathophysiological process of the development of heart failure from later stages when more severe heart failure has developed. It is suggested that the early phase of the disease is characterized by a stimulation of sympathetic nerve activity and an augmented secretion of atrial natriuretic peptide which may be able to suppress the renin-angiotensin-aldosterone system, prevent an increase in peripheral vascular resistance and preserve renal blood flow. In later stages of the disease with more profound circulatory impairment the beneficial actions of atrial natriuretic peptide are no longer present. This results in an increase of afterload, stimulated secretion of renin, and a reduction of renal blood flow.

References

1. Abboud FM, Thames MD, Mark AL (1981) Role of cardiac afferent nerves in regulation of circulation during coronary occlusion and heart failure. In: Abboud FM, Fozzard HA, Gilmore JP, Reid DJ (eds) Disturbances in neurogenic control of the circulation. American Physiological Society, Bethesda, pp 65–86

2. The CONSENSUS Trial Study Group (1987) Effects of enalapril on mortality in severe congestive heart failure: results of the Cooperative North Scandinavian Enalapril Survival Study (CONSENSUS). N Engl J Med 316:1429–1435
3. Donald DE, Shepherd JT (1978) Reflexes from the heart and lungs: physiological curiosities or important regulatory mechanisms. Cardiovasc Res 12:449–469
4. Elsner D, Kromer EP, Riegger AJG (1990) Effects of vagal blockade on neurohumoral systems in conscious dogs with heart failure. J Cardiovasc Pharmacol 15:586–591
5. Goodfriend TL, Elliot ME, Atlas SA (1984) Actions of synthetic atrial natriuretic factor on bovine adrenal glomerulosa. Life Sci 35:1675–1682
6. Greenberg TT, Richmond WH, Stocking RA, Gupta PD, Meehan KP, Henry JP (1973) Impaired atrial receptor responses in dogs with heart failure due to tricuspid insufficiency and pulmonary artery stenosis. Circ Res 32:424–433
7. Holmer SR, Riegger AJG, Notheis WF, Kromer EP, Kochsiek K (1987) Hemodynamic changes and renal plasma flow in early heart failure: implications for renin, aldosterone, norepinephrine, atrial natriuretic peptide and prostacyclin. Basic Res Cardiol 82:101–108
8. Kurtz A, Bruna RD, Pfeilschifter J, Taugner R, Bauer C (1986) Atrial natriuretic peptide inhibits renin release from juxtaglomerular cells by a cGMP-mediated process. Proc Natl Acad Sci USA 83:4769–4773
9. Mancia G, Romero JC, Shepherd JT (1975) Continuous inhibition of renin release in dogs by vagally innervated receptors in the cardiopulmonary region. Circ Res 36:529–535
10. Opgenorth TJ, Burnett JC, Granger JP, Scriven TA (1986) Effects of atrial natriuretic peptide on renin secretion in nonfiltering kidney. Am J Physiol 250:F798–801
11. Riegger AJG, Liebau G (1982) The renin-angiotensin-aldosterone system, antidiuretic hormone and sympathetic nerve activity in an experimental model of congestive heart failure. Clin Sci 62:465–469
12. Riegger AJG, Elsner D, Kromer EP (1989) Circulatory and renal control by prostaglandins and renin in low cardiac output in dogs. Am J Physiol 256:H1079–1086
13. Riegger AJG, Elsner D, Kromer EP et al. (1988) Atrial natriuretic peptide in congestive heart failure in the dog: plasma levels, cyclic guanosine monophosphate, ultrastructure of atrial myoendocrine cells, and hemodynamic, hormonal, and renal effects. Circulation 77:398–406
14. Thames MD, Schmid PG (1979) Cardiopulmonary receptors with vagal afferents tonically inhibit ADH release in the dogs. Am J Physiol 237:H299–304
15. Villarreal D, Freeman RH, Davis JO, Verburg KM, Vari RC (1986) Renal mechanisms for suppression of renin secretion by atrial natriuretic factor. Hypertension 8(Suppl II):28–35
16. Zucker IH, Earle AM, Gilmore JP (1977) The mechanisms of adaptation of left atrial stretch receptors in dogs with chronic congestive heart failure. J Clin Invest 60:323–331
17. Zucker IH, Share L, Gilmore JP (1979) Renal effects of left atrial distension in dogs with chronic congestive heart failure. Am J Physiol 236:H554–560

Author's address:

Prof. A. J. G. Riegger, M.D.
Medizinische Universitätsklinik
Josef-Schneider-Straße 2
W-8700 Würzburg, FRG

Modulation of baroreflex and baroreceptor function in experimental heart failure

I. H. Zucker and W. Wang

Department of Physiology and Biophysics, University of Nebraska College of Medicine, Omaha, Nebraska, USA

Summary: The reflex control of the circulation is clearly abnormal in heart failure. It has been known for many years that the baroreflex control of heart rate is depressed in both humans and animals with heart failure. The mechanisms for these abnormalities have not been well worked out. We have carried out experiments to determine the relative roles of the various components involved in the arterial baroreflex arc which may be abnormal in chronic heart failure. An experimental model of chronic heart failure was used which involved continuous ventricular pacing in dogs for periods of up to 6 weeks. This model is characterized by progressive increases in left atrial and left ventricular enddiastolic pressure with increases in resting heart rate and decreases in mean arterial pressure. The dogs become edematous, showing both pulmonary and peripheral edema and ascites. Exercise tolerance is also reduced. Three sets of experiments are described. In the first study, the activity from arterial baroreceptors was recorded in normal dogs and in dogs with heart failure. Carotid sinus pressure-receptor discharge curves were constructed along with pressure-diameter curves. Increasing carotid sinus pressure using either static or pulsatile pressure steps from below threshold to saturation levels caused an increase in discharge at each step. The curves generated in each group of dogs showed that the baroreceptor discharge sensitivity was significantly depressed in the dogs with heart failure. The peak slope of the curves as well as the threshold were significantly different from the normal dogs. There were no differences in carotid sinus compliance curves between the two groups of dogs. Perfusion of the carotid sinus with a dose of ouabain which did not constrict the carotid sinus (0.01 µg/ml) caused a shift in the pressure-discharge curve back to that seen in normal dogs. This dose of ouabain did not affect discharge sensitivity in normal dogs. These data suggest that an augmentation of Na-K ATPase in baroreceptor nerve endings in heart failure contributes to the poor discharge sensitivity. In the second series of experiments, the baroreflex control of heart rate was evaluated in dogs before and after heart failure had been induced. Both reflex tachycardia (in response to nitroglycerin) and reflex bradycardia (in response to phenylephrine) were depressed in dogs with heart failure. The use of cholinergic and β adrenergic blocking drugs indicated that both arms of the autonomic control of the heart were partly responsible for this depressed chronotropic response. The final series of experiments evaluated the baroreflex control of renal sympathetic nerve activity and mean arterial pressure in dogs with heart failure. The relationship between carotid sinus pressure and mean arterial pressure as well as renal nerve activity was depressed in dogs with heart failure. Electrical stimulation of the carotid sinus nerve reduced arterial pressure less in heart failure than in normal dogs. However, electrical stimulation of the carotid sinus nerve reduced renal sympathetic nerve activity to a similar degree in heart failure and normal dogs. Vagotomy caused an increase in the sensitivity of the baroreflex control of arterial pressure in the heart failure dogs, but not in the normal dogs. These data demonstrate that the abnormal baroreflex is likely to be mediated by alterations in arterial and cardiac receptor discharge, but not in the central regulation of sympathetic outflow. The control of the circulation in heart

* These studies were supported by a grant from the National Heart, Lung and Blood Institutes (# HL 38690) and from a Post-Doctoral Fellowship to Dr. Wang from the American Heart Association, Nebraska Affiliate.

failure is multifactorial and the abnormal reflex control of peripheral vascular resistance and heart rate contribute to the pathophysiology of this disease.

Key words: Heart failure; baroreflex; cardiac afferents; renal nerves; arterial pressure

Introduction

Several studies have now shown that the neurohumoral regulation of the cardiovascular system is abnormal in heart failure (9, 10, 12, 22, 23, 28). The arterial baroreflex plays an integral role in the short-term control of heart rate, peripheral vascular resistance, and the secretion of a variety of regulatory hormones. Baroreceptor denervation clearly results in acute hypertension and increased sympathetic nervous outflow (7, 18). Chronic baroreceptor denervation, while not resulting in hypertension, does cause an increase in the variability of both arterial pressure and heart rate (7, 13). Abnormal baroreflex function has been implicated as a causative or exacerbating factor in a variety of cardiovascular syndromes such as orthostatic hypotension (3, 6), the exercise-induced syncope that accompanies aortic stenosis (14), and the increased sympathetic tone characteristic of chronic, severe heart failure (11). In this review, we will describe experiments which were conducted with the goal of determining the mechanism(s) for abnormal arterial baroreflex control of the circulation in heart failure.

The baroreflex control of heart rate in conscious dogs with heart failure

The model of heart failure used in this and subsequent experiments is one which was originally described by Whipple et al. (27), and expanded upon by Coleman et al. (5). It involves chronic cardiac (ventricular) pacing at rates of approximately 250 bpm for a

Table 1. Res/ting hemodynamics and baroreflex sensitivity before and after 4–6 weeks of left ventricular pacing

	Pre-pace	Post-pace
LVSP (mm Hg)	116.0± 18.3 (7)	105.9± 9.5*
LVEDP (mm Hg)	4.6± 3.4 (7)	21.5± 6.6***
dP/dt$_{max}$ (mm Hg/s)	2250 ±272 (7)	1534 ±447 **
SAP (mm Hg)	121.9± 8.3 (13)	101.4± 8.3***
DAP (mm Hg)	80.9± 7.6 (13)	68.8± 7.9***
PP (mm Hg)	40.9± 6.5 (13)	32.6± 6.3***
MAP (mm Hg)	96.8± 7.6 (13)	80.8± 7.6***
LAP (mm Hg)	2.8± 3.5 (12)	22.2± 5.5***
HR (bpm)	77.1± 10.8 (13)	124.3± 13.0***
BRS-PE (ms/mm Hg)	32.0± 26.7 (13)	15.0± 14.8***
BRS-NG (ms/mm Hg)	16.6± 5.1 (13)	5.0± 2.7***

LVSP = left ventricular peak systolic pressure, LVEDP = left ventricular end diastolic pressure, dP/dt$_{max}$ = maximum of the first differentiation of left ventricular pressure. SAP = peak systolic arterial pressure, DAP = diastolic arterial pressure, PP = pulse pressure, MAP = mean arterial pressure, LAP = mean left atrial pressure, HR = heart rate. BRS-PE or BRS-NG = BRSs in response to phenylephrine or nitroglycerin injections, respectively. Data are expressed as mean ± SD (n dogs). *, **, ***: p values less then 0.05, 0.01, 0.005, respectively, when compared with pre-pace. [From (4), with permission.]

period of 4–6 weeks. Adult mongrel dogs were chronically instrumented for the measurement of arterial, left atrial and left ventricular pressures. In addition, pacing leads were sutured to the epicardial surface of the left ventricle and left atrium. After recovery from surgery (7–10 days) baseline hemodynamic measurements were taken in the conscious state with the dogs resting quietly on a laboratory table. After the control experiments

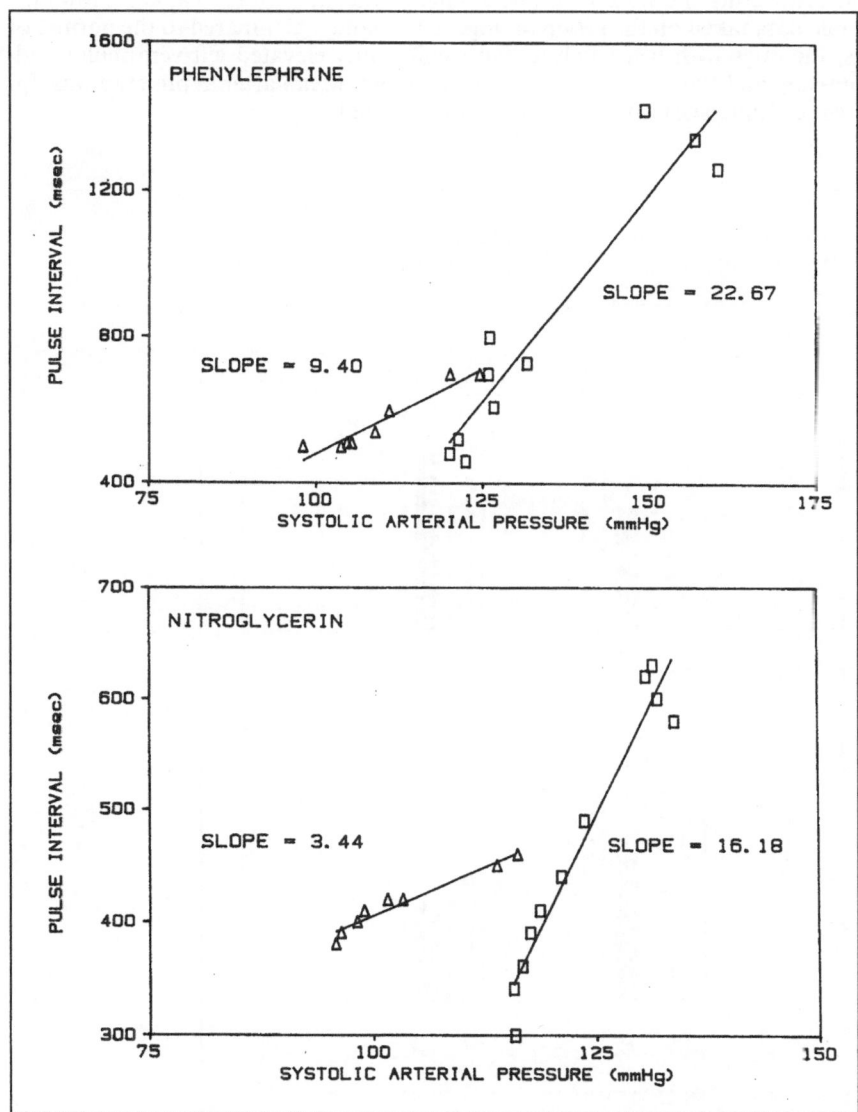

Fig. 1. A linear regression analysis of systolic arterial pressure against pulse interval for bolus injections of phenylephrine (top) and nitroglycerin (bottom) in a dogs before (squares) and after (triangles) heart failure induced by chronic ventricular pacing. [From (4), with permission.]

were done, the dogs were paced using a small Medtronics pacemaker (Model 5320) which was carried in the pocket of a mesh jacket worn by the dogs. Each dog was examined daily. Hemodynamic measurements were made approximately twice per week. When the dogs showed hemodynamic signs of heart failure the final experiment was done. Most dogs also showed significant pulmonary congestion and ascites after 4–6 weeks of pacing. In many dogs exercise tolerance was reduced, as evidenced by the dogs stopping to rest during the walk from the kennel to the laboratory. Table 1 shows the hemodynamic data taken on the group of dogs in this study. Compared to the normal or sham dogs, the dogs with heart failure had significantly elevated left-ventricular end-diastolic pressure and elevated mean left-atrial pressure. Mean arterial pressure was significantly reduced and heart rate was significantly elevated.

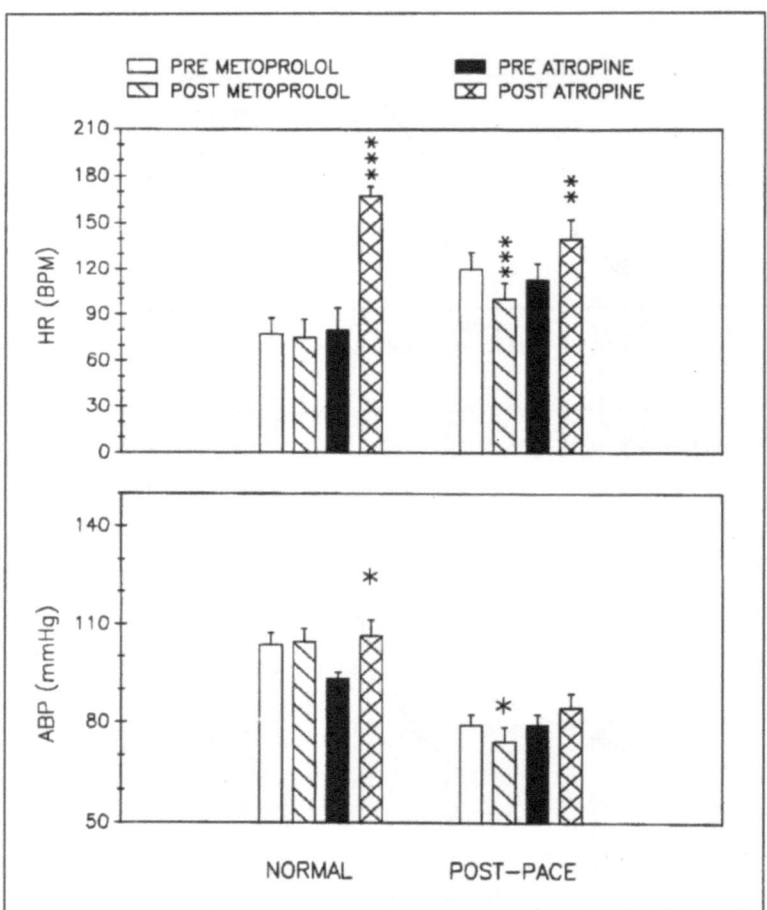

Fig. 2. Baseline heart rate (top) and arterial pressure (bottom) responses to autonomic blocking agents, metoprolol and atropine, in the normal and heart failure state. *, **, ***: p < 0.05, 0.01, 0.001, respectively, when compared with preautonomic blockade. Data are expressed as means ± SD. [From (4), with permission.]

The baroreflex was evaluated by administering bolus injections of nitroglycerin and phenylephrine. The technique of Smyth et al. (21) was used to determine the baroreflex sensitivity. Briefly, this entailed plotting the systolic arterial pressure against the subsequent pulse interval during both increases and decreases in arterial pressure. A linear regression was fit to these data and the slope of the regression was used as an index of baroreflex sensitivity. Figure 1 shows data from one dog studied before and after heart failure was induced (4). As can be seen, both nitroglycerin and phenylephrine slopes were depressed after heart failure. The autonomic components of this depressed baroreflex control of heart rate were determined. In this regard, the autonomic control of basal heart rate should be dissociated from the baroreflex mediated change in vagal and sympathetic outflow. Figure 2 shows the effects of autonomic blockade with atropine

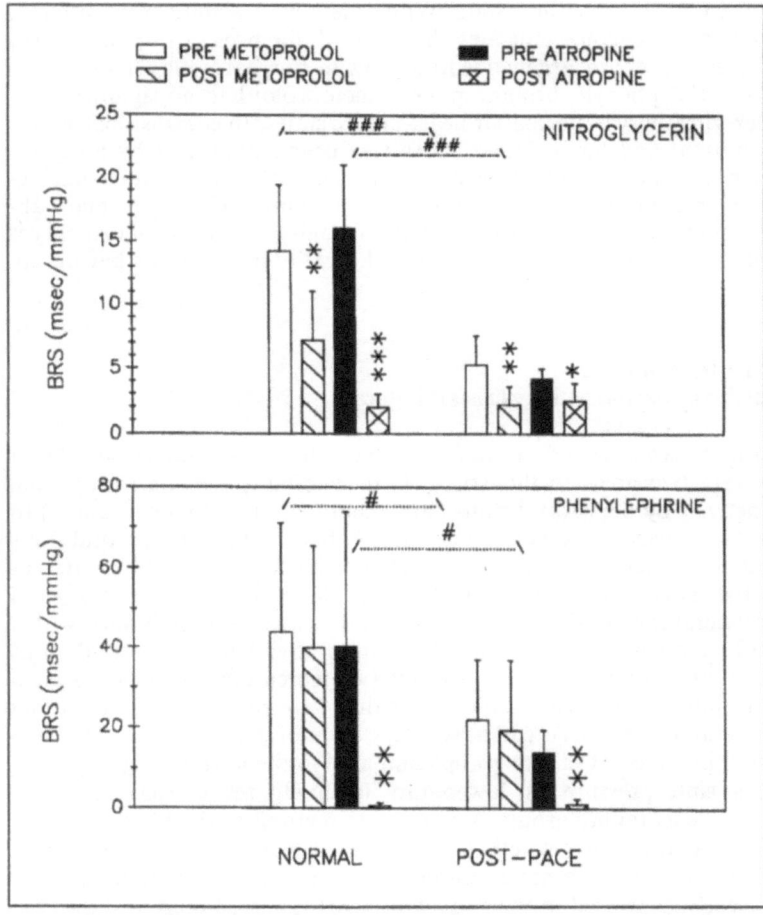

Fig. 3. Baroreflex responses to metoprolol and atropine in dogs in the normal and heart failure state during nitroglycerin induced hypotension (top) and phenylephrine induced hypertension (bottom). Baroreflex sensitivity is expressed as ms/mm Hg. *, **, ***: $p < 0.05, 0.01, 0.001$, respectively, when compared with pre-autonomic blockade. #, ##, ###: $p < 0.05, 0.01, 0.001$, respectively when compared with the normal state. Data are expressed as means $\pm$ SD. [From (4), with permission.]

and the cardio-specific β-blocker metoprolol on resting heart rate and arterial blood pressure. As can be seen, in the normal state metoprolol had no effect on resting heart rate, but atropine had a marked effect. In contrast, in the heart failure state, metoprolol reduced heart rate significantly and atropine increased heart rate only slightly. These data strongly suggest that dogs in heart failure have an elevated cardiac sympathetic outflow and a reduced vagal outflow, both of which contribute to the elevated resting heart rate in heart failure. Figure 3 shows the baroreflex sensitivity in the normal and heart-failure states for nitroglycerin and phenylephrine. As can be seen, both metoprolol and atropine reduced baroreflex sensitivity in normal and heart-failure states during nitroglycerin administration. Metoprolol depressed baroreflex sensitivity by $47.6 \pm 26.3\%$ (mean $\pm$ SD) in the normal state, and by $63.6 \pm 58.5\%$ in the heart-failure state. Atropine decreased the baroreflex sensitivity by $86.7 \pm 7.8\%$ in the normal state, and by $39.5 \pm 30.2\%$ in the heart-failure state. While these were significantly different ($p < 0.05$), an analysis of covariance indicates that these differences in response in the normal and heart-failure states are largely due to the low resting baroreflex sensitivity in the heart-failure state. For phenylephrine responses, metoprolol had no significant influence on baroreflex sensitivity in normal or heart-failure states. In contrast, baroreflex sensitivity in both normal and heart-failure states was nearly abolished by atropine. These data provide the first description of the autonomic control of heart rate in pacing-induced heart failure. In contrast to other studies of heart failure (9), the primary abnormality is seen during baroreceptor unloading with nitroglycerin. This abnormality is largely due to a decrease in sympathetic activation in heart failure when the baroreceptors are unloaded.

Baroreflex control of arterial pressure and peripheral sympathetic nervous activity in heart failure

This series of experiments was carried out in anesthetized dogs with and without heart failure (23). There were two goals to this study: 1) to determine the control of renal sympathetic nerve activity by the carotid sinus baroreceptors in heart failure, and 2) to determine if the abnormal baroreflex was due to a CNS abnormality. One carotid sinus was vascularly isolated and perfused with a Krebs-Henseleit solution. All other afferent pathways were ablated. This included bilateral section of the vagi and aortic nerves and section of the contralateral carotid sinus nerve. The carotid sinus was conditioned with a static pressure of 100 mm Hg for approximately 30 min, after which a carotid sinus pressure-mean arterial pressure curve was constructed by increasing carotid sinus pressure in a stepwise fashion. Figure 4 shows the curves that were generated in the normal group and in the heart failure group. As can be seen, the slope of the baroreflex curve was significantly depressed in the heart failure group compared to the normal dogs. In addition, when the carotid sinus pressure was lowered to 50 mm Hg, mean arterial pressure did not increase in the heart failure group. A similar attenuation of the baroreflex was observed when renal sympathetic nerve activity is plotted against carotid sinus pressure, as is shown in Fig. 5. While not as dramatic a difference as was seen in Fig. 4, the slope of this relationship is clearly depressed in the dogs with heart failure. Figure 6 shows the percent change in mean arterial pressure in response to electrical stimulation of the carotid sinus nerve with varying frequencies, voltages and durations of stimulation in normal and heart failure dogs. As was the case for pressurizing the carotid sinus, the response to electrical stimulation was significantly less in the dogs with heart failure compared to the normal dogs. Interestingly, when the relationship between renal nerve ac-

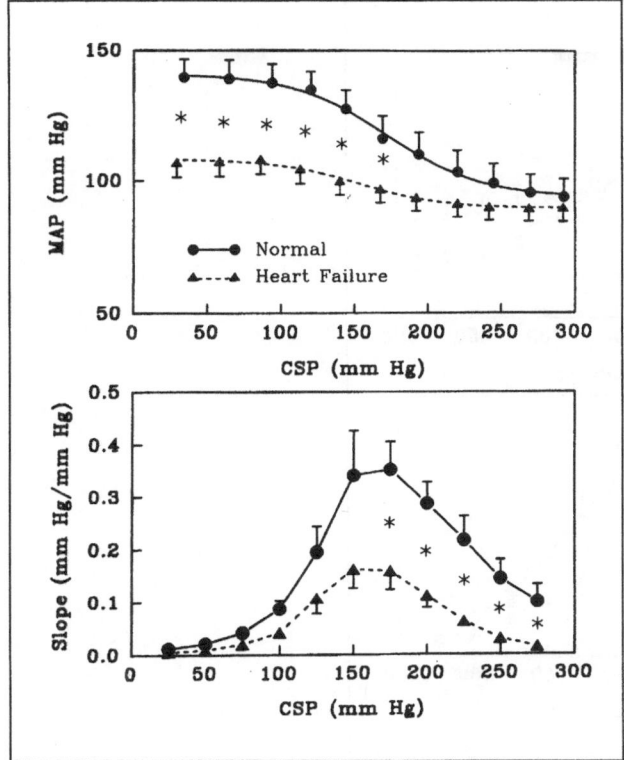

Fig. 4. The mean data of carotid sinus pressure-mean arterial pressure relationships and their respective slopes in normal and heart failure dogs. *=significant difference between normal and heart failure dogs. [From (23), with permission.]

tivity and carotid sinus nerve stimulation was examined (Fig. 7) there was no difference between the groups. What these data strongly suggest is that the abnormal baroreflex resides either within the afferent endings or at the vascular smooth muscle, but not within the CNS since when the receptors are bypassed by electrical stimulation, the output of the CNS is normal in dogs with heart failure. There are several limitations to this study which temper our conclusions slightly. One, of course, is the fact that the dogs were anesthetized. While it is possible that dogs with heart failure respond to anesthesia differently, there are several studies in the literature which confirm the depressed baroreflex in conscious dogs using various models of heart failure (12, 22, 23, 28). Secondly, the use of electrical stimulation of the carotid sinus nerve will stimulate afferents from the carotid bodies as well as baroreceptor afferents. While this is undoubtedly true, the prominent depressor and renal nerve inhibition seen in these dogs during electrical stimulation is primarily mediated by baroreceptor stimulation. Thirdly, it is possible that sympathetic nervous activity targeted to other beds may behave differently than renal nerve activity. This is certainly possible since sympathetic nervous outflow is not homogeneous (26). The answer to this question will have to await further experimentation.

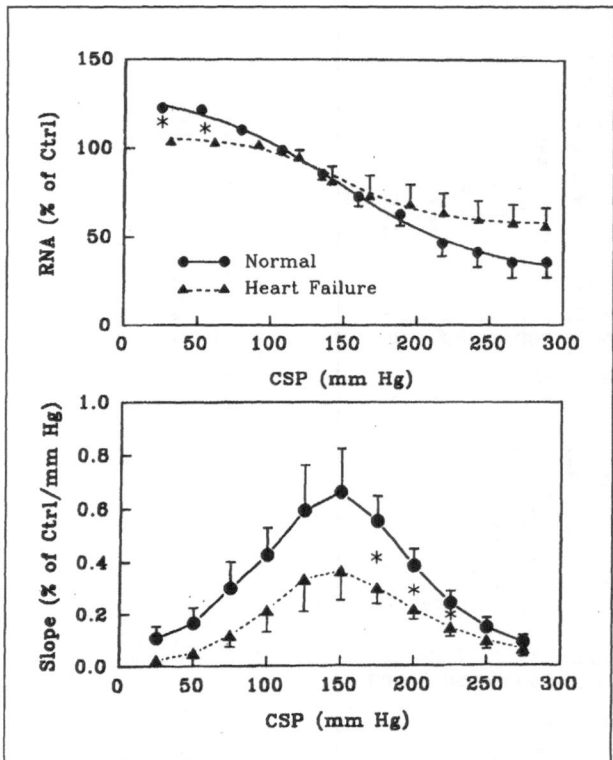

Fig. 5. Mean data of carotid sinus pressure-renal nerve activity relationships and their respective slopes in normal and heart-failure dogs. * = significant difference between the normal and heart failure groups. [From (23), with permission.]

Lastly, it is possible that the use of only one carotid sinus with the vagi cut attenuates the baroreflex more in the heart-failure dog than it does in the normal dog. More recent studies in which the baroreflex response to carotid sinus pressurization was evaluated in normal and heart-failure dogs with and without the vagi suggests that input from vagal afferents may be responsible, in part, for the depressed baroreflex in heart failure. Figure 8 shows the relationship between electrical stimulation of the carotid sinus nerve and mean arterial pressure in normal and heart failure dogs before and after bilateral vagotomy. The responses shown with the vagi intact were carried out after aortic nerve section. As can be seen, the baroreflex was similar after vagotomy in the normal dog, however the baroreflex sensitivity was markedly enhanced after vagotomy in the dog with heart failure, even though the baroreflex was blunted in the dog with heart failure compared to the normal dogs. In recent studies by Dibner-Dunlap and Thames (8) using the same mode of heart failure it was found that vagotomy had no effect on the baroreflex slope by relating the percent change in aortic nerve activity to the change in mean arterial pressure in heart-failure dogs, but that it increased the slope in sham-operated dogs. However, in this same study, vagotomy reduced the gain of the renal nerve activity – mean arterial pressure relationship in both groups of dogs. The reasons

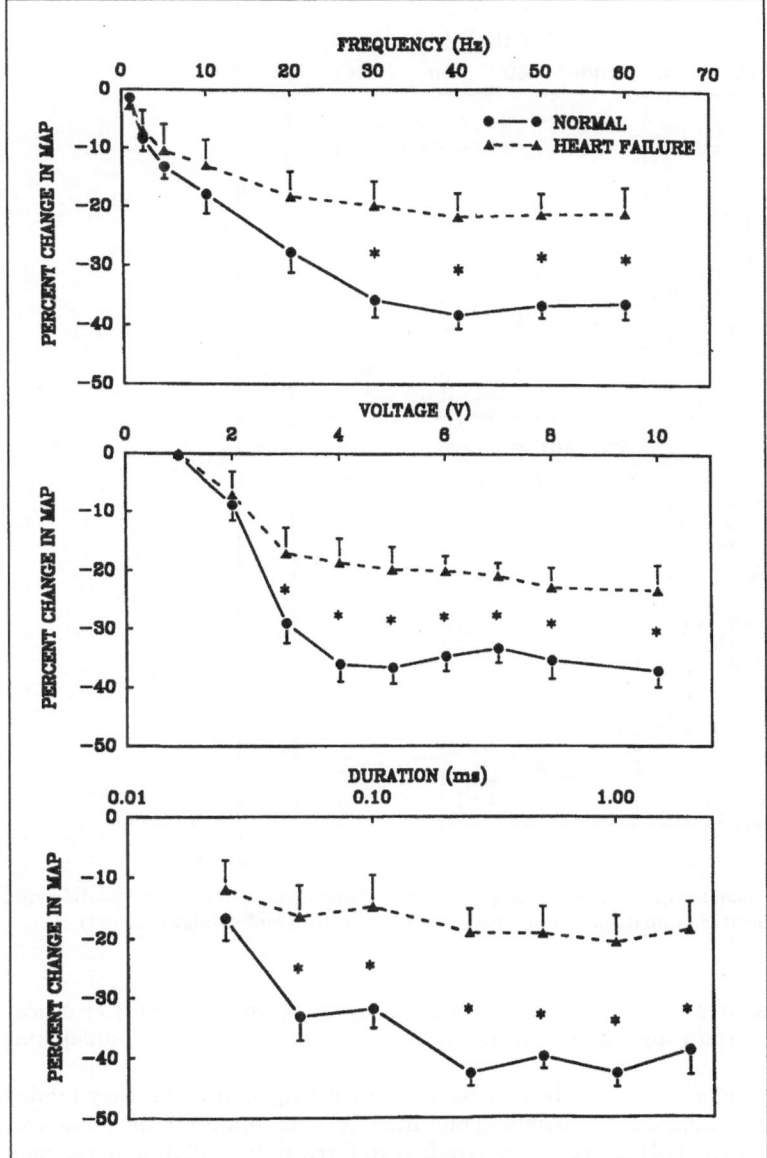

Fig. 6. Mean data of mean arterial pressure responses to electrical stimulation of the carotid sinus nerve with varying frequencies, voltages or durations in normal and heart failure dogs. * = significant difference between normal and heart failure dogs. [From (23), with permission.]

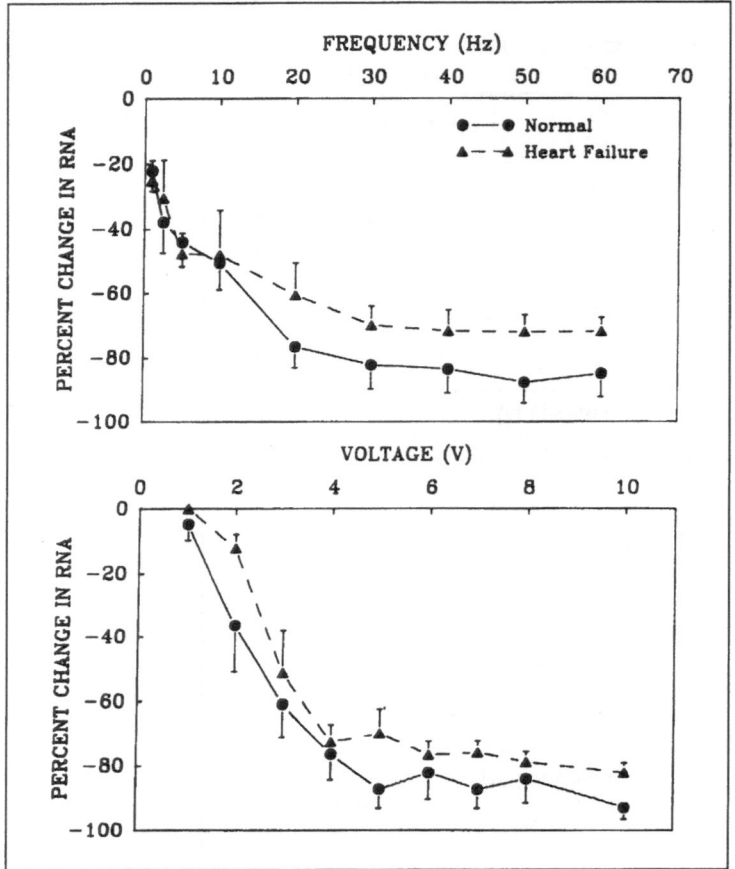

Fig. 7. Mean data of renal sympathetic nerve responses to electrical stimulation of the carotid sinus nerve in normal and heart failure dogs with increasing frequency (top) and voltage (bottom). [From (23), with permission.]

for the differences in our two studies are not readily apparant, however, electrical stimulation of the carotid sinus nerve was not done in the study of Dibner-Dunlap and Thames (8).

The notion that augmented input from cardiopulmonary vagal afferents may inhibit the baroreflex in heart failure is an intriguing one and has some support in the literature. For instance, Mark et al. (14) has shown a paradoxical forearm vasodilation in patients with aortic stenosis who undergo strenuous exercise. Mitral stenosis patients respond normally. Cardiac prostaglandin synthesis is increased in animals with dilated hearts (15). It has been shown that both prostacyclin and arachidonic acid stimulate cardiac afferents which, in turn, inhibit the baroreflex (16, 17). It is, therefore, possible that this mechanism could be responsible for augmenting cardiac receptor input in heart failure. Additionally, it is possible that mechanical stimuli from afferents in the dilated heart would be augmented, especially those of unmyelinated c-fiber afferents which do not show acute resetting as readily as do myelinated fibers (20).

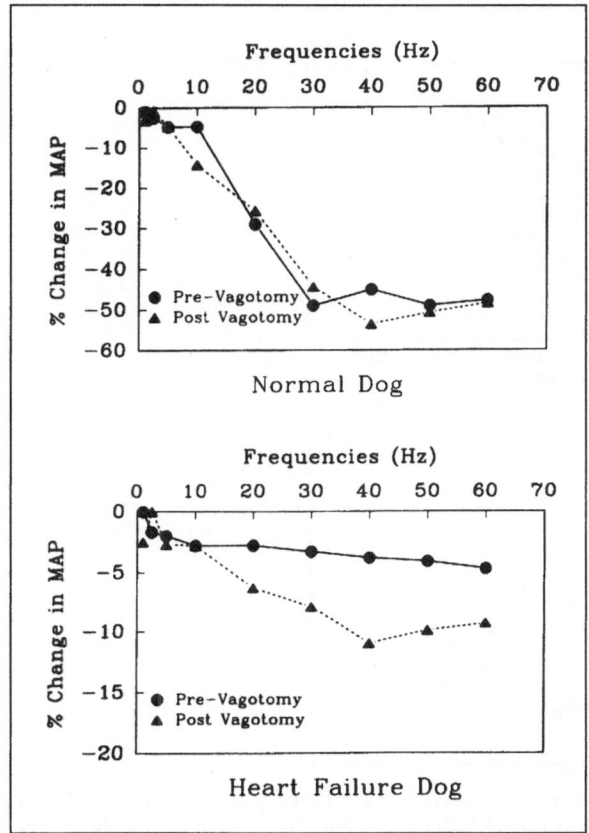

Fig. 8. The relationship between electrical stimulation of the carotid sinus nerve and the percent change in arterial pressure in a normal dog and in a heart-failure dog, before and after bilateral vagotomy

Baroreceptor discharge sensitivity in heart failure

One location in the baroreflex arc which remains a prime candidate for producing a reduction in the baroreflex sensitivity is the baroreceptor itself. We undertook a series of experiments to determine if baroreceptor discharge sensitivity is abnormal in dogs with pacing-induced heart failure. We recorded action potentials from carotid sinus baroreceptors in vascularly isolated carotid sinuses (25). In addition, we measured carotid sinus diameter by sonomicrometry to determine compliance of the carotid sinus in the two groups of dogs. As can be seen in Fig. 9, the pressure-discharge relationship in the heart failure dogs was significantly depressed compared to the normal dogs. The pressure threshold was elevated from 91.0 ± 5.0 (mean $\pm$ SEM) mm Hg in the normal dogs to 119.1 ± 4.4 mm Hg in the heart-failure dogs. The peak slope was significantly reduced from 0.63 ± 0.06 spikes/s/mm Hg in the normal dogs, to 0.40 ± 0.04 spikes/s/mm Hg in the heart-failure dogs. There were no significant differences in the compliance curves of the sinuses in the two groups of dogs. However there was a sig-

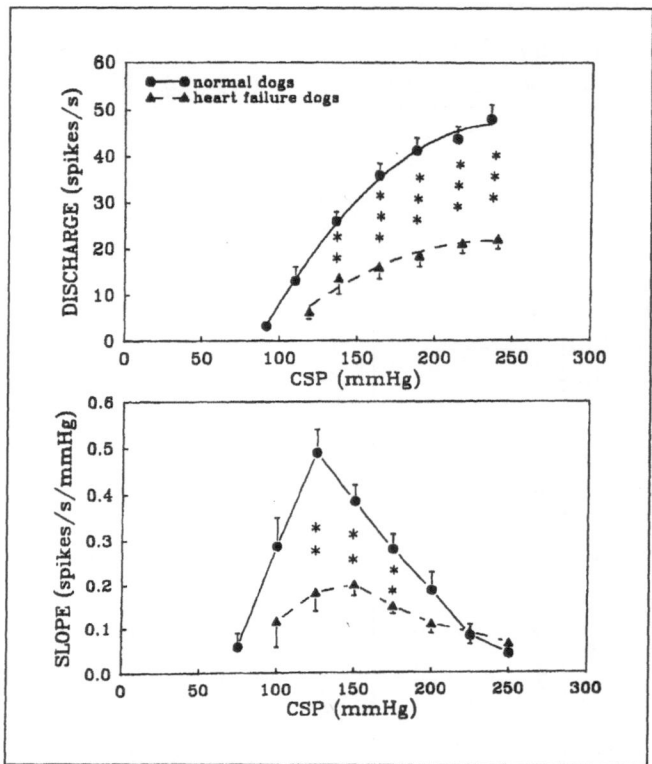

Fig. 9. Carotid sinus pressure (CSP, mm Hg)-baroreceptor discharge (spikes/sec) curves (upper panel) in normal and heart-failure dogs. Lower panel shows the slope (spikes/s/mm Hg) of the curves in the upper panel plotted vs CSP, ** $p < 0.01$, *** $p < 0.001$, comparing normal and heart failure dogs. [From (25), with permission.]

nificant decrease in the strain sensitivity in the heart-failure dogs. Perfusion of the carotid stinus with a Krebs-Henseleit solution containing 0.01 µg/ml of ouabain shifted the pressure-discharge curve upwards and to the left in the heart failure group. There was no such effect in the normal dogs (Fig. 10). At this concentration ouabain had no effect on carotid sinus diameter or compliance.

As further evidence for depressed baroreceptor discharge in heart failure, we analyzed the phenomenon of postexcitatory depression (PED) in normal and heart failure dogs (24). PED refers to the period of baroreceptor silence that occurs following the release of a pressure step (Fig. 11). It has been shown that the duration of PED is linearly related to the pressure step (1) and that PED can be abolished by administration of a cardiac glycoside (2), thereby implicating activation of a Na-K ATPase mediated Na pump as the cause of PED. We reasoned that if there was an increase in Na-K ATPase activity in heart failure, then the relationship between the pressure step and the duration of PED should be altered in heart failure. Figure 12 shows the results of this experiment. There was a linear increase in the duration of PED up to pressure steps of about 80 mm Hg in heart failure dogs, however, this relationship was nearly flat in the normal dogs.

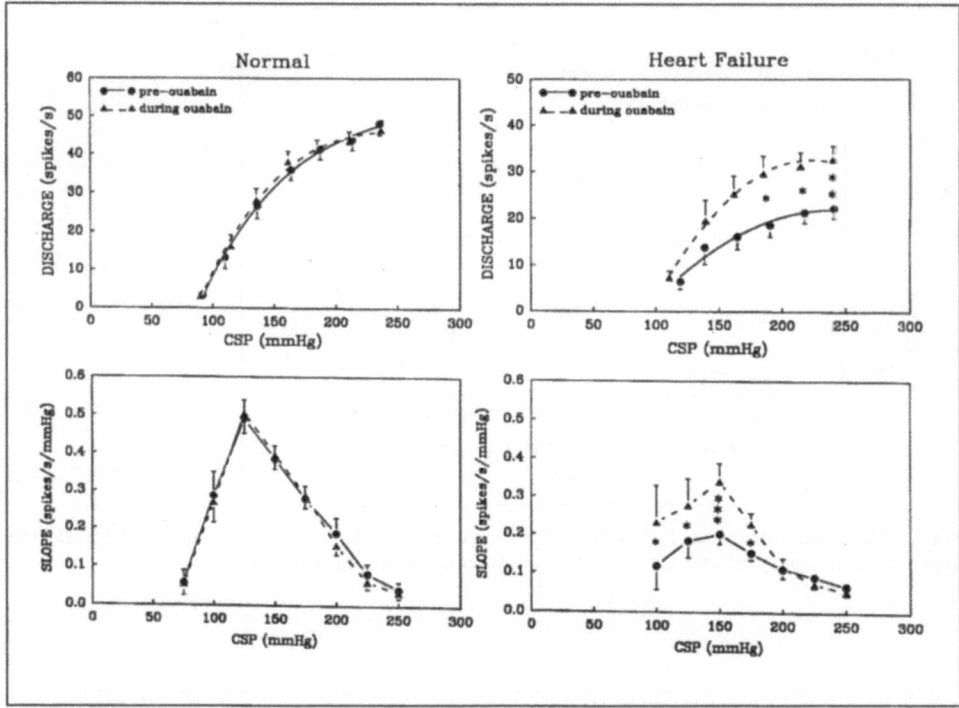

Fig. 10. Curves showing the effects of ouabain (0.01 µg/kg) perfusion of the carotid sinus on carotid sinus pressure (CSP, mm Hg)-discharge (spikes/s; upper panels) and CSP-slope (spikes/s/mm Hg; lower panels) relations in normal (left panels) and heart-failure (right panels) dogs. * $p < 0.05$, ** $p < 0.01$, *** $p < 0.001$ comparing preouabain vs postouabain. [From (25), with permission.]

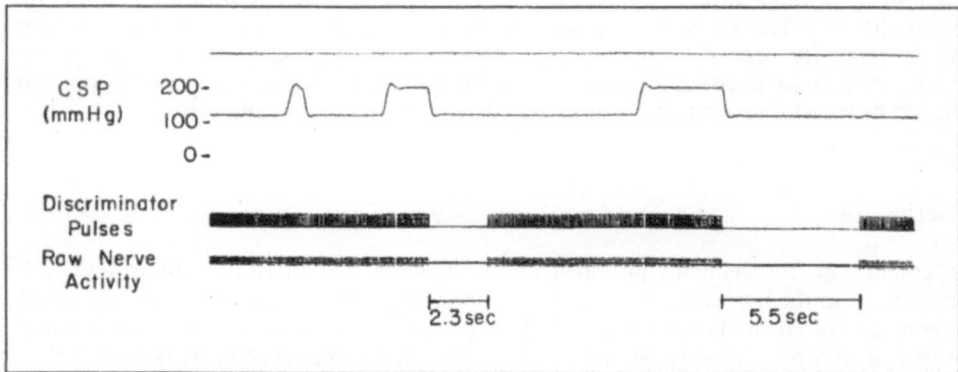

Fig. 11. An original recording from a normal dog showing receptor discharge when the duration of the pressure step is varied at a constant step amplitude. CSP = carotid sinus pressure. [From (24), with permission.]

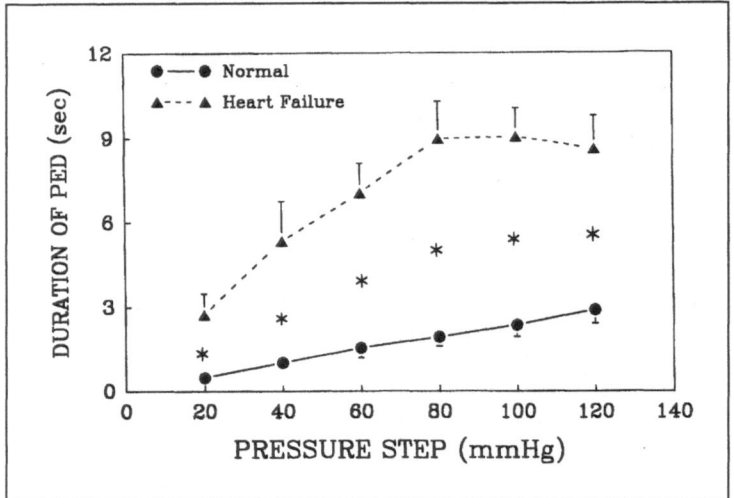

Fig. 12. Mean data for the pressure step vs duration of PED relationship in normal and heart failure dogs. * = significantly different from each other. [From (24), with permission.]

The above pressure-discharge data is consistent with the view that baroreceptor discharge is depressed in this model of heart failure and that a probable mechanism is an increase in Na-K ATPase activity in the receptor ending or in the cells of the carotid sinus wall. It is not clear what mechanism(s) would lead to an increase in Na-K ATPase activity in heart failure, however, in this and other models of heart failure, plasma aldosterone concentration is increased (19); this could contribute to an increase in Na-K ATPase synthesis in the cell bodies of the baroreceptors or in the endothelial and/or smooth muscle cells of the carotid sinus. We have obtained preliminary evidence that high levels of aldosterone (200–500 pg/ml) do, indeed, inhibit baroreceptor discharge sensitivity (29). This phenomenon may not, however, be related to an increase in Na-K ATPase activity since it occurs within 15 min and is not blocked by ouabain. In any event, an increase in sodium pumping in the baroreceptor endings could hyperpolarize the receptor membrane which, in turn, would decrease discharge sensitivity.

Conclusions

In conclusion, the evidence provided above suggests that there are abnormalities at several loci in the baroreflex arc. The receptor endings themselves are clearly abnormal, having a reduced discharge sensitivity. It is possible that the autonomic regulation of heart rate and peripheral resistance are abnormal in this model of heart failure. It does not appear that there is a central abnormality, at least as far as the control of renal sympathetic nerve activity is concerned. Many issues still remain unresolved as far as the baroreflex is concerned. Is there uniform depression of all baroreceptor endings such as C and A fibers? Are cardiac receptors altered in heart failure? Is there depression of αmediated vasoconstriction in heart failure? Finally, what is the role of other neurohumoral substances in modulation of the baroreflex in heart failure? It is important that these issues be addressed in a sequential fashion in future work.

Acknowledgements. The authors express their appreciation to Ms. Johnnie Hackley and Mrs. Pam Curry for their excellent technical assistance.

References

1. Bronk DW, Stella G (1935) The response to steady pressures of single end organs in the isolated carotid sinus. Am J Physiol 110:708–714
2. Brown AM, Saum WR, Tuley FH (1976) A comparison of aortic baroreceptor discharge in normotensive and spontaneously hypertensive rats. Circ Res 39:488–496
3. Chen HI, Chow LH, Wang DJ (1988) Closed-loop analysis of the reflex function in orthostatic hypotension. Chinese J Physiol 31:31–42
4. Chen J-S, Wang W, Bartholet T, Zucker IH (1991) Analysis of baroreflex control of heart rate in conscious dogs with pacing-induced heart failure. Circulation 83:260–267
5. Coleman HN, Taylor RR, Pool P, Whipple GH, Covell JW, Ross J Jr, Braunwald E (1971) Congestive heart failure following chronic tachycardia. Am Heart J 81:790–798
6. Convertino VA, Doerr DF, Eckberg DL, Fritsch JM, Vernikos-Danellis J (1990) Head-down bed rest impairs vagal baroreflex responses and provokes orthostatic hypotension. J Appl Physiol 68:1458–1464
7. Cowley AW Jr, Liard JF, Guyton AC (1973) Role of the baroreceptor reflex in daily control of arterial blood pressure and other variables in dogs. Circ Res 32:564–576
8. Dibner-Dunlap ME, Thames MD (1989) Baroreflex control of renal sympathetic nerve activity is preserved in heart failure despite reduced arterial baroreceptor sensitivity. Circ Res 65:1526–1535
9. Eckberg DL, Drabinsky M, Braunwald E (1971) Defective cardiac parasympathetic control in patients with heart failure. New Engl J Med 285:877–883
10. Ellenbogen KA, Mohanty PK, Szentpetery S, Thames MD (1989) Arterial baroreflex abnormalities in heart failure: reversal after orthotopic cardiac transplantation. Circulation 79:51–58
11. Ferguson DW, Berg WJ, Sanders JS, Roach PJ, Kempf JS, Kienzle MG (1989) Sympathoinhibitory responses to digitalis glycosides in heart failure patients. Direct evidence from sympathetic neural recordings. Circulation 80:65–77
12. Higgins CB, Vatner SF, Eckberg DL, Braunwald E (1972) Alterations in baroreceptor reflex in conscious dogs with heart failure. J Clin Invest 51:715–724
13. Jacob HJ, Alper RH, Brody MJ (1989) Lability of arterial pressure after baroreceptor denervation is not pressure dependent. Hypertension 14:501–510
14. Mark AL, Kioschos JM, Abboud FM, Heistad DD, Schmid P (1973) Abnormal vascular responses to exercise in patients with aortic stenosis. J Clin Invest 52:1138–1146
15. Newman WH, Frankis MB, Halushka PV (1983) Increased myocardial release of prostacyclin in dogs with heart failure. J Cardiovasc Pharmacol 5:194–201
16. Panzenbeck MJ, Tan W, Hajdu MA, Cornish KG, Zucker IH (1989) PGE_2 and arachidonate inhibit the baroreflex in conscious dogs via cardiac receptors. Am J Physiol 256:H999–H1005
17. Panzenbeck MJ, Tan W, Hajdu MA, Zucker IH (1988) Intracoronary infusion of prostaglandin I_2 attenuates arterial baroreflex control of heart rate in conscious dogs. Circ Res 53:860–868
18. Peuler JD, Patel KP, Morgan DA, Whiteis CA, Lund DD, Pardini BJ, Schmid PG (1989) Altered peripheral noradrenergic activity in intact and sinoaortic denervated Dahl rats. Can J Physiol Pharmacol 67:442–449
19. Riegger AJG, Liebau G (1982) The renin-angiotensin-aldosterone system, antidiuretic hormone and sympathetic nerve activity in an experimental model of congestive heart failure in the dog. Clin Sci 62:465–469

20. Schultz HD, Pisarri TE, Coleridge HM, Coleridge JCG (1985) Absence of acute resetting by C-fiber baroreceptors in the carotid sinus of dogs. Fed Proc 44:1033
21. Smyth HS, Sleight P, Pickering GW (1969) Reflex regulation of arterial pressure during sleep in man: a quantitative method of assessing baroreflex sensitivity. Circ Res 24:109–121
22. Vatner SF, Higgins CB, Braunwald E (1974) Sympathetic and parasympathetic components of reflex tachycardia induced by hypotension in conscious dogs with and without heart failure. Cardiovas Res 8:155–161
23. Wang W, Chen J-S, Zucker IH (1991) Carotid sinus baroreceptor reflex in dogs with experimental heart failure. Circ Res 68:1294–1301
24. Wang W, Chen J-S, Zucker IH (1991) Postexcitatory depression of baroreceptors in dogs with experimental heart failure. Am J Physiol 260:H1160–H1165
25. Wang W, Chen J-S, Zucker IH (1990) Carotid sinus baroreceptor sensitivity in experimental heart failure. Circulation 81:1959–1966
26. Weaver LC, Fry HK, Meckler RL (1984) Differential renal and splenic nerve responses to vagal and spinal afferent inputs. Am J Physiol 246:R78–R87
27. Whipple GH, Sheffield LT, Woodman EG, Theophilis C, Freidman S (1962) Reversible congestive heart failure due to rapid stimulation of the normal heart. Proc New Engl Cardiovas Soc 20:39
28. White CW (1981) Abnormalities in baroreflex control of heart rate in canine heart failure. Am J Physiol 240:H793–H799
29. Zucker IH, Wang W (1990) Aldosterone reduces baroreceptor discharge in the dog. Circulation 82:III-10

Authors' address:

Prof. Irving H. Zucker, Ph.D.
Department of Physiology and Biophysics
University of Nebraska College of Medicine
600 S. 42nd Street
Omaha, Nebraska 68198-4575, USA

Does converting enzyme inhibition change the neuronal and extraneuronal uptake of catecholamines?

P. Dominiak[1] and A. Blöchl[2]

[1] Department of Pharmacology, Medical University of Lübeck, FRG
[2] Department of Pharmacology, University of Illinois, Chicago, USA

Summary: In previous studies concerning the sympathetic outflow during converting enzyme inhibition, no significant changes after chronic treatment could be observed. Therefore, we investigated the effects of the long-acting converting enzyme inhibitor ramipril on the neuronal and extraneuronal uptake of SHR. Ramipril was administered either i.v. or orally to SHR, whereas desipramine or corticosterone were additionally infused to block the neuronal or extraneuronal uptake of catecholamines. As an index of sympathetic outflow, plasma noradrenaline and adrenaline concentrations were determined during preganglionic stimulation of the spinal cord using HPLC and ELCD. Blood pressure of SHR was measured in a carotid artery and was significantly decreased in the ramipril treated group under resting and stimulating conditions. Ramipril did not influence stimulated sympathetic outflow. However, in acute and chronic experiments ramipril led to an additive effect to desipramine concerning stimulated circulating catecholamines. Similar results could be obtained after blocking the uptake-2 with corticosterone. ^{3}H-NA-uptake into the hearts of SHR was significantly diminished by about 10% after chronic ramipril administration. It is suggested that ramipril is able to decrease the neuronal and extraneuronal uptake of catecholamines by an unspecific effect due to the comparably high lipophilicity. The blood pressure lowering effect of ramipril is not supported by an inhibition of presynaptic noradrenaline release.

Key words: Converting enzyme inhibition; spontaneously hypertensive rats (SHR); sympathetic outflow; neuronal and extraneuronal uptake

Introduction

Angiotensin II (Ang II) is capable of releasing noradrenaline from sympathetic varicosities via presynaptic Ang II receptors and of adrenaline from adrenal medulla (10). The inhibition of the Ang II biosynthesis by converting enzyme inhibitors should, therefore, consequently lead to a decrease in catecholamine release, as was demonstrated by (8) in acute experiments on pithed rabbits using captopril as an inhibitor, or by a decrease in circulating noradrenaline in patients with congestive heart failure after acute oral administration of captopril (15).

In contrast to the acute effects of converting enzyme inhibition on catecholamine release, we observed no significant changes in catecholamine biosynthesis, storage and release in spontaneously hypertensive rats (SHR) having received chronic treatment in order to investigate various converting enzyme inhibitors (2, 3).

Several mechanisms could contribute to the almost unchanged sympathetic outflow in SHR after chronic converting enzyme inhibition: an accumulation of Ang I and bradykinin whereby both peptides are able to influence the catecholamine release (12), or interaction with the uptake or a degradation of both noradrenaline and adrenaline.

In the present study, we have investigated the acute and chronic effects of the long-acting converting enzyme inhibitor ramipril on the neuronal and extraneuronal uptake of SHR.

Methods

Animals

Male spontaneously hypertensive rats (SHR, strain: SHR/NCrl BR, Ivanovas, Kißlegg) at the age of about 12 weeks (200 g) were used for the experiments. The animals were housed in a plastic cage (Makrolon) and given water and a standard diet (Altromin) ad libitum.

Drugs

Ramipril was administered either intravenously (0.1 mg/kg) or orally (1 mg/kg/d, 14 days) by gavage to achieve acute or chronic inhibition of the converting enzyme. Controls received the same volume of water.

To block the neuronal uptake of catecholamines, desipramine (100 ng/kg/min) was additionally infused during the stimulation experiments, whereas corticosterone (33 µg/kg/min i.v.) served as an inhibitor for the extraneuronal uptake. Ang II (10 ng/kg/min) was also administered i.v. during the stimulation experiments.

Stimulation experiments

SHR were pithed by a steel rod (diameter: 1.5 mm), according to (5), which was coated with enamel except for the length of the thoracolumbar spinal cord (Th4-Th12 segment). The steel rod served as a positive electrode. Both vagus nerves were cut at the neck and the neuromuscular junction was blocked by administering D-tubocurarin (3 ng/kg i.v.) 45 min prior to the stimulation experiments. Sympathetic outflow was induced by preganglionic electrical stimulation (50 mA, 3.3 Hz, 1 ms, 3 min) and assessed by measuring circulating noradrenaline and adrenaline at the end of each stimulation period in blood samples obtained from a PE-50 catheter which was inserted into the left carotid artery. The drugs mentioned above were given to both ramipril- and control-treated SHR and the stimulations were repeated.

Blood pressure measurements

During the experimental procedures, blood pressure and heart rate were measured in the right carotid artery through a PE-50 catheter, using a Statham P 23 Db pressure transducer and a Gould-Brush system for monitoring. Drugs were injected via a PE-10 catheter placed into a femoral vein.

Determination of circulating catecholamines

At the end of each stimulation period, blood samples were taken from the left carotid artery and mixed with heparine (5000 I.U.) and centrifugated at 4° C. 0.2 m reduced glutathione and 0.25 m EDTA were added to the yielded plasma and the samples were kept frozen ($-70°$ C) until assayed according to (4). After thawing, a glutathione solution [consisting of 300 mm EDTA and 50 mm reduced glutathione (pH 7.0)] was added to the plasma and then adsorbed into the alumina. Desorbtion was performed by perchloric acid (200 mm), and after centrifugation the supernatant was injected into the chromatographic system consisting of a reversed phase Machery and Nagel column (Nucleosil; flow rate: 1 ml/min) and an electrochemical detector (Waters M 450).

Neuronal uptake of ^{3}H-noradrenaline

To determine the neuronal uptake, 5 µCi/kg body-weight ^{3}H-noradrenaline was injected into a tail vein of both control- and chronic ramipril-treated SHR. Thirty min after injection the hearts were removed and homogenized at 4° C. After alumina adsorption radioactivity was determined in a liquid scintillation counter. Uptake of tritiated noradrenaline was calculated by using a standard ^{3}H-NA curve. As a positive control a third group of SHR received desipramine (100 ng/kg) i.v. prior to ^{3}H-noradrenaline injections.

Results

Acute experiments

A) Blood pressure: Ramipril (0.1 mg/kg), injected 30 min prior to the stimulation experiments, significantly lowered systolic and diastolic blood pressure before and after stimulation with 3.3 Hz (Table 1). In recuperation, additionally infused desipramine had no further effect on blood pressure. However, during preganglionic stimulation of the sympathetic nerves, desipramine increased mainly diastolic blood pressure (Table 1). In ramipril-treated animals, desipramine only enhanced systolic blood pressure during electrical stimulation. Ang II infusion increased primarily the diastolic blood pressure under all experimental conditions.

B) Circulating catecholamines: As we anticipated, stimulation-dependent noradrenaline overflow was significantly enhanced when desipramine was administered (Fig. 1). Sur-

Table 1. Stimulation-dependent blood pressure changes in SHR after *acute* administration of ramipril: influence of desipramine and ANG II

		0 SBP/DBP$\pm$SEM	DIP SBP/DBP$\pm$SEM	DIP+ANG II SBP/DBP$\pm$SEM
	Control	84/ 49$\pm$ 3.4/7.0	94/ 55$\pm$ 4.9/3.5	110/ 63$\pm$ 4.9/3.0
	Ramipril	70/ 30$\pm$ 4.4/3.2*	67/ 30$\pm$ 4.8/3.7**	70/ 38$\pm$ 6.3/5.4**
3.3 Hz {	Control	181/119$\pm$12/7.5	200/139$\pm$14/5.8	217/149$\pm$18/6.2
	Ramipril	128/ 73$\pm$ 5.7/7.3**	140/ 77$\pm$ 7.1/8.2**	146/ 94$\pm$ 7.4/9.1**

SBP = systolic blood pressure; DBP = diastolic blood pressure; DIP = additionally infused desipramine (100 ng/kg $\times$ min); ANG II = additionally infused angiotensin II (10 ng/kg $\times$ min). Ramipril was injected intravenously (0.1 mg/kg) 30 min prior to the stimulation experiments; stimulation parameters: 3.3 Hz, 50 mA, 1 ms, 3 min; significance values: * = $p > 0.05$, ** = $p > 0.01$, Ramipril vs control; n = 6 SHR per each group.

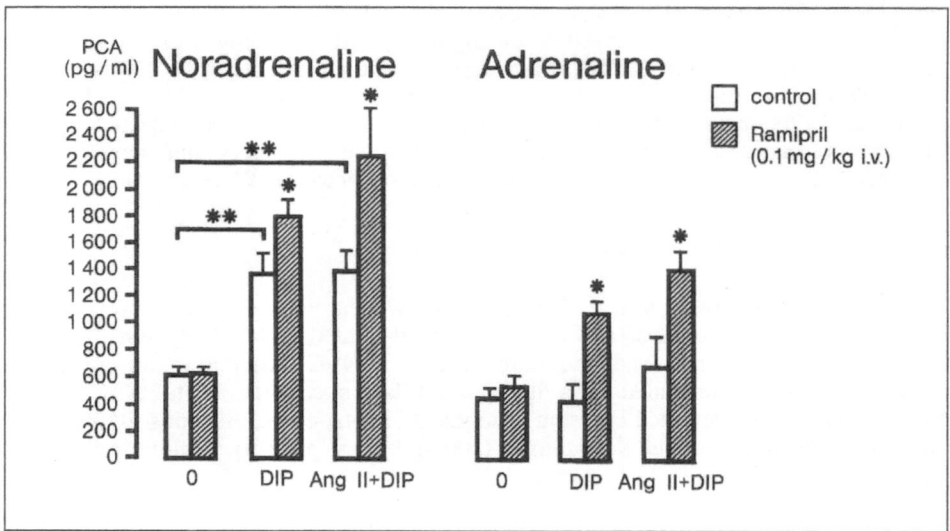

Fig. 1. Effects of acute inhibition of the converting enzyme with ramipril (0.1 mg/kg i.v.) on stimulated sympathetic outflow as assessed by determination of plasma noradrenaline and adrenaline concentrations during preganglionic electrical stimulation of the thoracolumbar spinal cord of pithed SHR. Desipramine was additionally infused (100 ng/kg × min i.v.) to block the neuronal uptake of catecholamines. Ang II was administered i.v. (10 ng/kg × min) in addition to desipramine. Abbreviations: DIP = desipramine; Ang II = angiotensin II; PCA = plasma catecholamine concentration; 0 = before DIP and Ang II. Stimulation parameters: frequency = 3.3 Hz; duration = 3 min; amperage = 50 mA; width = 1 ms. Significance values: * = p < 0.05; ** = p < 0.01

prisingly, in the ramipril-treated group desipramine infusion led to a further significant increase in circulating noradrenaline and adrenaline (Fig. 1). In comparison to desipramine, Ang II showed no considerable changes in stimulated catecholamine release (Fig. 1).

Chronic experiments

Desipramine
A) blood pressure: As was demonstrated by the acute experiments, ramipril significantly decreased resting and stimulation-dependent blood pressure (Table 2). No significant changes in blood pressure were observed when desipramine and/or Ang II were additionally administered (Table 2).

B) Circulating catecholamines: Ramipril did not significantly change the stimulated noradrenaline overflow into plasma; however, adrenaline release showed an increase of about 100% (Fig. 2). Desipramine effects on stimulated circulating catecholamines were similar to those observed in acute experiments (Fig. 2).

Corticosterone
A) blood pressure: Corticosterone, as an uptake-2 blocking agent, did not influence stimulated blood pressure in the control and ramipril-treated group. Therefore, a representation in graphical or tabular form was not attempted.

Table 2. Stimulation-dependent blood pressure changes in SHR after *chronic* administration of ramipril: influence of desipramine and ANG II

		0 SBP/DBP ± SEM	DIP SBP/DBP ± SEM	DIP + ANG II SBP/DBP ± SEM
	Control	81/ 45 ± 3.7/1.9	80/ 41 ± 7.9/3.5	83/ 53 ± 6.2/5.8
	Ramipril	60/ 26 ± 3.2/0.8**	60/ 23 ± 3.2/1.9**	63/ 23 ± 3.7/2.1*
3.3 Hz	Control	249/160 ± 10/3.5	242/156 ± 6.1/2.5	255/161 ± 8.9/3.5
	Ramipril	134/ 86 ± 6.4/6.0***	140/ 96 ± 6.0/15**	131/ 83 ± 6.2/11**

SBP = systolic blood pressure; DBP = diastolic blood pressure; DIP = additionally infused desipramine (100 ng/kg × min); ANG II = additionally infused angiotensin II (10 ng/kg × min). Ramipril was orally administered by gavage (1 mg/kg/d) over 14 days; stimulation parameters: 3.3 Hz, 50 mA, 1 ms, 3 min; significance values: * = $p > 0.05$, ** = $p > 0.01$, *** = $p > 0.001$; Ramipril vs control; n = 6 SHR per each group.

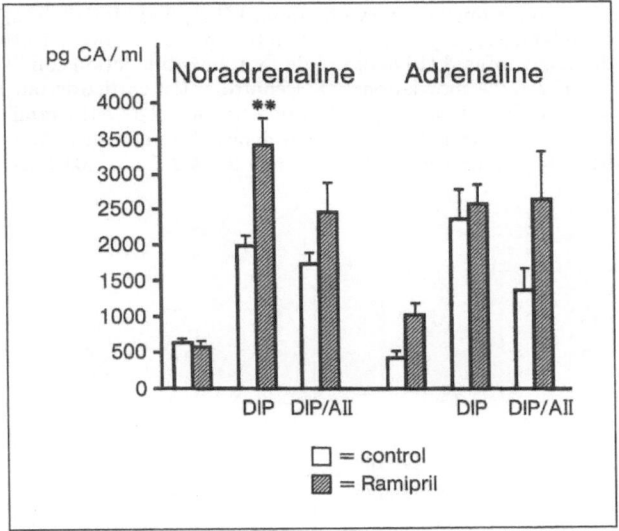

Fig. 2. Effects of chronic inhibition of the converting enzyme with ramipril (1 mg/kg/d for 14 days) on stimulated sympathetic outflow. For abbreviations and stimulation conditions see Fig. 1

B) Circulating catecholamines: Corticosterone infusion significantly increased stimulated noradrenaline and adrenaline concentrations in plasma (Fig. 3). Chronic ramipril treatment led to a further significant noradrenaline overflow, but not to a further increase of adrenaline concentration during corticosterone infusion (Fig. 3).

³H-noradrenaline uptake

As is depicted in Fig. 4, chronic ramipril administration over 14 days diminished slightly yet significantly the uptake of ³H-noradrenaline into the varicosities of the hearts of

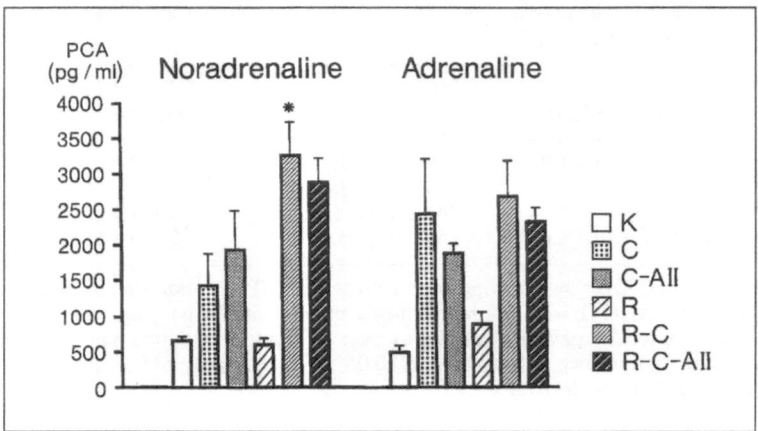

Fig. 3. Effects of chronic inhibition of the converting enzyme with ramipril (1 mg/kg/d for 14 days) on extraneuronal uptake of catecholamines, represented by infusion of corticosterone (33 µg/kg × min i.v.). Ang II was additionally infused (10 ng/kg × min i.v.). For stimulation conditions and significance values see Fig. 1. Abbreviations: K = control; C = corticosterone; C-AII = corticosterone + Ang II; R = ramipril; R-C = ramipril + corticosterone; R-C-AII = ramipril + corticosterone + Ang II. Depicted significance is R-C vs C. Not depicted significances: C vs K = p < 0.05 and R vs RC = p < 0.01 for noradrenaline, C vs K and R vs RC = p < 0.01 for adrenaline

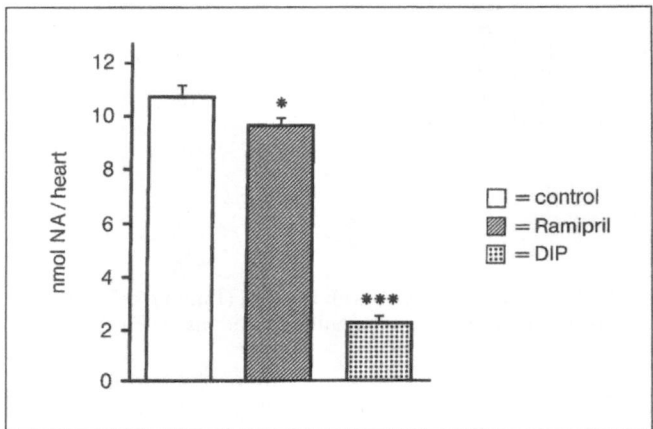

Fig. 4. Uptake of ^{3}H-noradrenaline (nmol NA/heart) into the heart of SHR chronically treated with ramipril (1 mg/kg/d, for 14 days). For positive comparison, desipramine (DIP) (100 ng/kg i.v.) was injected into a third group of SHR prior to the ^{3}H-noradrenaline administration. Significance values: * = p < 0.05; *** = p < 0.001

SHR by about 10%. For positive comparison, the uptake-1 blocking agent desipramine (100 ng/kg) was injected into a third group of SHR prior to the ^{3}H-noradrenaline administration. This resulted in an about 80% inhibition of ^{3}H-NA uptake into the hearts (Fig. 4).

Discussion

In terms of a first analysis, our recent results concerning a nearly unchanged sympathetic outflow during converting enzyme inhibition (2, 3) appear contradictory to the observations of a decrease in sympathetic activity (1, 16). The discrepancies may be due to the different experimental procedures used by the different authors. Whereas we measured the stimulated peripheral sympathetic outflow as a parameter for the peripheral catecholamine release, the other groups directly determined sympathetic nerve activity by measuring the nerve spikes as a parameter for central sympathetic activity. Because some compounds may chemically influence the synapse by inhibiting the reuptake, the noradrenaline release could be diminished, but the circulating amine, however, may be unchanged or enhanced by administering the same drug. In making a statement about the interactions of a substance to the sympathetic varicosity, we prefer an animal model for peripheral catecholamine release as described here.

Our present results demonstrate that converting enzyme inhibition by ramipril lead to significantly enhanced effects of desipramine and corticosterone on stimulation-dependent noradrenaline and adrenaline concentrations in peripheral plasma of spontaneously hypertensive rats. Desipramine binds specifically to the neuronal uptake carrier (9, 11) and inhibits the noradrenaline uptake, whereas corticosterone is able to block the nonspecific uptake of catecholamines, mostly of adrenaline (7).

Since neuronal uptake is the main inactivation pathway for noradrenaline (about 70%), and the affinity of noradrenaline for the uptake carrier is more pronounced when compared to adrenaline (13, 14), the inhibition of the uptake 1 could significantly contribute to an increase in stimulated noradrenaline overflow. In our experiments the additive effect of ramipril to desipramine ranged between 27% and 70% (acute and chronic experiments) with respect to stimulated noradrenaline. However, concerning ^{3}H-noradrenaline, the uptake blocking effect of ramipril was only about 10%. The discrepancy may be explained by an observation of the additive action of ramipril to corticosterone: ramipril further enhanced stimulation-dependent noradrenaline increase during corticosterone infusion, but not that of adrenaline.

However, the experiments could demonstrate a clear-cut difference between the post-synaptic effects of converting enzyme inhibition, namely, a significant decrease in resting and sympathetically stimulated blood pressure and the presynaptic actions described here, indicating that the antihypertensive effects of converting enzyme inhibitors are independent of those due to presynaptic sympathetic interactions.

Since ramipril was significantly less potent in inhibiting the neuronal uptake compared to desipramine, the effect may be interpreted as an unspecific one, due to the comparably high lipophilicity of ramipril (6).

In summary, the additive effects of ramipril on uptake-1 and uptake-2 inhibition cannot fully explain the clear-cut increase of stimulation-dependent noradrenaline increase during desipramine and corticosterone infusions. It is also likely that the metabolism of noradrenaline by monoamineoxidase and/or catechol-0-methyl transferase could be partially blocked by ramipril. Further investigations should consider a certain inhibition of catecholamine metabolism.

References

1. Berecek KH, Kirk KA, Nagahama S, Oparil S (1987) Sympathetic function in spontaneously hypertensive rats after chronic administration of captopril. Am J Physiol 252:H796–H806
2. Dominiak P, Elfrath A, Türck D (1987) Effects of chronic treatment with ramipril, a new ACE blocking agent, on presynaptic sympathetic nervous system of SHR. Clin Exp Hypertens A-Theor 9:369–373
3. Dominiak P, Elfrath A, Türck D (1987) Biosynthesis of catecholamines and sympathetic outflow in spontaneously hypertensive rats (SHR) after chronic treatment with CE-blocking agents. J Cardiovasc Pharmacol 10 (Suppl 7):S122–S124
4. Erikson BM, Persson BA (1982) Determination of catecholamines in rat heart tissue and plasma samples by liquid chromatography with electrochemical detection. J Chromatogr 228:143–154
5. Gillespie JS, Muir TC (1967) A method of stimulating the complete sympathetic outflow from the spinal cord to blood vessels in the pithed rat. Br J Pharmac Chemother 30:78–87
6. Gohlke P, Urbach H, Schölkens B, Unger Th (1989) Inhibition of converting enzyme in the cerebrospinal fluid of rats after oral treatment with converting enzyme inhibitors. J Pharmacol Exp Ther 249:609–616
7. Grohmann M, Trendelenburg U (1988) The handling of five amines by the extraneuronal deaminating system of the rat heart. Naunyn-Schmiedeberg's Arch Pharmacol 337:159–163
8. Majewski H, Hedler L, Schurr C, Starke K (1984) Modulation of noradrenaline release in the pithed rabbit: a role for angiotensin II. J Cardiovasc Pharmacol 6:888–896
9. Maxwell RA, Keenan DP, Chaplin E, Roth B, Eckhardt SB (1969) Molecular features affecting the potency of tricyclic antidepressants and structurally related compounds as inhibitors of the uptake of tritiated norepinephrine by rabbit aortic strips. J Pharmacol Exp Ther 66:320–329
10. Peach MJ (1977) Renin-angiotensin system: biochemistry and mechanism of action. Physiol Rev 57:313–370
11. Schömig E, Michael-Hepp J, Bönisch H (1988) Inhibition of neuronal adrenaline uptake (uptake$_1$) and desipramine binding by N-ethylmaleimide (NEM). Naunyn-Schmiedeberg's Arch Pharmacol 337:633–636
12. Starke K, Taube HD, Borowski E (1977) Presynaptic receptor systems in catecholaminergic transmission. Biochem Pharmacol 26:259–268
13. Trendelenburg U (1980) A kinetic analysis of the extraneuronal uptake and metabolism of catecholamines. Rev Physiol Biochem Pharmacol 87:33 ff
14. Trendelenburg U (1986) The metabolizing systems involved in the inactivation of catecholamines. Naunyn-Schmiedeberg's Arch Pharmacol 332:201–207
15. Wenting GJ, Man in't Veld AJ, Woitliez AJ, Derk FHM, Schalekamp MADH (1984) Captopril in treatment of severe acute and chronic heart failure. Progress in Pharmacology, 5/3: 107–112, Fischer Verlag, Stuttgart
16. Xiang J-Z, Linz W, Becker H, Ganten D, Lang RE, Schölkens B, Unger Th (1985) Effects of converting enzyme inhibitors: ramipril and enalapril on peptide action and sympathetic neurotransmission in the isolated heart. Eur J Pharmacol 113:215–223

Authors' address:

Prof. Dr. P. Dominiak
Institut für Pharmakologie
Medizinische Universität zu Lübeck
Ratzeburger Allee 160
W-2400 Lübeck, FRG

Part IV: Therapeutical Principles from a Pathophysiological Point of View

Compensatory mechanisms for cardiac dysfunction in myocardial infarction *

G. Ertl, P. Gaudron, C. Eilles, W. Schorb, and K. Kochsiek

Medizinische Klinik und Klinik und Poliklinik für Nuklearmedizin,
Universität Würzburg, FRG

Summary: Loss of contractile myocardial tissue by myocardial infarction would result in depressed cardiac output if compensatory mechanisms would not be operative. Frank-Straub-Starling-mechanism and increased heart rate and contractility due to sympathetic stimulation are unlikely to chronically compensate for cardiac dysfunction. Structural left ventricular dilatation may be compensatory, but results in increased wall stress and, ultimately, in progressive dilatation and heart failure. In patients with myocardial infarction, we have shown left-ventricular dilatation in dependence of infarct size and time after infarction. Dilatation is compensatory first and normalizes stroke volume. However, left ventricular dilatation progresses without further hemodynamic profit and, thus, may participate in development of heart failure.

Key words: Myocardial infarction; heart failure; natural history; remodeling; cardiac function

Introduction

Irreversible injury to larger parts of myocardium requires compensation by residual functioning myocytes to maintain cardiac output. Basically, four mechanisms may be considered for cardiac compensation: 1) The Frank-Straub-Starling-mechanism, which has been shown to be operative to maintain stroke volume by residual myocardium after experimental coronary artery occlusion (19). An elevated sympathetic tone induced indirectly by cardiac dysfunction may increase, 2) contractility and 3) heart rate and, thus, stroke volume and cardiac output, respectively (26). 4) For geometric reasons, structural ventricular dilatation may result in increased stroke volume at the same level of circumferential fiber shortening (12).

Hypercontraction of residual myocardium

It is tempting to assume that a loss of contractile myocardium is compensated by hypercontraction of residual myocardium spared from the infarct. Only 13% of all patients, however, showed significant hyperkinesia of residual myocardium during acute myocardial infarction (11). This was a rather unexpected result of the "Thrombolysis and angioplasty in acute myocardial infarction" study, since in animal experiments hyperkinesia of residual myocardium was a consistent finding (19, 37, 38). No relation existed between infarct size and hyperactivity of residual myocardium (18, 31). We have studied

* Work included in this manuscript was supported by the Deutsche Forschungsgemeinschaft (Er 100/3-3, Ko 210/9-2)

global and regional left ventricular function in patients 3–5 days and 3–4 weeks after a first myocardial infarction. By tomographic radionuclide ventriculography ("gated blood pool single-photon-emission computed tomography") standardized scores were obtained for regional function amplitude and phase (5). Positive scores, representative for statistically significantly increased amplitude by comparison with normal control persons, were found neither at 3–5 days nor at 4 weeks post myocardial infarction (5). Thus, hypercontraction is unlikely to be a mechanism for chronic compensation of cardiac dysfunction.

Elevated heart rate

Tachycardia is frequently observed in patients with myocardial infarction in the acute phase (23). Later on, heart rate levels off if overt heart failure does not develop. Thus, elevated heart rate appears not to be a relevant mechanism for chronic compensation of cardiac dysfunction, but rather is an indicator of decompensation.

Structural left-ventricular dilatation

The close relation of cardiac size, symptoms of heart failure, and prognosis has led to the conception that "structural dilatation" is the morphologic and pathophysiologic substrate of cardiac decompensation. One single angiographically determined endsystolic left ventricular volume has been shown to be a powerful indicator of prognosis post myocardial infarction (40). In contrast, a larger ventricle would expell a larger stroke volume than a smaller ventricle at the same circumferential fiber shortening, if only for geometric reasons (12). Figure 1 shows for a spheric model that the larger sphere needs a circumferential fiber shortening of 1.1 cm to expell a stroke volume of 100 cc, while the smaller sphere needs 3.2 cm fiber shortening. Thus, while clinical observations suggest a detrimental role of ventricular dilatation in cardiac dysfunction, theoretical considerations suggest a potential compensatory effect of an increased cardiac size.

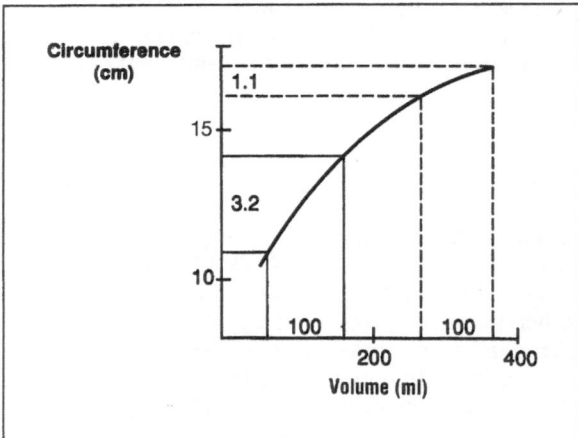

Fig. 1. Geometric dependence of stroke volume on cavity size and circumferential fiber shortening in a spheric model. The larger sphere needs less fiber shortening to expell the same stroke volume

The phenomenon of left-ventricular dilatation post myocardial infarction

Based on observations of Linzbach, Hort reported in 1965 on left-ventricular dilatation post experimental myocardial infarction (14). The purpose of his study was to diagnose myocardial infarction by left-ventricular dilatation. Thus, he expected and found a close relation between the incidence of myocardial infarction and left-ventricular enlargement. By reperfusion studies in rats, Hort demonstrated the dependence of left-ventricular volume on duration of coronary occlusion and, thus, myocardial infarct size. Later on, Pfeffer and coworkers followed this animal model under different suppositions. Pfeffer's group showed that left-ventricular volume depended on infarct size and time interval after coronary ligation. They suggested that left-ventricular dilatation was progressive over time (29).

Expansion of the healing infarct has been known for a long time to have an adverse influence on prognosis (4). Dilatation of noninfarcted residual myocardium was consistently found in patients with infarct expansion by echocardiographic studies (21). Only on the basis of expansion of residual myocardium may left-ventricular dilatation result in increased stroke volume (12).

Hypertrophy of residual myocardium

Noteworthy, global left-ventricular weight did not decrease post myocardial infarction, despite considerable weight loss by scarring (29). This could only be explained by an increase in weight of residual myocardium. A number of experimental studies showed hypertrophy of residual myocardium (1, 2, 32, 33). Ginzton and coworkers (10) recently documented in echocardiographic studies in 32 of 45 patients an increase in left-ventricular mass index with a positive correlation to ejection fraction. Morphologic investigations proved growth of thickness and length of residual myocytes ("concentric and eccentric hypertrophy") post myocardial infarction in rats (2).

Wall stress in residual myocardium

Thus, myocardial infarct expansion may occur and be accompanied by expansion and hypertrophy of residual myocardium. The mechanism of dilatation and hypertrophy of residual myocardium is not known in detail. According to Laplace's law, however, dilatation will result in an increase in, and hypertrophy in a decrease in wall stress (Fig. 2). Olivetti and coworkers (25), based on hemodynamic and morphometric studies in rats, calculated an increased diastolic wall stress in residual myocardium to 7.2-fold of normal, as early as 2 days after extensive infarction. We have observed an increase in length of residual myocardium after coronary occlusion in dogs for 1 h which persisted after reperfusion (34). Hypertrophy is unlikely at this time and an elevated wall stress must be assumed. This is particularly the case for diastole, since in the acute phase of large infarcts end-diastolic pressure is elevated (34).

It is conceivable, therefore, that early dilatation of non-infarcted myocardium, due to increased diastolic pressure progresses to structural dilatation accompanied by normalization of diastolic pressure. Increased wall stress due to increased volume, if not normalized by adequate hypertrophy, could represent a stimulus for further and thus progressive dilatation.

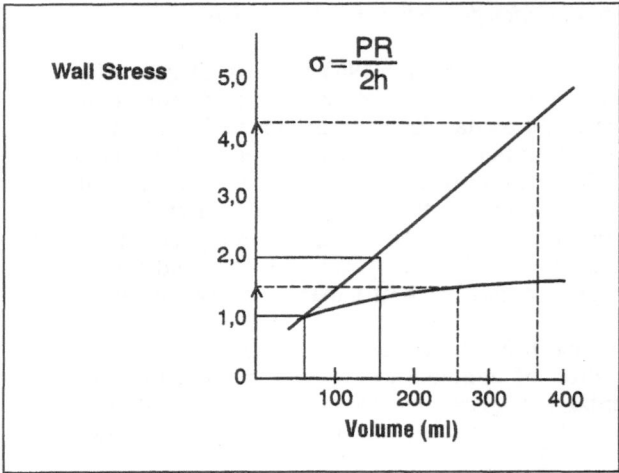

Fig. 2. Relationship between cavity size and wall stress. The larger cavity size results in increased wall stress, especially in diastole, in patients with acute infarctions when pressure is increased. Reduced pressure (P) or increased wall thickness (h) would reduce wall stress

Relation of left-ventricular size and stroke volume in patients with myocardial infarction

We prospectively investigated, in 29 non-selected patients with a first myocardial infarction, development of left-ventricular volume and its hemodynamic consequences (7). Left-ventricular volume was measured by gated single-photon-emission computed tomography (tomographic radionuclide ventriculography). This technique has proven reliable as an investigator-independent, non-invasive method to determine left-ventricular volumes, as validated by comparison with angiocardiography (7, 8). Left-ventricular ejection fraction was measured by conventional planar radionuclide ventriculography, cardiac output and pressures by Swan-Ganz catheter. We considered it essential to measure left-ventricular volumes, stroke volume, and ejection fraction by independent methods since the major goal of the study was to determine potential biologic interdependences among these variables. All studies were performed 4 days and 4 weeks after myocardial infarction. Sequential measurements of creatinphosphokinase were used to estimate myocardial infarct size, and patients were prospectively assigned to a "small", "moderate" or "large" infarct size group. Patients with large infarcts had a lower ejection fraction than patients with small infarcts during the period of observation. Left-ventricular volume was similar in both groups 4 days post infarct, however, it increased in patients with large infarcts, but decreased in patients with small infarcts. Thus, left-ventricular end-diastolic and end-systolic volumes were significantly larger at 4 weeks in patients with "large" infarcts than in patients with "small" infarcts. Left-ventricular stroke volume was depressed 4 days after large infarcts, but increased during 4 weeks. Thus, increase in left-ventricular volume in patients with large infarcts was accompanied by an increase in stroke volume. Not yet published results suggest that during further observation, left ventricles increased without improval of stroke volume (7a). The primarily compensatory left-ventricular dilatation progresses to an unfavorable dilatation without hemodynamic benefit, but carries the burden of increased wall stress and energy demand. Since "wedge pressure" (representative of left-ventricular filling pressure) did not change, left-ventricular dilatation was likely to be structural and not based on a pressure/volume relation (7). Other groups have studied the time-course of left-ventricular dilatation and reported a small increase in left-ventricular volume as early as 11 days, with further dilatation after 6 months or 10.5 months, respectively (15, 39). In accordance with our experimental results (34), others observed left-ventricular dilation hours after acute infarction (35) and considered it a compensatory mechanism which may maintain stroke volume in presence of depressed left-ventricular function.

Gadsboll and coworkers (6) have shown a relation of incidence of symptoms of heart failure and left-ventricular dilatation 1 year after myocardial infarction. Further studies over a longer period of time will have to show whether left-ventricular dilatation will be a major cause of heart failure and mortality in these patients independent of other risk factors and of progression of coronary heart disease.

Therapeutic interventions

Trials have been started to look for therapeutic interventions to support compensatory mechanisms post myocardial infarction and to avoid heart failure. The strong relation of left-ventricular dilatation to myocardial infarct size suggests that measures to reduce infarct size might prevent dilatation. In fact, analysis of data of the GISSI (Gruppo Italiano per lo Studio dello Streptochinasi nell' Infarte Miocardico) trial showed smaller left-ventricular volumes in patients who underwent thrombolytic therapy than in the control group both, at hospital discharge and 6 months later (20). Smaller studies revealed controversial results (17, 39). Infarct expansion is limited by reperfusion established too late to reduce infarct size (13).

Besides reducing infarct size, reperfusion might change stiffness of reperfused myocardium and, thus, load on residual myocardium (3, 24). Early functional aneurysm is related to an adverse prognosis (22). Very early reperfusion, however, results in a decrease in myocardial stiffness by maintaining cellular integrity and function of myocardium (16). Finally, myocardial stiffness when increased too much may disturb diastolic function to an extent that balances improvement of systolic function (3).

Pfeffer and coworkers have recently shown in an experimental model in rats that an ACE-inhibitor may delay left-ventricular dilatation and reduce mortality in the animals (28, 30). Gaudron and associates (9) reported that rats on high-sodium diet had larger left-ventricular volumes than animals on low sodium. Pfeffer and coworkers (27) and Sharpe and coworkers (36) showed left-ventricular dilatation in patients with anterior infarctions and depressed left-ventricular function. An ACE-inhibitor (captopril) could delay this process. Further studies are under way using ACE-inhibitors to test the possibility of their retarding left-ventricular dilatation, preventing heart failure, and reducing mortality in patients post myocardial infarction.

Acknowledgements. We thank Carmen Zeller and Ingrid Wendl for technical assistance, and Elisabeth Fischer for typing the manuscript.

References

1. Anversa P, Beghi C, McDonald SL, Levicky V, Kikkawa Y, Olivetti G (1984) Morphometry of right ventricular hypertrophy induced by myocardial infarction in the rat. Am J Pathol 116:504–513

2. Anversa P, Beghi C, Kikkawa Y, Olivetti G (1986) Myocardial infarction in rats: infarct size, myocyte hypertrophy, and capillary growth. Circ Res 58:26–37
3. Bogen DK, Rabinowitz SA, Needleman A, McMahon TA, Abelmann WH (1980) An analysis of the mechanical disadvantage of myocardial infarction in the canine left ventricle. Circ Res 47:728–741
4. Eaton LW, Weiss JL, Bulkley BH, Garrison JB, Weisfeldt MD (1979) Regional cardiac dilatation after acute myocardial infarction. N Engl J Med 300:57–62
5. Eilles Chr, Gaudron P, Ertl G (1990) Regional left ventricular function during remodeling post myocardial infarction. Eur Heart J 11(Abstract Suppl):365
6. Gadsboll N, Hoilund-Carlsen P-F, Badsberg JH, Stage P, Marving J, Lonborg-Jensen H (1989) Late ventricular dilatation in survivors of acute myocardial infarction. Am J Cardiol 64:961–966
7. Gaudron P, Eilles C, Ertl G, Kochsiek K (1990) Early remodeling of the left ventricle in patients with myocardial infarction. Eur Heart J 11:139–146
7a. Gaudron P, Eilles C, Ertl G, Kochsiek K (1991) Compensatory and non-compensatory left ventricular dilatation after myocardial infarction: time course, hemodynamic consequences at rest and exercise. Am Heart J (in press)
8. Gaudron P, Eilles Ch, Reiser E, Ertl G, Kochsiek K (1990) Subacute adaption of left ventricular size and hemodynamics to loss of contractile mass in patients with myocardial infarction-remodeling. In: Jacob R, Seipel L, Zucker HJ (eds) Cardiac Dilatation: Pathogenesis, Morphology, Hemodynamic and Energetic Consequences. Fischer, Stuttgart New York, pp 109–122
9. Gaudron P, Pfeffer JM, Pfeffer MA (1986) Chronic modifications of dietary sodium after ventricular dilatation in rats with myocardial infarction (abstract). J Am Coll Cardiol 7:206
10. Ginzton LE, Conant R, Rodrigues DM, Laks MM (1989) Functional significance of hypertrophy of the noninfarcted myocardium after myocardial infarction in humans. Circulation 80:816–822
11. Grines CL, Topol EJ, Califf RM, Stack RS, George BS, Kereiakes D, Boswick JM, Kline E, O'Neill WW, TAMI Study Group (1989) Prognostic implications and predictors of enhanced regional wall motion of the noninfarct zone after thrombolysis and angioplasty therapy of acute myocardial infarction. Circulation 80:245–253
12. Gülch RW, Jacob R (1988) Geometric and muscle physiological determinants of stroke volume as evaluated on the basis of model calculations. Basic Res Cardiol 83:476–485
13. Hochman JS, Choo H (1987) Limitation of myocardial infarct expansion by reperfusion independent of myocardial salvage. Circulation 75:299–306
14. Hort W (1965) Ventrikeldilatation und Muskelfaserdehnung als früheste morphologische Befunde beim Herzinfarkt. Virchows Arch path Anat 339:72–82
15. Jeremy RW, Allman KC, Bantovitch G, Harris PhJ (1989) Patterns of left ventricular dilatation during the six months after myocardial infarction. J Am Coll Cardiol 13:304–310
16. Kurnik PB, Courtois MR, Ludbrook PA (1988) Diastolic stiffening induced by acute myocardial infarction is reduced by early reperfusion. J Am Coll Cardiol 12:1029–1036
17. Lavie CJ, O'Keefe JH, Chesebro JH, Clements JP, Gibbons RJ (1990) Prevention of late ventricular dilatation after acute myocardial infarction by successful thrombolytic reperfusion. Am J Cardiol 66:31–36
18. Lefkowitz CA, Gallagher KP, Pace DP, Wright LA, Krause LD, Buda AJ (1987) Compensatory augmentation of normal regional function following coronary occlusion: relation to myocardial area at risk and extent of ischemic dysfunction. J Am Coll Cardiol 9:92A
19. Lew WYW, Chen Z, Guth B, Covell JW (1985) Mechanism of augmented segment shortening in nonischemic areas during acute ischemia of the canine left ventricle. Circ Res 56:351–358
20. Marino P, Zanolla L, Zardini P (1989) Effect of streptokinase on left ventricular modeling and function after myocardial infarction: the GISSI (Gruppo Italiano per lo Studio della Streptochinasi nell' Infarto Miocardico) trial. J Am Coll Cardiol 14:1149–1158
21. McKay RG, Pfeffer MA, Pasternak RC, Markis JE, Come PC, Nakao S, Alderman JD, Ferguson JJ, Safian RD, Grossman W (1986) Left ventricular remodeling following myocardial infarction: a corollary to infarct expansion. Circulation 74:693–702

22. Meizlisk JL, Berger HJ, Michael P, Errigo D, Levy W, Zaret BL (1984) Functional left ventricular aneurysm formation after acute anterior transmural myocardial infarction. Incidence, natural history, and prognostic implications. N Engl J Med 311:1001–1006
23. Meltzer LE, Kitchell JB (1966) The incidence of arrhythmias associated with acute myocardial infarction. Progr Cardiovasc Dis 9:50
24. Mirski I (1979) Elastic properties of the myocardium: a quantitative approach with physiological and clinical applications. In: Berne R, Sperelakis N (eds) Handbook of physiology, section 2. The cardiovascular system, vol 1. Williams & Wilkins, Baltimore, pp 497–531
25. Olivetti G, Capasso JM, Sonnenblick EH, Anversa P (1990) Side-to-side slippage of myocytes participates in ventricular wall remodeling acutely after myocardial infarction in rats. Circ Res 67:23–34
26. Peterson DF, Kasper RL, Bishop VS (1974) Reflex tachycardia due to temporary coronary occlusion in the conscious dog. Circ Res 34:226–232
27. Pfeffer MA, Lamas GA, Vaughan DE, Parisi AF, Braunwald E (1988) Effect of captopril on progressive left ventricular dilatation after anterior myocardial infarction. N Engl J Med 19:80–86
28. Pfeffer JM, Pfeffer MA, Braunwald E (1985) Influence of chronic captopril therapy on the infarcted left ventricle of the rat. Circ Res 57:84–95
29. Pfeffer MA, Pfeffer JM, Fishbein MC, Fletcher PJ, Spadaro J, Kloner RA, Braunwald E (1979) Myocardial infarct size and ventricular function in rats. Circ Res 44:503–512
30. Pfeffer MA, Pfeffer JM, Steinberg C, Finn P (1985) Survival after an experimental myocardial infarction: beneficial effects of long-term therapy with captopril. Circulation 72:406–412
31. Rigaud M, Rocha P, Boskat J, Farcot JC, Bardet J, Bourdarias JP (1979) Regional left ventricular function assessed by contrast angiography in acute myocardial infarction. Circulation 60:130–139
32. Rubin SA, Fishbein MC, Swan HJC (1983) Compensatory hypertrophy in the heart after myocardial infarction in the rat. J Am Coll Cardiol 1:1435–1441
33. Sasayamas S, Gallagher KP, Kemper WS, Franklin D, Ross J (1981) Regional left ventricular wall thickness early and late after coronary occlusion in the conscious dog. Am J Physiol 240:H293–299
34. Schorb W, Bauer B, Ertl G (1990) Early dilatation of non-ischaemic myocardium after coronary occlusion and reperfusion (abstract). Eur Heart J 11(Suppl):33
35. Seals A, Pratt CM, Makmarian JJ, Tadros S, Kleiman N, Roberts R, Verani MS (1988) Relation of left ventricular dilatation during acute myocardial infarction to systolic performance, diastolic dysfunction, infarct size and location. Am J Cardiol 61:224–229
36. Sharpe N, Murphy J, Smith M, Hannan S (1988) Treatment of patients with symptomless left ventricular dysfunction after myocardial infarction. Lancet I:255–259
37. Theroux P, Franklin D, Ross J, Kemper WS (1974) Regional myocardial function during acute coronary occlusion and its modification by pharmacologic agents in the dog. Circ Res 34:896–908
38. Theroux P, Ross J, Franklin D, Kemper WS, Sasayama S (1976) Regional myocardial function in the conscious dog during acute coronary occlusion and responses to morphine, propranolol, nitroglycerine and lidocaine. Circulation 53:302–314
39. Warren SE, Royal HD, Markis JE, Grossman W, McKay RG (1988) Time course of left ventricular dilation after myocardial infarction: influence of infarct-related artery and success of coronary thrombolysis. J Am Coll Cardiol 11:12–19
40. White MD, Norris RM, Brown MA, Brandt PW, Whitlock RML, Wild ChrJ (1987) Left ventricular end-systolic volume as the major determinant of survival after recovery from myocardial infarction. Circulation 76:44–51

Authors' address:

Priv.-Doz. Dr. G. Ertl
Med. Klinik der Universität
Josef-Schneider-Straße 2
W-8700 Würzburg, FRG

The effect of decreased left-ventricular afterload on cardiac performance in the normal and hypertrophied rat heart

G. Kissling and M. Brändle

Physiologisches Institut II der Universität Tübingen, FRG

Summary: The effect of left-ventricular afterload on cardiac performance was investigated in normotensive Wistar rats and in spontaneously hypertensive rats (10 months old) with a left-ventricular hypertrophy of 54%. The measurements were performed on a modified heart-lung preparation in which left-ventricular afterload could be adjusted arbitrarily. In the heart in situ, left-ventricular afterload limits not only the mechanical conditions of the contraction, but also influences coronary perfusion pressure. With decreasing afterload stroke volume and pressure-volume work initially increases. Simultaneously coronary resistance decreases considerably so that coronary flow increases, although coronary perfusion pressure is reduced. However, when perfusion pressure falls short of a critical value, coronary flow cannot be maintained despite maximal coronary dilatation and stroke volume decreases, i.e., stroke volume, pressure-volume work and coronary flow run through an optimum with decreasing afterload. A reduction in coronary perfusion pressure below a certain value yields acute heart failure in all preparations. The minimal aortic mean pressure without reaching cardiac insufficiency was in the spontaneously hypertensive rats with 65 mm Hg significantly higher than in the control animals with 35 mm Hg, although the minimal coronary resistance was identical in both groups. The elevated critical coronary perfusion pressure of the spontaneously hypertensive rats can be explained by the increased O_2-demand of the hypertrophied hearts.

Key words: Left-ventricular afterload; coronary perfusion pressure; coronary flow; coronary resistance; efficiency of the heart

Introduction

From a muscle-physiological point of view, a reduction in left-ventricular afterload seems to be favorable for the treatment of cardiac insufficiency. However, in the heart in situ left-ventricular afterload limits not only the external mechanical conditions of the heartbeat, but also influences coronary perfusion pressure and hence coronary flow. Both processes interact: with increasing afterload, stroke volume decreases due to the external mechanical condition; simultaneously, myocardial contractility is increased due to the enhanced coronary perfusion pressure (1, 2), which in turn tends to increase the stroke volume. On the other hand, due to muscle-physiological laws, a decrease in left-ventricular afterload should result in an enhanced stroke volume. However, the simultaneous diminution in coronary perfusion pressure induces a decrease in contractility, which in turn causes a decrease in stroke volume.

On the strength of these considerations, it can be expected that stroke volume runs through an optimum with decreasing left-ventricular afterload. The extent to which the relations between left-ventricular afterload and stroke volume are modified by cardiac hypertrophy is unknown. Therefore, in the present investigations, we have examined the influence of left-ventricular afterload on cardiac performance in the normal and hyper-trophied rat heart in detail.

Methods

The investigations were performed on a modified heart-lung preparation of the rat which allows a primary adjustment of left-ventricular afterload. Measurements were performed on seven normotensive Wistar rats (body weight 381 ± 23 g; left-ventricular weight

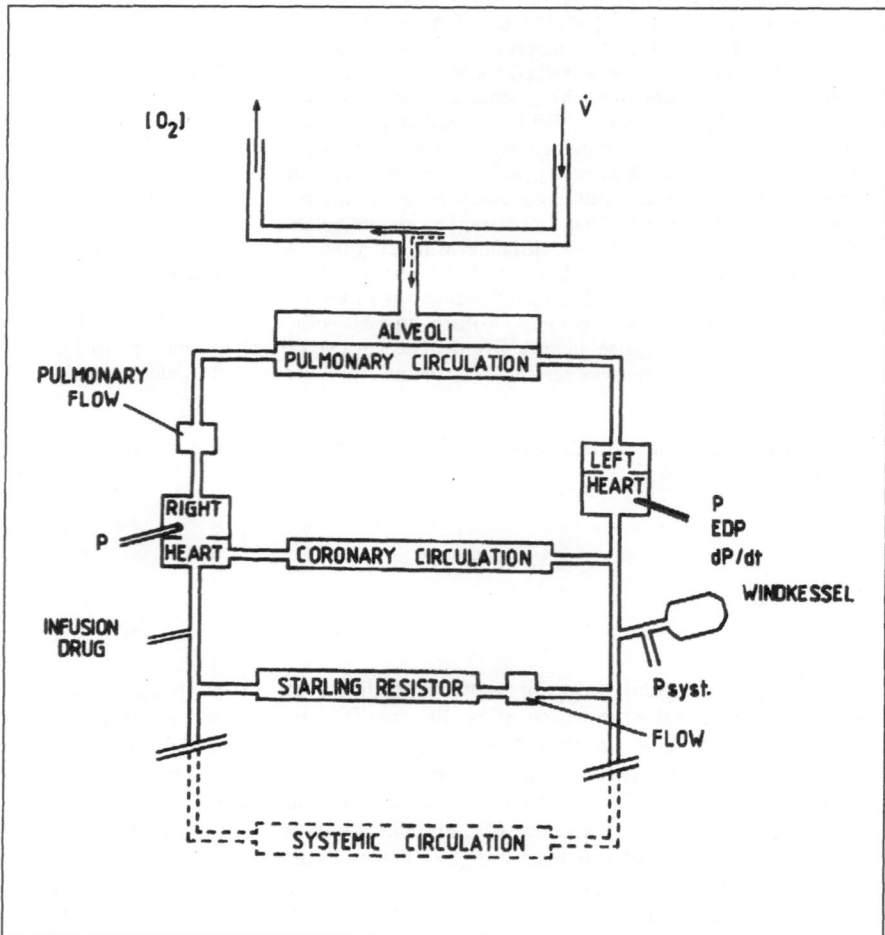

Fig. 1. Schematic presentation of the modified heart-lung preparation. The entire systemic circula-tion is reduced to the coronary circulation and to a shunt circuit between the aortic root and the vena cava inferior, whereas pulmonary circulation remains intact. Left-ventricular afterload can be adjusted arbitrarily via a Starling resistor in the shunt circuit. For further explanation see text

840 ± 59 mg) and on seven spontaneously hypertensive rats (Aoki-Okamoto strain, body weight 395 ± 20 g; left ventricular weight 1291 ± 77 mg) at 10 months of age with a left-ventricular hypertrophy of 54%.

Figure 1 shows a scheme of the experimental set up. After opening the chest under urethane anesthesia (1.2 g/kg b.w.) and after removing the pericardium an electromagnetic flow probe was placed around the pulmonary artery trunk. Subsequently, the aortic root as well as both caval veins were ligated, and the aortic root was connected to the vena cava inferior via a shunt circuit with a Starling resistor. In order to smooth aortic blood pressure amplitude the aortic root was additionally connected to a "Windkessel". Left-ventricular afterload could be adjusted arbitrarily via the Starling resistor in the shunt circuit. Pulmonary flow and the flow in the shunt circuit, as well as left- and right-ventricular pressures and the pressure in the aortic root were measured. Since under steady state conditions the left and the right ventricle eject the same volume, the left-ventricular stroke volume could be measured by means of the pulmonary flow. Coronary flow was calculated from the difference between pulmonary flow and the flow in the shunt circuit. Total peripheral resistance, coronary resistance, and the resistance in the shunt circuit were calculated from the mean aortic pressure and the respective flow.

The O_2-consumption of the preparation was determined by means of the difference in O_2-concentration between the inspired and expired air and the respiration volume per minute. The efficiency of the heart was calculated from the pressure-volume work and the O_2-consumption.

At the end of each experiment the diastolic pressure-volume relationships of the left ventricle were measured in the beating heart (3, 4). The enddiastolic pressure-volume relationship was used to determine the respective enddiastolic ventricular volume from the measured enddiastolic pressure of each beat. Left-ventricular wall stress was calculated assuming a thick-wall sphere (5); using the formula

$$\sigma = \frac{p}{[(v+w)/v]^{2/3} - 1},$$

where: p = ventricular pressure; v = internal ventricular volume; w = wall volume, and whereby myocardial specific weight is considered to be 1 g/cm^3.

Results and discussion

In our experiments the maximum rate of stress development ($d\sigma/dt_{max}$) depends on the mean aortic pressure (Fig. 2), although it is obtained in the isovolumic pre-ejection period and, therefore, should not be influenced by the afterload. Since $d\sigma/dt_{max}$ may be considered as a measure of myocardial contractility, the linear and continuous increase in $d\sigma/dt_{max}$ with increasing mean aortic pressure reflects simply the dependence of myocardial contractility on coronary perfusion pressure (1, 2). In the spontaneously hypertensive rats $d\sigma/dt_{max}$ is significantly reduced and depends less on aortic pressure (Fig. 2).

On the other hand, at a given aortic pressure the hypertrophied hearts eject a significantly greater stroke volume than the control hearts (Fig. 3). With decreasing aortic pressure, stroke volume increases at first in both groups, runs through an optimum and decreases again at a low aortic pressure. However, the optimum of the hypertrophied hearts lies at a higher aortic pressure than that of the control hearts. A reduction in aortic pressure below a certain value yields acute heart failure in all preparations. The minimal

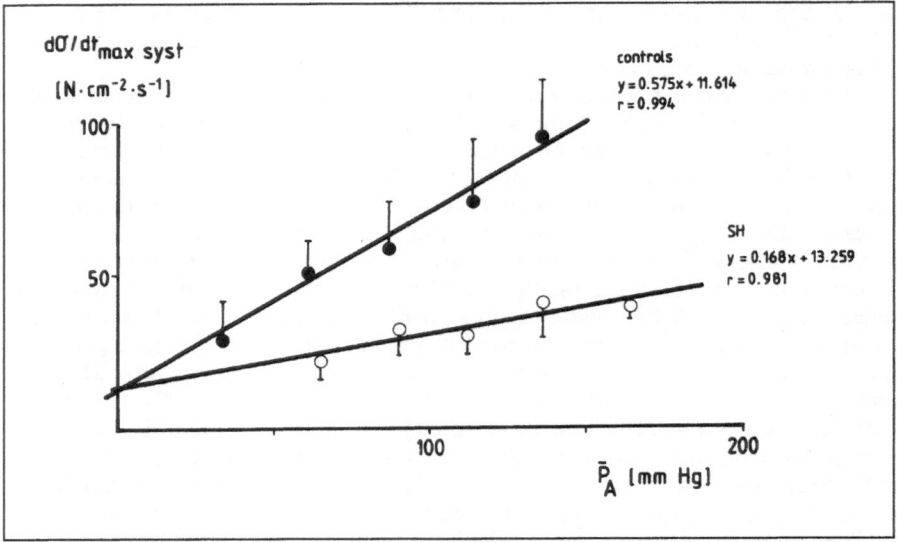

Fig. 2. Relations between maximum rate of stress development ($d\sigma/dt_{\text{max syst}}$) and mean aortic pressure ($\bar{P}_A$) in control animals (●) and in spontaneously hypertensive rats (○). Mean values and standard deviation are shown

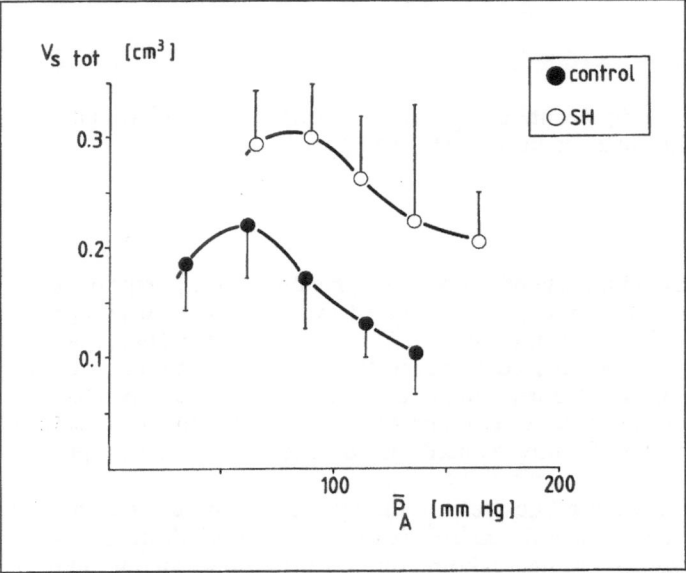

Fig. 3. Dependence of left ventricular stroke volume ($V_{s\ tot}$) on mean aortic pressure ($\bar{P}_A$) in control animals (●) and in spontaneously hypertensive rats (○). Mean values and standard deviation are shown

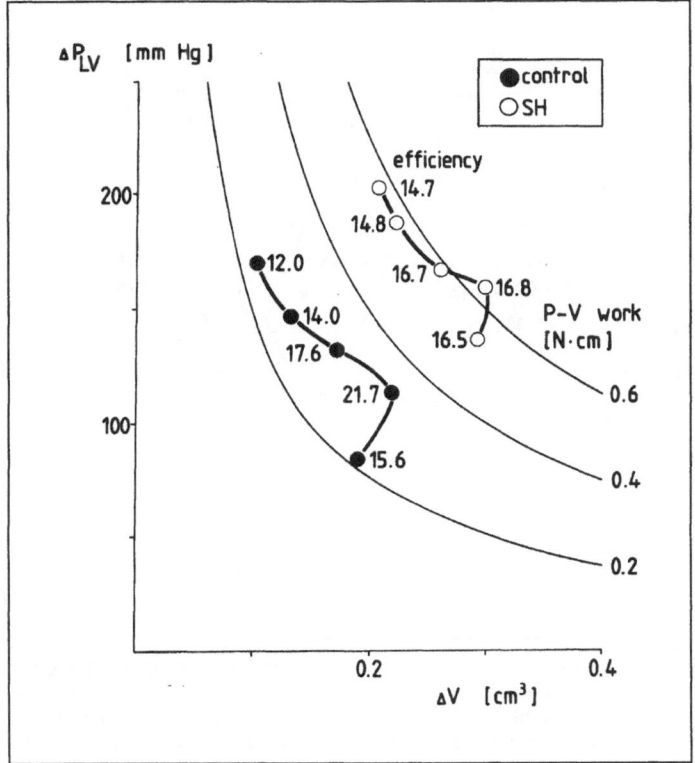

Fig. 4. The summarizing graph shows the influence of left-ventricular afterload on left-ventricular pressure, stroke volume and pressure-volume work. The ordinate represents left-ventricular pressure, averaged over the change in ventricular volume during the ejection period, the abscissa represents stroke volume. The respective hyperbolic lines connect values with identical pressure-volume work. The numbers indicate the efficiency calculated from pressure-volume work and O_2-consumption. Mean values are of control animals (●) and of spontaneously hypertensive rats (○)

aortic mean pressure, without reaching cardiac insufficiency, was in the hypertensive rats with 65 mm Hg significantly higher than in the control animals with 35 mm Hg.

The changes in left-ventricular pressure, stroke volume, and pressure-volume work, which were observed during alteration of left-ventricular afterload, are summarized in Fig. 4. The ordinate represents left-ventricular pressure averaged over the change in ventricular volume during the ejection period, and the abscissa represents stroke volume. The respective hyperbolic lines connect values with identical pressure-volume work. The hypertrophied hearts produce a significantly greater pressure-volume work than the controls. Although the developed pressure is significantly enhanced in the hypertrophied hearts, left-ventricular wall stress is not increased. In both groups left-ventricular pressure-volume work increases at first with decreasing afterload, runs through an optimum, and decreases at a low afterload. The optimum in pressure-volume work lies, for the hypertrophied hearts, at a significantly higher pressure value than for the controls. The numbers in Fig. 4 indicate the calculated mean-values of efficiency. The most

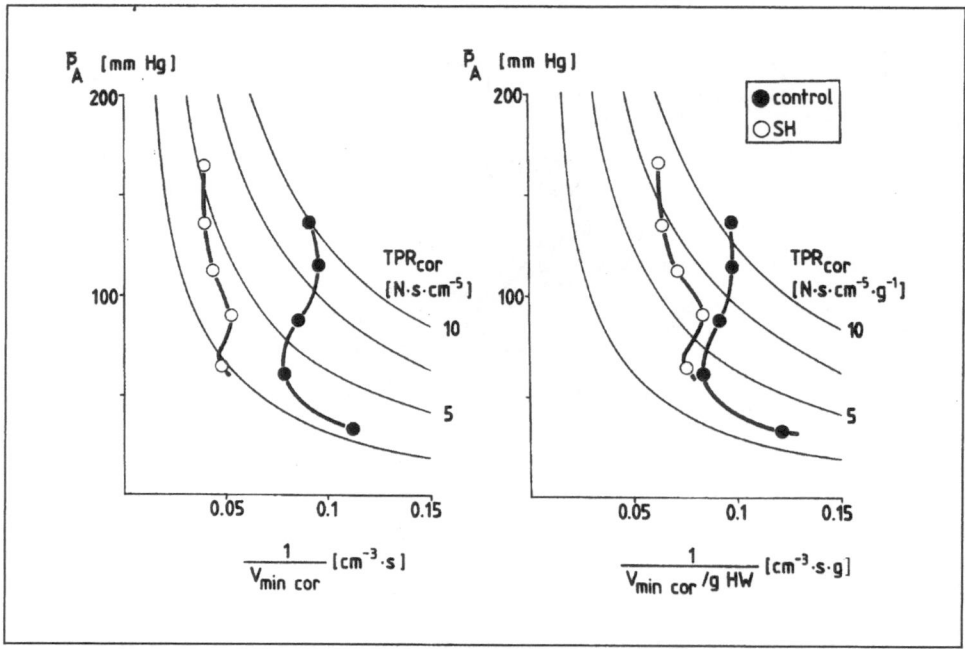

Fig. 5. Influence of left-ventricular afterload on coronary perfusion pressure, coronary flow, and coronary resistance. Lefthand side: absolute values of coronary flow; righthand side: flow values related to heart weight. The ordinate represents mean aortic pressure, the abscissa represents the reciprocal value of coronary flow. The respective hyperbolic lines connect values with identical resistance. Mean values of control animals (●) and of spontaneously hypertensive rats (○)

favorable efficiency is found to be at the optimum of the pressure-volume work in each case.

The relations between coronary perfusion pressure, coronary flow, and coronary resistance are shown in Fig. 5. The ordinate represents mean aortic pressure, the abscissa represents the reciprocal value of coronary flow. The product of perfusion pressure and reciprocal flow yields the Ohmic resistance. The respective hyperbolic lines connect values with identical resistance. On the left part of Fig. 5 the curves are based on absolute values of coronary flow, on the right part on values related to heart weight. Note that the reciprocal value of flow is shown, i.e., a shift to the left represents an increase in flow, and a shift to the right represents a decrease. As can be seen on the lefthand side of Fig. 5, in control animals coronary flow runs through an optimum with decreasing mean aortic pressure. Simultaneously, coronary resistance is reduced markedly. At a mean aortic pressure of about 60 mm Hg the coronary arteries are maximally dilated, so that a further decrease in aortic pressure cannot initiate a change worth mentioning in coronary resistance, whereas coronary flow shows a considerable reduction. At a high perfusion pressure the absolute values of coronary flow are significantly increased in the hypertrophied hearts and the absolute values of coronary resistance are significantly reduced. At a perfusion pressure of about 65 mm Hg the coronary arteries of the hypertrophied hearts are also maximally dilated and the absolute value of coronary resistance is even somewhat smaller than in the controls. A further reduction in perfusion pressure necessarily leads to a marked decrease in coronary flow. However, O_2-demand of the hypertrophied hearts is greater than in controls due to the increased muscle mass and due to the enhanced pressure-volume work, so that a further reduction in coronary flow cannot be tolerated. Therefore, the hypertrophied hearts reach acute heart failure when the mean aortic pressure is decreased below 65 mm Hg.

The right part of Fig. 5 shows the correlation between mean aortic pressure and coronary flow related to heart weight. Even when muscle mass is taken into consideration the coronary flow is found to be increased in the hypertrophied hearts and the minimal coronary resistance is identical in spontaneously hypertensive rats and in controls.

Conclusions

In contrast to the isolated muscle, in the heart in situ, left-ventricular afterload influences not only the external mechanical conditions of the contraction, but also coronary perfusion pressure and, hence, the O_2-supply of the heart. With increasing left-ventricular afterload the external mechanical conditions predominate and stroke volume decreases despite an optimal O_2-supply. With decreasing afterload, stroke volume increases due to the external mechanical conditions. At first, coronary flow and O_2-supply are maintained since coronary resistance decreases simultaneously. However, when the perfusion pressure falls short of a critical value, coronary flow cannot be maintained, despite maximal vasodilatation, and stroke volume decreases. The result of both interacting processes is that stroke volume runs through an optimum with decreasing afterload. In our experiments the minimal coronary resistance was identical in spontaneously hypertensive rats and in controls. Nevertheless, the critical minimal aortic pressure lies in the hypertrophied hearts at a higher value, since the O_2-demand of the hypertrophied hearts is greater. It can be expected that in hypertrophied hearts which additionally have restricted coronary reserve the critical coronary perfusion pressure is enhanced so that even a moderate reduction in left-ventricular afterload which involves necessarily a simultaneous reduction in coronary perfusion pressure must almost certainly impair cardiac performance.

References

1. Arnold G, Kosche F, Neitzert A, Lochner W (1968) The importance of the perfusion pressure in the coronary arteries for the contractility and the oxygen consumption of the heart. Pflügers Arch Ges Physiol 299:339–356
2. Cross CE, Rieben PA, Salisbury PF (1961) Influence of coronary perfusion and myocardial edema on pressure-volume diagram of left ventricle. Amer J Physiol 201:102–108
3. Kissling G, Gassenmaier T, Wendt-Gallitelli MF, Jacob R (1977) Pressure-volume relations, elastic modulus, and contractile behaviour of the hypertrophied left ventricle of rats with Goldblatt II hypertension. Pflügers Arch Ges Physiol 369:213–221
4. Kissling G, Takeda N, Vogt M (1985) Left ventricular end-systolic pressure-volume relationships as a measure of ventricular performance. Basic Res Cardiol 80:594–607
5. Sandler H, Dodge HT (1963) Left ventricular tension and stress in man. Circ Res 13:91–104

Authors' address:

Prof. Dr. G. Kissling
Physiologisches Institut II
Gmelinstraße 5
W-7400 Tübingen, FRG

Function and structure
of the failing left ventricular myocardium
in aortic valve disease before and after valve replacement *

H. P. Krayenbuehl, O. M. Hess, E. S. Monrad, J. Schneider [1], G. Mall [2], and M. Turina [3]

Division of Cardiology, Medical Policlinic, Institute of Pathology [1]
and Clinic of Cardiovascular Surgery [3], University Hospital Zurich, Switzerland,
and Institute of Pathology, University of Heidelberg [2], FRG

Summary: Left ventricular (LV) cineangiography and endomyocardial biopsies were performed preoperatively in 49 patients (pts) with aortic stenosis (AS) and 35 pts with aortic insufficiency (AI). LV failure (group 1) was present in 15 pts with AS and 17 pts with AI. In these pts ejection fraction (EF) was < 57% and either cardiac index was < 2.5 L/min/m² and/or LV end-diastolic pressure was > 20 mm Hg. Macroscopic LV hypertrophy was assessed by angiographic muscle mass (LMMI, g/m²). Morphometric evaluation of LV biopsies included the determination of muscle fiber diameter (MFD, μ), percent interstitial fibrosis (IF, %), volume fraction of myofibrils (VFM, %) and the calculation of LV fibrous content (FC, g/m²). Pts of group 1 and 2 were restudied 22.5 and 24.0 months, respectively, after successful aortic valve replacement. Preoperatively, group 1 pts had a significantly higher LMMI, MFD, and FC than did the patients in group 2 (non-failing group consisting of 34 pts with AS and 18 with AI). IF and VFM did not differ. After surgery EF increased significantly from 44% to 59% in group 1, whereas it remained unchanged in group 2 (66%). Although in both groups LMMI and MFD decreased significantly these quantities were increased after surgery in group 1 as compared to group 2. IF, VFM, and FC did not change significantly in group 1 after valve replacement. There was no difference in these latter three quantities between groups 1 and 2 after surgery. It is concluded that 1) macroscopic and microscopic hypertrophy is more marked in the failing than in the non-failing left ventricle, 2) left ventricular pump function is not related to percent interstitial fibrosis, and 3) at an intermediate time after aortic valve replacement pts with previously failing left ventricle show considerable improvement of ejection performance, but residual hypertrophy persists.

Key words: Aortic valve disease; heart failure; left ventricular hypertrophy; interstitial fibrosis; aortic valve replacement

Introduction

Chronic pressure and/or volume overload in aortic valve disease is associated with marked left ventricular angiographic (1–3) as well as cellular hypertrophy (4, 5). This process of secondary hypertrophy is accompanied by an increase in interstitial tissue. Are the microscopic alterations different in patients with preserved and depressed left ventricular function? Comparing intraoperative transmural biopsies from patients with compensated and decompensated aortic stenosis, Schwarz et al. (6) found a reduced volume fraction of myofibrils in those with depressed left ventricular function. In

* This work was supported by a grant of the Swiss National Science Foundation

patients with aortic insufficiency and a massively impaired left ventricular ejection fraction of 32%, volume fraction of myofibrils was smaller and muscle fiber diameter was larger than in patients with aortic insufficiency and only a moderately depressed ejection fraction of 48% (7). The purpose of the present study was to evaluate left ventricular morphometric structure from endomyocardial biopsies in patients with aortic valve disease with compensated and failing left ventricles, and to report changes of morphometric variables at an intermediate time after aortic valve replacement.

Patients and methods

Forty-nine patients with pure or predominant aortic stenosis (AS) and 35 patients with aortic insufficiency (AI) were studied hemodynamically prior to surgery. Left ventricular cineangiography and endomyocardial biopsies using a transseptal technique were performed (5). Coronary arteriography was carried out in all patients with aortic stenosis and in those with aortic insufficiency who were older than 37 years. In none of these patients was coronary artery narrowing of more than wall irregularities present. The patients were divided in two groups. In group 1 with left ventricular failure there were 15 patients with AS and 17 with AI. Left ventricular failure was said to be present when ejection fraction (EF) was $< 57\%$ and either cardiac index (CI) was < 2.5 L/min/m^2 and/or left ventricular end-diastolic pressure (LVEDP) was > 20 mm Hg. In the non-failing group (group 2) there were 34 patients with AS and 18 with AI. In these patients EF was $\geq 57\%$, CI ≥ 2.5 L/min/m^2 and LVEDP ≤ 20 mm Hg. Eleven patients of group 1 and 19 of group 2 were recatheterized 22.5 and 24.0 months, respectively, after successful aortic valve replacement.

Left ventricular quantitative angiography and assessment of angiographic muscle mass was carried out as reported previously (5). Morphometric evaluation of left ventricular endomyocardial biopsies included the determination of muscle fiber diameter (MFD), percent interstitial fibrosis (IF), volume fraction of myofibrils (VFM), and the calculation of left ventricular fibrous content (FC) (5).

Results

Because left ventricular morphometric structure was not different between patients with aortic stenosis and aortic insufficiency in both the failing and the non-failing group, only the pooled data of groups 1 and 2 are reported. Patients in group 1 were older than patients in group 2 (55.7 vs 48.2 years, $p < 0.02$). Figure 1 shows EF, CI and LVEDP in groups 1 and 2. Left ventricular muscle mass index (LMMI) was 234 g/m^2 in group 1 and 161 g/m^2 in group 2 ($p < 0.001$, Fig. 1). MFD amounted to 32.5 μ in group 1 and to 29.6 μ in group 2 ($p < 0.02$). IF and VFM did not differ in the two groups (Fig. 2). FC was 49.9 g/m^2 in group 1 and 30.6 g/m^2 in group 2 ($p < 0.001$). The increased FC in group 1 was due to the larger LMMI in group 1 as compared to that in group 2.

After valve replacement in group 1 EF increased from 44 to 59% ($p < 0.005$) and LVEDP decreased from 26.3 to 11.0 mm Hg ($p < 0.001$) (Fig. 3). CI increased slightly, but not significantly. LMMI decreased markedly from 236 to 146 g/m^2 ($p < 0.001$). MFD decreased in group 1 from 34.4 to 29.6 μ ($p < 0.001$), whereas IF, VFM, and FC did not change significantly after valve replacement (Fig. 4).

In the patients with a non-failing left ventricle prior to surgery (group 2) EF and CI did not change postoperatively (Fig. 5). LVEDP decreased from 13.7 to 9.2 mm Hg

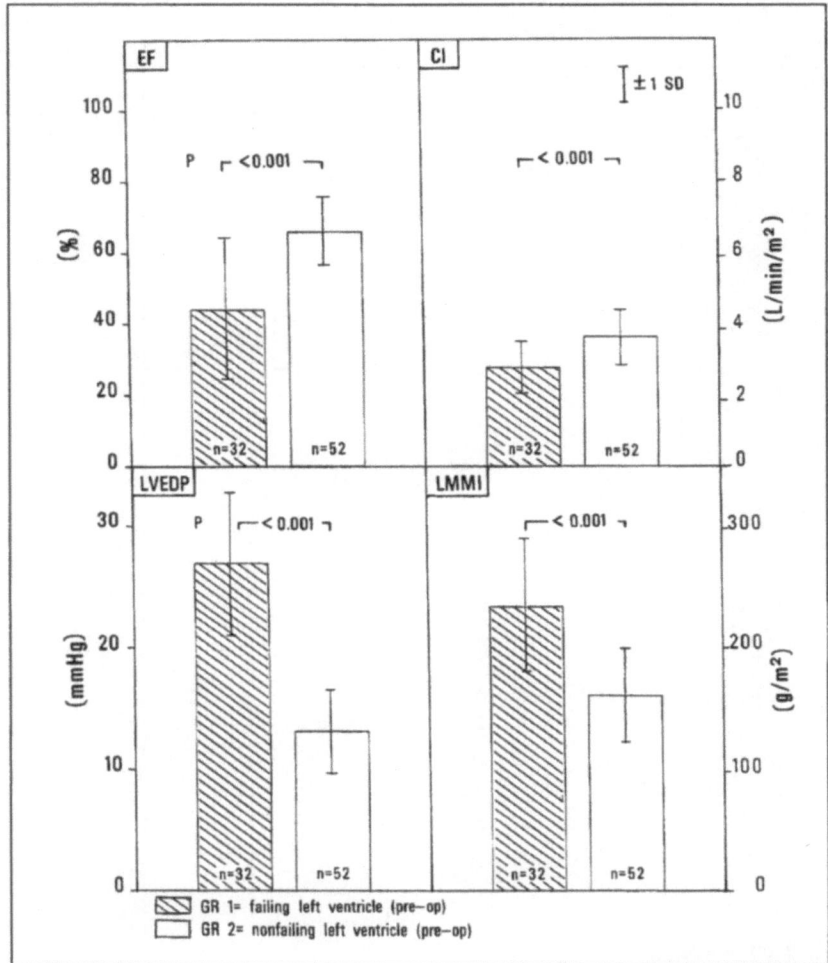

Fig. 1. Preoperative hemodynamic data in aortic valve disease. EF = left ventricular ejection fraction; CI = cardiac index; LVEDP = left ventricular end-diastolic pressure; LMMI = left ventricular muscle mass index; p values were obtained by unpaired Student's *t*-test

(p < 0.001) and LMMI from 162 to 103 g/m² (p < 0.001) (Fig. 5). MFD decreased from 29.4 to 26.9 μ (p < 0.025) and IF increased from 19.7 to 23.5% (p < 0.05) (Fig. 6). VFM did not change, whereas there was a decrease of fibrous content from 32.6 to 24.7 g/m² (p < 0.05).

Figure 7 depicts the hemodynamics in the two groups at the postoperative catheterization. EF, CI, and LVEDP did not differ. LMMI was, however, still significantly larger in group 1 than in group 2 (p < 0.01). Similarly, cellular hypertrophy as evaluated from MFD was greater (p < 0.05) in group 1 than in group 2 (Fig. 8).

At the postoperative study, there was no difference between group 1 and group 2 with respect to EF, VFM, IF and FC.

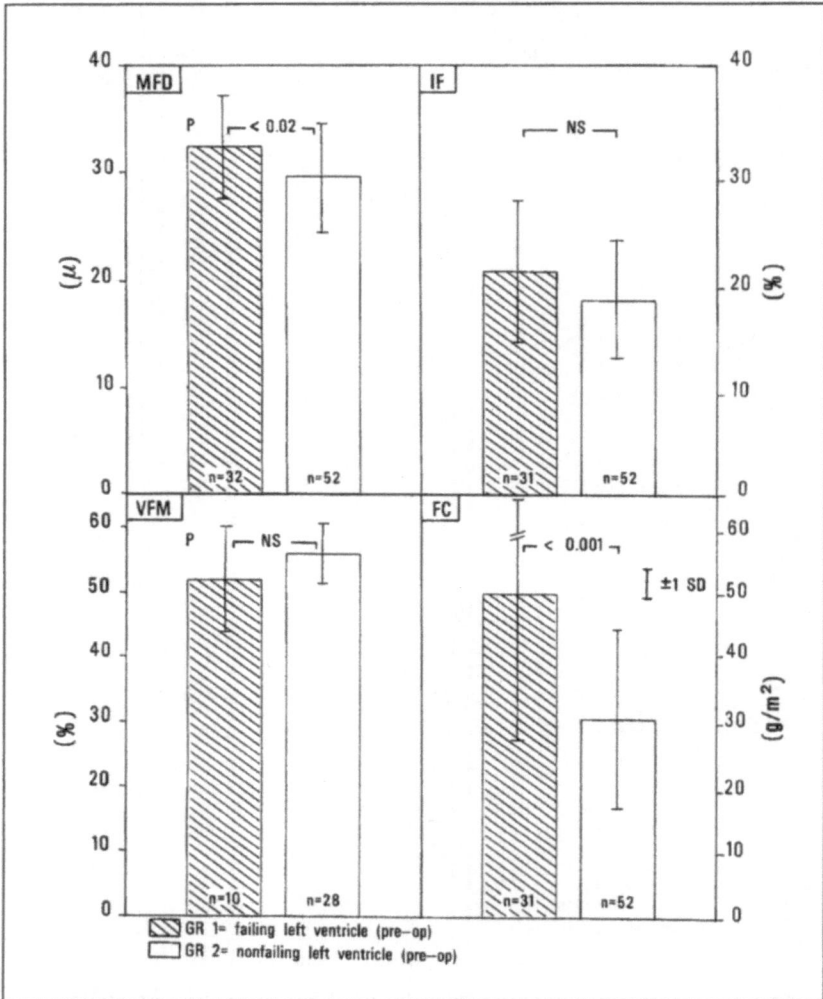

Fig. 2. Preoperative morphometric data in patients with aortic valve disease. MFD = muscle fiber diameter; IF = percent interstitial fibrosis; VFM = volume fraction of myofibrils; FC = left ventricular fibrous content (LMMI × IF/100). The p values were obtained by unpaired Student's *t*-test

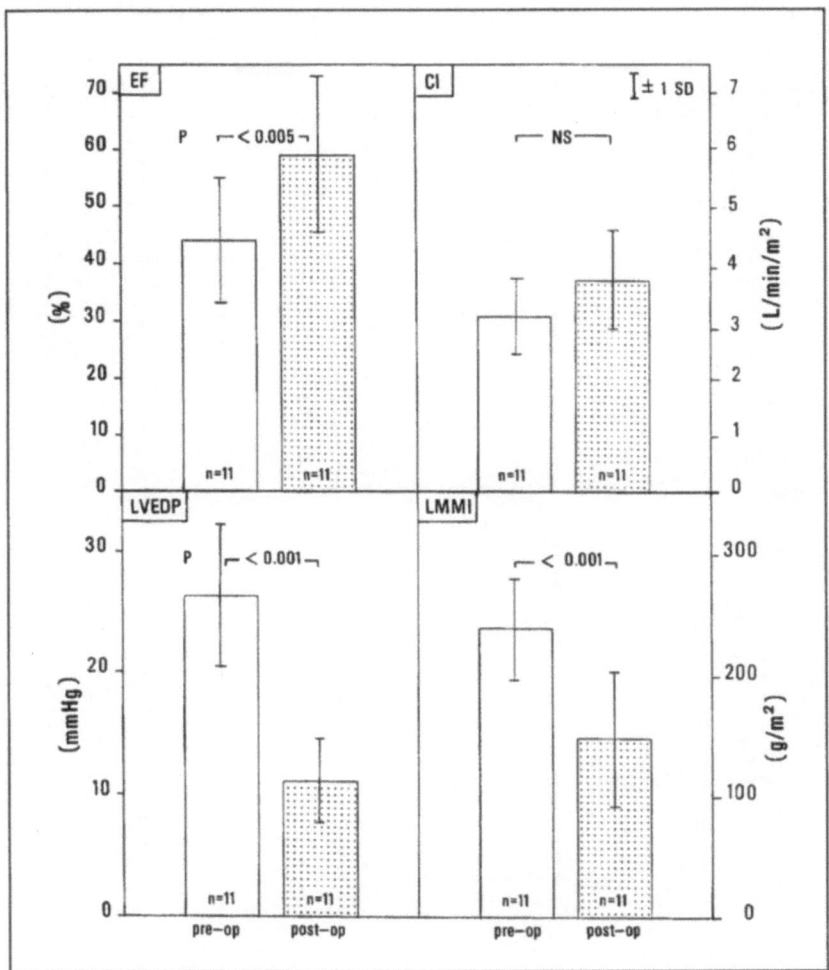

Fig. 3. Pre- and postoperative hemodynamic data in a subset of patients with aortic valve disease who had preoperative left ventricular failure. Abbreviations as in Fig. 1. The p values were obtained by paired Student's *t*-test

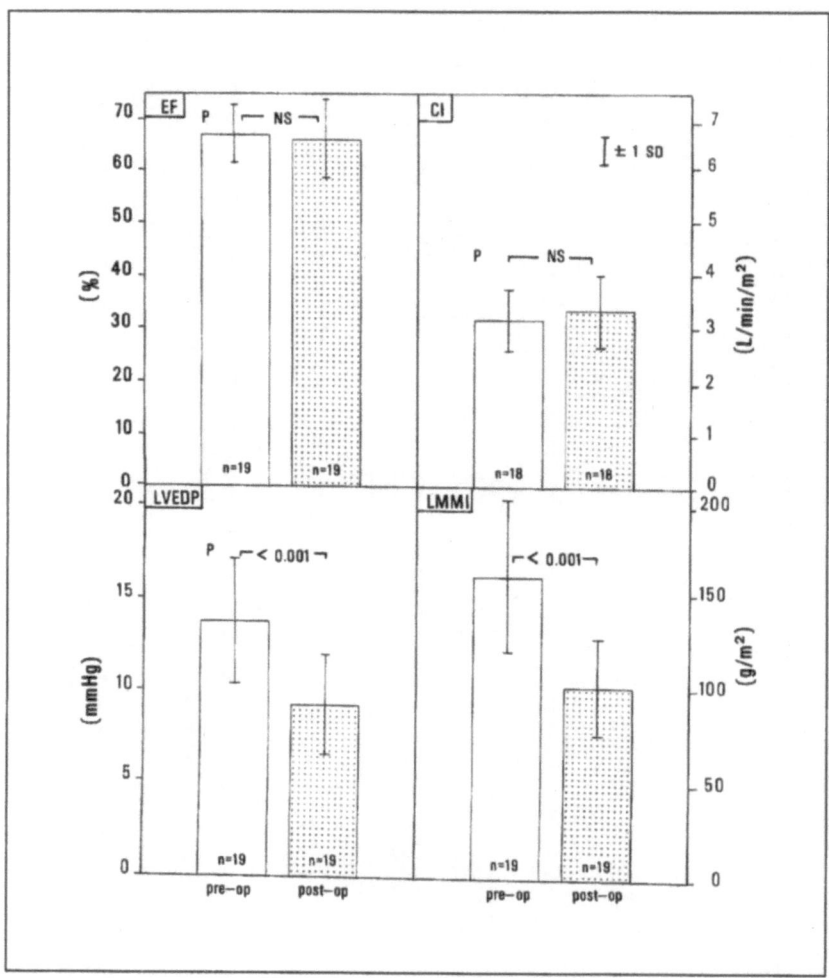

Fig. 4. Pre- and postoperative morphometric data in a subset of patients with aortic valve disease who had preoperative left ventricular failure. The abbreviations are the same as in Fig. 2. The p values were obtained by paired Student's *t*-test

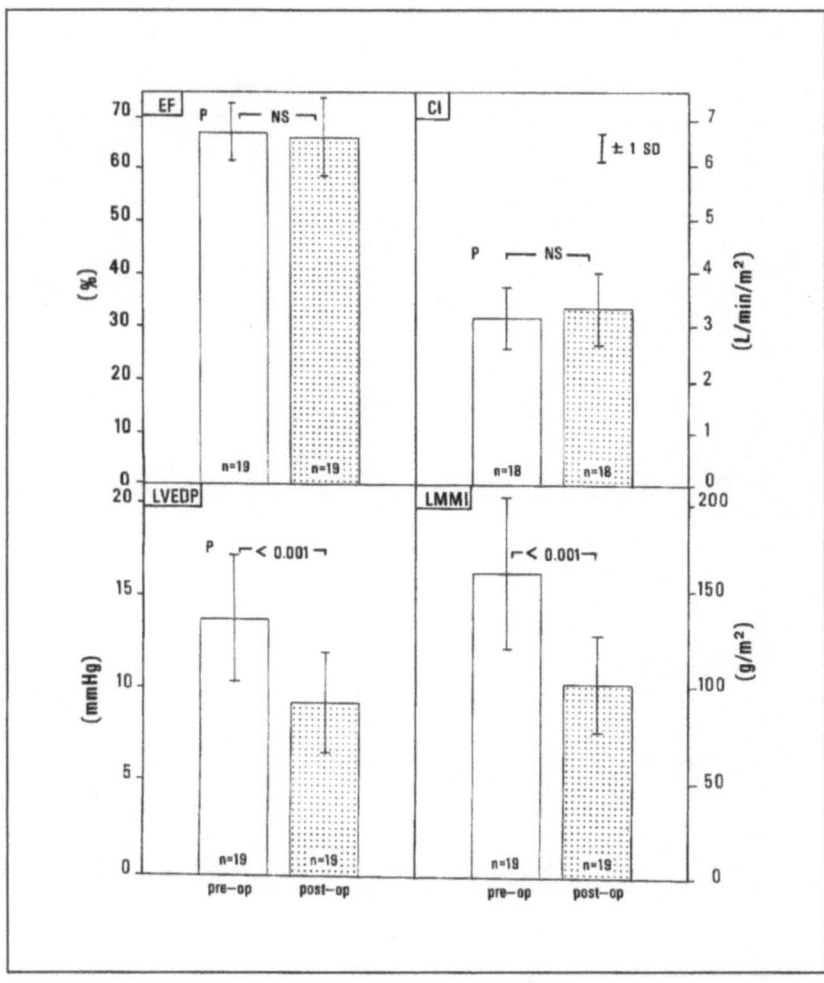

Fig. 5. Pre- and postoperative hemodynamic data in a subset of patients with aortic valve disease and preoperative non-failing left ventricle. The abbreviations are the same as in Fig. 1. The p values were obtained by paired Student's *t*-test

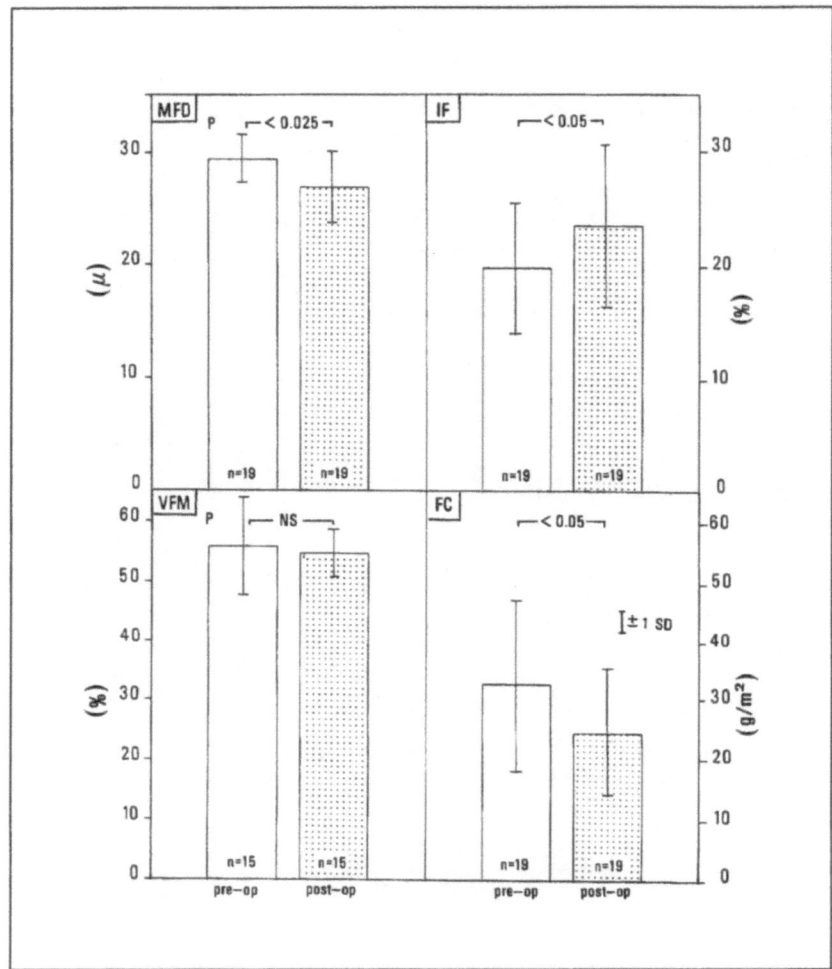

Fig. 6. Pre- and postoperative morphometric data in a subset of patients with aortic valve disease and preoperative non-failing left ventricle. The abbreviations are the same as in Fig. 2. The p values were obtained by paired Student's *t*-test

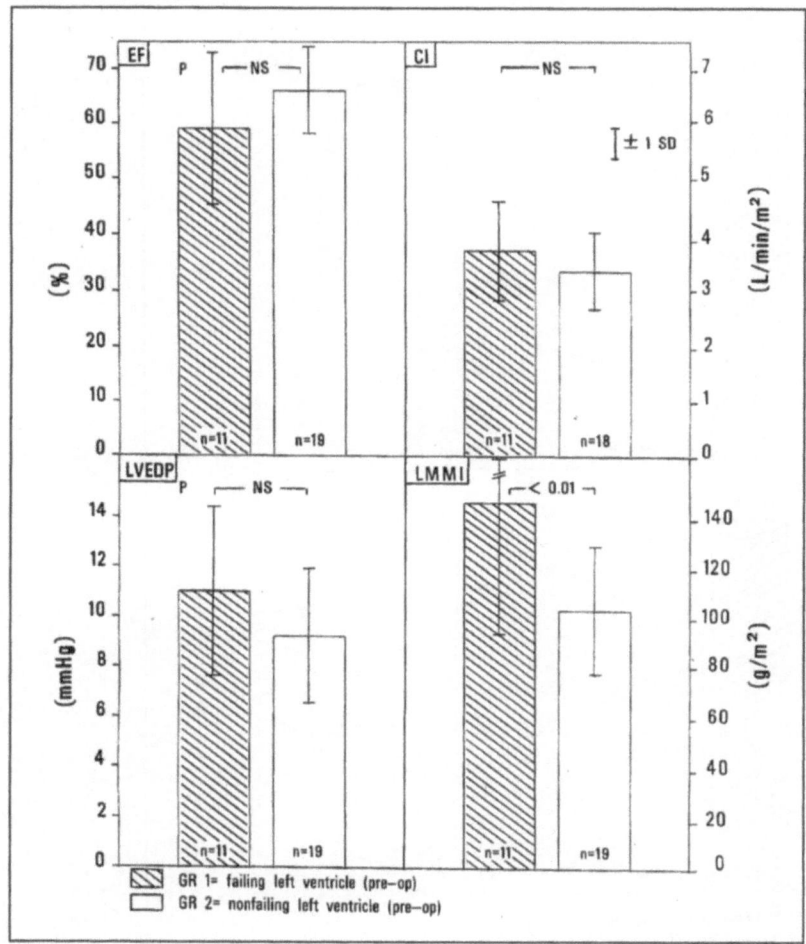

Fig. 7. Hemodynamic data at the postoperative catheterization in patiens with aortic valve disease who had a failing (GR 1) or a non-failing (GR 2) left ventricle at the preoperative study. Abbreviations as in Fig. 1. The p values were obtained by unpaired Student's t-test

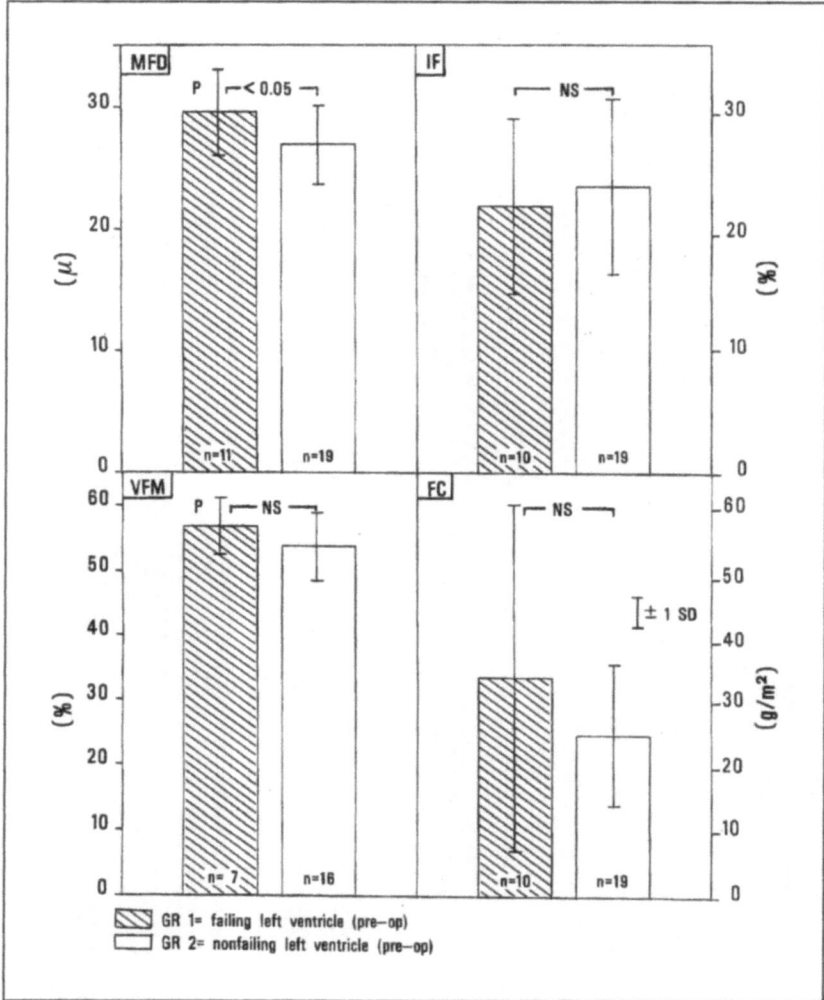

Fig. 8. Postoperative morphometric data in patients with aortic valve disease who had a failing (GR 1) or a non-failing (GR 2) left ventricle at the preoperative study. Abbreviations as in Fig. 2. The p values were obtained by unpaired Student's *t*-test

Discussion

This study has shown that in patients with aortic valve disease and hemodynamically defined left ventricular failure macroscopic and microscopic hypertrophy is more marked than in patients with compensated left ventricular function. Left ventricular pump function was not related to percent interstitial fibrosis. This observation is in agreement with the findings of others in aortic stenosis (6) and aortic insufficiency (7). In contrast to these authors (6, 7), volume fraction of myofibrils was not depressed in our patients with left ventricular failure. The reason for this discrepancy is not clear, but might be related to patient selection. It should be noted that the patients with aortic insufficiency of Perennec et al. (7) who had an unfavorable postoperative outcome were in a more advanced stage of left ventricular dysfunction, their ejection fraction being only 32%. Because in our patients with preoperatively depressed left ventricular function, but no intracellular depletion of myofibrils, there was postoperative restoration of ejection fraction in contrast to those of Perennec et al. (7), one might speculate whether the reduction of volume fraction of myofibrils represents a stage of no recuperable contractile dysfunction. On the other hand, it is evident from our study that reduction of volume fraction of myofibrils is not a prerequisite for some milder form of hemodynamic left ventricular failure. In these instances a functional rather than an anatomical derangement of the myofibrils is likely to be at the origin of left ventricular dysfunction.

Finally, this investigation emphasizes that there is residual macroscopic and microscopic left ventricular hypertrophy 2 years after aortic valve replacement. This residual hypertrophy is more marked in patients who have elicited preoperative left ventricular failure.

References

1. Gould KL, Kennedy JW, Frimer M, Pollack GH, Dodge HT (1976) Analysis of wall dynamics and directional components of left ventricular contraction in man. Am J Cardiol 38:322–331
2. Gunther S, Grossman W (1979) Determinants of ventricular function in pressure-overload hypertrophy in man. Circulation 59:679–688
3. Herreman F, Ameur A, De Vernejoul F, Bourgin JG, Gueret P, Guerin F, Degeorges M (1979) Pre- and post-operative hemodynamic and cineangiographic assessment of left ventricular function in patients with aortic regurgitation. Am Heart J 98:63–72
4. Schaper J, Schwarz F, Hehrlein F (1981) Ultrastructural changes in human myocardium with hypertrophy due to aortic valve disease and their relationship to left ventricular mass and ejection fraction. Herz 6:217–225
5. Hess OM, Ritter M, Schneider J, Grimm J, Turina M, Krayenbuehl HP (1984) Diastolic stiffness and myocardial structure in aortic valve disease before and after valve replacement. Circulation 69:855–865
6. Schwarz F, Schaper J, Kittstein D, Flameng W, Walter P, Schaper W (1981) Reduced volume fraction of myofibrils in myocardium of patients with decompensated pressure overload. Circulation 63:1299–1304
7. Perennec J, Herreman F, Cosma H, Ilers F, Djigouadi Z, Degeorges M, Hatt PY (1988) Relationship of myocardial morphometry in aortic valve regurgitation to myocardial function and post-operative results. Bas Res Cardiol 83:10–23

Authors' address:

Prof. H. P. Krayenbuehl, M.D.
Medical Policlinic
Division of Cardiology
University Hospital
CH-8091 Zurich

Protective effect of ACE- and kininase-inhibitor on the onset of cardiomyopathy *

M. Nagano, M. Kato, M. Nagai, and J. Yang

Department of Internal Medicine, Aoto Hospital,
Jikei University School of Medicine, Tokyo, Japan

Summary: Attempts at treating idiopathic cardiomyopathy have been made both clinically and experimentally using the cardiomyopathic Syrian hamster. In recent years, the angiotensin converting enzyme (ACE) inhibitor has attracted considerable attention as an agent to treat heart failure. We administered the ACE inhibitor captopril to the cardiomyopathic hamster. In this study, 15 mg/kg body weight of captopril was administered to the cardiomyopathic hamster J2N at 5 weeks of age for 10 weeks; age matched J2N hamsters were used as non-treated control animals. At the end of captopril administration, blood was collected from the ventral aorta. Serum malondialdehyde (MDA), serum CPK, aldolase and LDH were determined, and myosin isoenzyme patterns of the extirpated myocardium were compared. Additionally, ECGs were compared and the fibrotic ratio of both ventricles determined. Serum MDA, CPK, and aldolase increased significantly in the cardiomyopathic hamster, whereas these indices were significantly inhibited in the hamster treated with captopril. The pathological ECG findings and the ventricular V3 predominant myosin isoenzyme patterns of the J2N were also much improved in the captopril group. However, the improvement in these parameters by enalapril administration was less than that seen with captopril. These results suggested that the effect of captopril is not only due to decrease of the angiotensin II level, but also due to increase in tissue kinin and vasodilatory prostaglandin which play an important role in the beneficial effect of captopril.

Key words: Cardiomyopathic hamster J2N; angiotensin converting enzyme; ACE-inhibitor; captopril; enalapril

Introduction

There are various vasodilators and cardioprotective drugs on the market worldwide; for example: Ca-channel blockers, α-1 receptor blocker, β-receptor blocker, prostaglandin, bradykinine, coenzyme Q_{10} and l-carnitine. These drugs have been tried for the therapy of cardiomyopathy, especially idiopathic dilated cardiomyopathy.

Up to now, also various cardioprotective drugs have been tried for treatment of cardiomyopathic Syrian hamster (1, 2). Of these drugs, some are also reported to be clinically effective.

Basic research has been undertaken using the cardiomyopathic Syrian hamster and the effectivity of these drugs has been rigorously examined. Although these drugs have shown some degree of experimental effectiveness, no effect has been observed on inhibiting the progress of cardiac degeneration. For several years now, alteration of the renin

* This work was supported in part by a research grant for intractable diseases from the Ministry of Health and Welfare 1989 and 1990, Japan.

angiotensin aldosterone system (3) in cardiac failure has been proposed an attractive hypothesis and if proven, one could propose that the angiotensin converting enzyme (ACE) inhibitor might be useful in the failing cardiomyopathic patient (4, 5).

In this study, we present evidence of the protective effect of the ACE-inhibitors captopril and enalapril in the cardiomyopathic Syrian hamster J2N.

Materials and methods

Cardiomyopathic Syrian hamster J2N

The J2N cardiomyopathic hamster (6) has been developed in our laboratory for 5 years. This new colony has been raised under normal environmental conditions to preserve the original genetic traits, without cannibalism. Care has been taken to preserve the animals pathological cardiac changes, its large body weight and its high reproduction rate.

Breeding the cardiomyopathic Syrian hamster: An F1 female (brown) hamster, obtained by breeding a male BIO 14.6 with a female golden hamster (brown), was crossbred again with a male BIO 14.6. The F2 female (white) obtained was bred with the same BIO 14.6 male, and the F3 white hamster thus obtained was cardiomyopathic with pathological and normal ECG. This cardiomyopathic hamster had a higher reproduction rate than the BIO 14.6 and also a body weight of nearly 150 g. This hamster was named J1N cardiomyopathic hamster. A female J1N with pathological ECG was crossbred with another line BIO 14.6 male. After three generations, the cardiomyopathic hamster J2N with pathological ECG and high CPK activity in serum was obtained.

Figure 1a shows the J2N hamster; the one on the right is a 50-week old hamster without cardiomyopathy, i.e., a normal white control animal. The one on the left is a car diomyopathic hamster. This 50-week-old hamster has severe edema with ascites due to cardiac failure.

Figure 1b shows cross-sections of their hearts. The left one is normal, and the right one is of the J2N cardiomyopathic hamster. The ventricular wall of J2N is very thin in comparison to the ventricular wall of the normal animal. Moreover, both ventricles of the J2N are severely dilated.

In the J2N hamster the abnormalities of muscle arrangement, degeneration, interstitial fibrosis, and many patchy myocardial necrosis are well visualized.

The pathological finding in the ECG were, for example: left axis deviation; QS pattern in II, III, aV_F, V1, V2 and V3–4; pulmonary P, ST-depression and arrhythmia, each scored 1 or 2. In a hamster with an ECG score of over 5, the cardiac damage is severely advanced (6). In a hamster with a score of 1–2, there is only minimal histological cardiac damage. The ECG score corresponds to the histological findings from the hearts. If the ECG score was more than 2, histological damage was hardly noticeable. Those with scores higher than 3 showed the falling off and degeneration of the myocardium and fibrosis of the intestitium.

Figure 2a shows the comparison of the ventricular myosin isoenzyme pattern of the normal white and cardiomyopathic J2N hamster. The one on the left is the normal myosine isoenzyme pattern of both ventricles, and the one on the right is the isomyosin from the cardiomyopathic heart. In the group of cardiomyopathic hamster, the isomyosin pattern of the ventricle remarkably shifted towards V3 (6).

We compared serum CPK and aldolase activities in both animal groups (Fig. 2b). In the normal control animal group, serum CPK and aldolase did not rise, and they showed

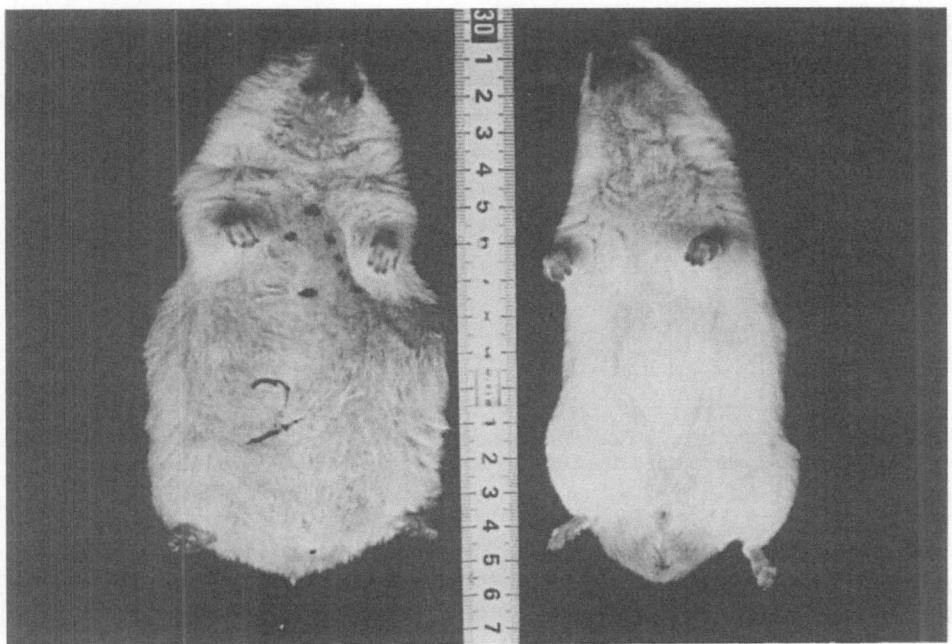

Fig. 1 a. The cardiomyopathic hamster J2N (left) and normal control white hamster (right), both 50 weeks old

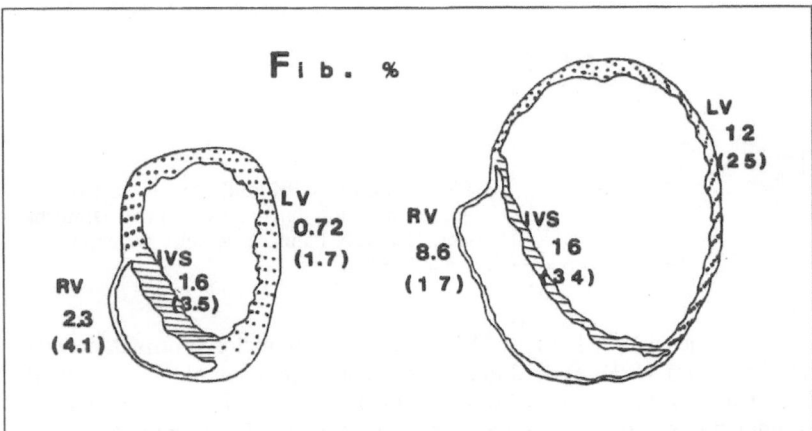

Fig. 1 b. The cross-section of J2N (right) and control (left) hamster. Both ventricles of the J2N are markedly dilated and the ventricular wall is very thin

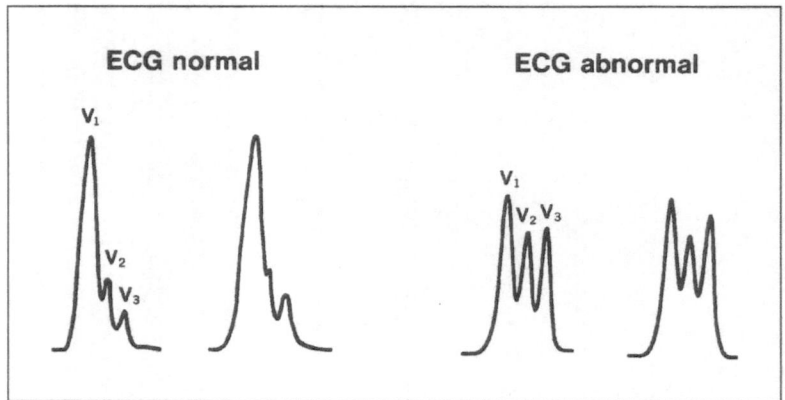

Fig. 2a. The ventricular myosin isoenzyme pattern of the J2N and normal white hamsters. The ventricular myosin isoenzyme pattern of the J2N hamster remarkably shifted towards V3

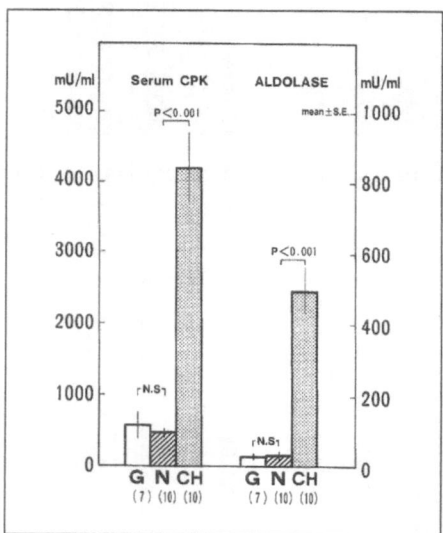

Fig. 2b. Serum CPK and aldolase activities. G: golden hamster; N: normal control white hamster; CH: J2N hamster. Results are expressed as means ± SEM

the same levels as in the golden hamster, but in the J2N hamster group there was a remarkable rise in serum CPK and aldolase (7). The sarcolemmal Ca^{2+} activated ATPase and Na^{+}-Ca^{2+} exchange in cardiomyopathic heart were also damaged, in comparison to the golden hamster or to the white hamster without cardiac damage (7).

Administration of ACE-inhibitor

In this experiment 15 mg/kg body weight of captopril and 1.5 mg/kg of enalapril were administered orally to the cardiomyopathic hamster J2N at 5 weeks of age. Captopril was given for 10 weeks and enalapril for 15 weeks.

Age-matched J2N hamster were used as non-treated control animals. At 5 weeks of age the cardiomyopathic hamster J2N did not yet exhibit cardiac damage.

Results and discussion

Figure 3a shows the serum CPK and aldolase activities of golden hamster, non-treated cardiomyopathic hamster, and of cardiomyopathic hamster treated with captopril. In the non-treated hamster, serum CPK activity rose to above 2000 mu/ml, compared to the captopril group where it only rose to 680 mu/ml. Captopril remarkably inhibited the CPK release. Aldolase activity showed almost the same tendency.

In the non-treated J2N hamster, an elevated level of serum MDA as superoxide-substance was observed, but this rise was also remarkably inhibited by the captopril treatment (Fig. 3b).

Figure 4 shows the comparison of the ventricular myosin isoenzyme patterns of cardiomyopathic hamsters with and without captopril treatment. In the group of J2N non-treated with captopril, the isomyosin patterns of the ventricles remarkably shifted towards V3. The captopril treated group displayed nearly identical ventricular myosin isoenzyme patterns to those of the normal ECG hamster and golden hamster.

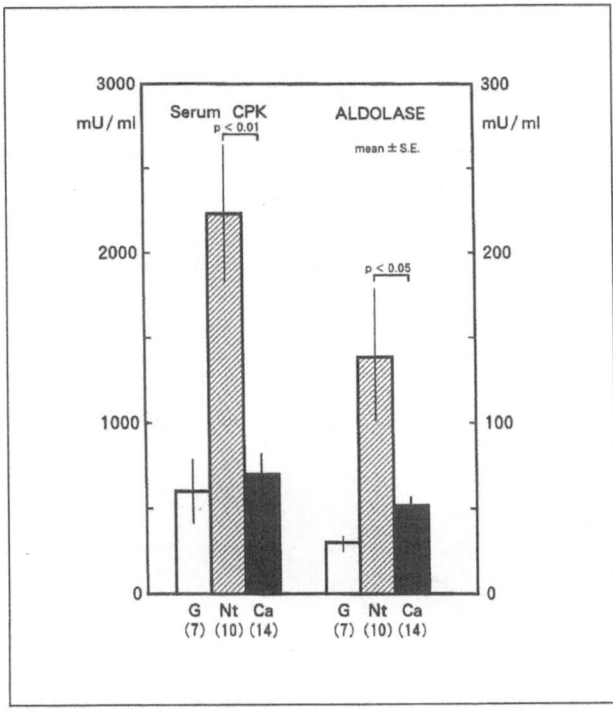

Fig. 3a. Serum CPK and aldolase activities of J2N cardiomyopathic hamster treated with and without captopril in comparison to golden hamster. G: golden hamster; Nt: non-treated; Ca: captopril treated. Results are expressed as means ± SEM

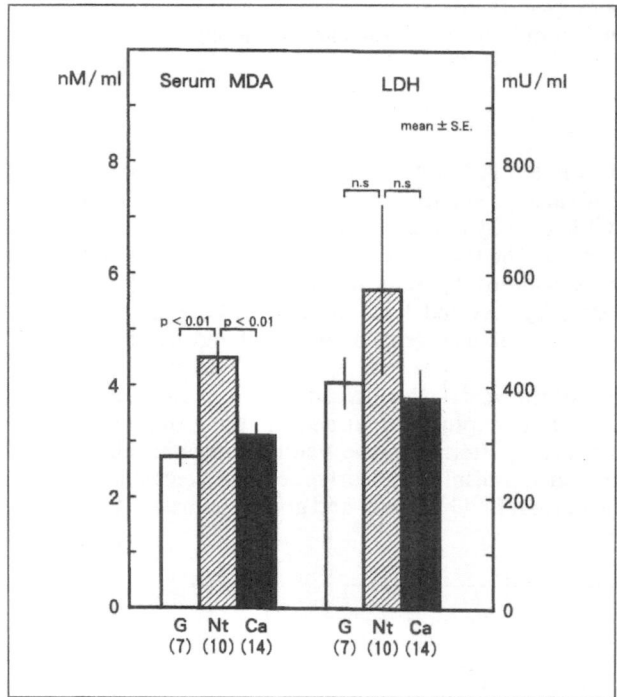

Fig. 3 b. Serum MDA level of the J2N cardiomyopathic hamster treated with and without captopril. Results are expressed as mean ± SD

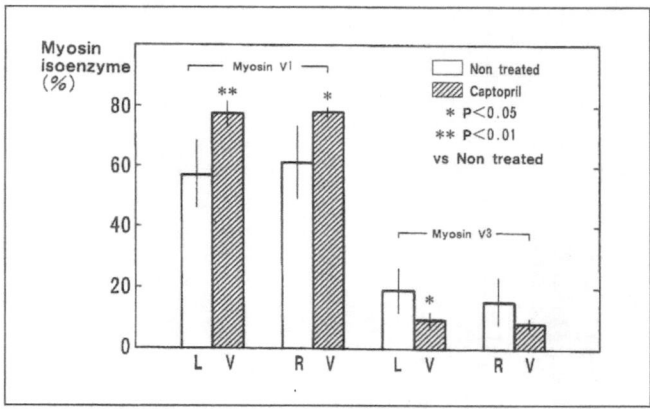

Fig. 4. The percent of the ventricular myosin isoenzyme, V1 and V3 in the J2N hamster treated with captopril and those not treated. (Number of non-treated: 10; treated: 14). Values are mean ± SD

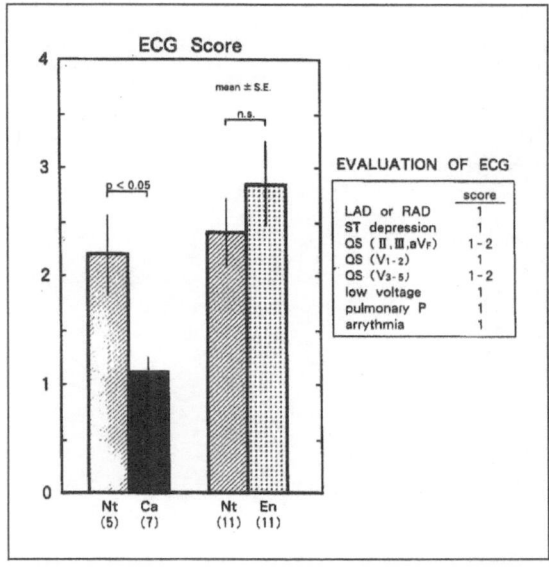

Evaluation of ECG table:

	score
LAD or RAD	1
ST depression	1
QS (II, III, aVr)	1 - 2
QS (V₁₋₂)	1
QS (V₃₋₅)	1 - 2
low voltage	1
pulmonary P	1
arrythmia	1

Fig. 5. The correlation between histological myocardial damage and ECG score

That is so say, the captopril administration provided good prophylaxis against myocardial damage in cardiomyopathic hamsters from the aspect of myocardial structural protein.

The ECG of the J2N at the end of this experiment revealed severe myocardial damage, left axis deviation, abnormal Q-wave, and arrhythmia. The hamster given captopril, however, showed no such findings, and exhibited similar ECGs to those of the control hamsters.

The histological myocardial damage shows a positive correlation with the ECG score (6). Figure 5 shows the ECG score as the grade of the myocardial damage in the captopril group and in the non-treated group. In the captopril group the ECG score is inhibited in comparison to the ECG score of non-treatment group.

In support of these ECG findings, myocardial tissue damage in the non-treatment group was observed to be severe (Fig. 6 bottom), but in the captopril-treated hamster only minimal damage was observed in the upper picture.

In general, the fibrotic ratio in the normal non-treated hamster had a mean value of 3.5% (6). The fibrotic ratio of the heart in the non-treated hamster had a mean value of 8.0%, and in the captopril-treated hamster this ratio was 4.5%. Thus captopril protect against myocardial cell damage in cardiomyopathic hamsters.

However, in our experiment with enalapril, we did not observe the effect of cardiac protection in the cardiomyopathic hamster compared to the captopril treatment.

MDA, which was inhibited by the captopril treatment, was not inhibited by enalapril administration. In the non-treated cardiomyopathic hamster, a reduction in myosin isoenzyme V1 and an increase in isoenzyme V3 of the ventricle were observed (8). The captopril group displayed very similar ventricular myosin isoenzyme patterns as the normal hamster. But in the enalapril group the myosin isoenzyme pattern of the ventricle shifted towards V3, compared to the non-treated cardiomyopathic animal.

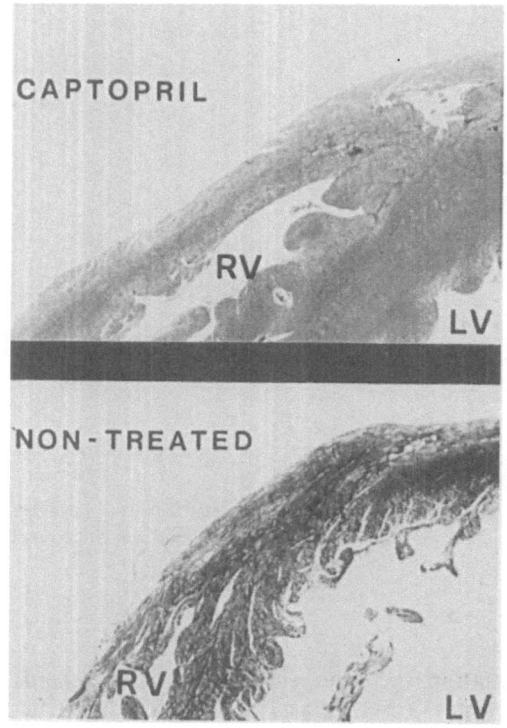

Fig. 6. The histopathological findings in the hearts of the J2N hamsters non-treated (lower photo) and those treated with captopril (upper)

The shift of myosin isoenzyme towards V3 was not inhibited by the enalapril treatment.

We have not observed the cardioprotective effect of enalapril in J2N in comparison with the captopril treatment (Fig. 5). Captopril inhibited the ECG score, compared to the ECG score of the non-treatment group.

The mechanism by which captopril may protect cardiac cell damage and fibrosis of cardiomyopathic heart is very interesting. The mechanism of the captopril effect includes the following (3, 9): 1) The inhibition of ACE reduces the rate of conversion of angiotensin I to angiotensin II. The falling angiotensin II level and the decrease in plasma aldosterone causes a decrease in peripheral vascular resistance and a decrease in sodium retention, leading to a drop in afterload. In addition, the decrease of angiotensin II reduces cardiac hypertrophy. 2) There is an increase in vasodilative prostaglandin and in tissue active kinin derivates. The increase in tissue levels of kinin may result in increased vasodilatation and stimulation of prostaglandin biosynthesis. The increased prostaglandin and tissue bradykinin induce a reduction of afterload.

In our experiment with enalapril, we did not observe a positive effect in cardiac protection of the cardiomyopathic hamster in comparison with captopril.

Enalapril's mechanism of action is limited to its inhibiting effect on the ACE-system. Enalapril has almost no bradykinin-stimulating or prostaglandin-formation promoting effects (9).

At the present time, it is not known whether the inhibiting effect of captopril on cardiomyopathy is due to suppression of angiotensin II via the ACE inhibitor action, or whether the increase in vasodilatory prostaglandin and active kinin is important.

These results suggest that the effect of captopril is due not only to decrease of the angiotensin II level, but also due to increase in active kinin and vasodilatory prostaglandin, both of which play an important role in the beneficial effect of captopril.

Acknowledgements. We would like to thank Miss Hitomi Iwasaki for excellent technical assistance.

References

1. Jasmin G, Solymoss B (1978) Prevention of hereditary cardiomyopathy in the hamster by verapamil and other agents. Proc Soc Exp Biol Med 149:193–198
2. Jasmin G, Proschek L (1987) Pathogenesis of the hamster hereditary cardiomyopathy. A pharmacologic appraisal. In: Kawai C, Abelmann WI (eds) Pathogenesis of Myocarditis and Cardiomyopathy. University of Tokyo Press, pp 79–89
3. Dzau VJ, Pratt RE (1988) Renin-angiotensin system: biology, physiology, and pharmacology. In: Fozzard H, Heaber H, Jennings RB, Katz AM, Morgan HE (eds) The Heart and Cardiovascular System. Raven Press NY, pp 1631–1662
4. Ahgostini PG, de Cesare N, Doria E, Polese A, Tomborini G, Guazzi MD (1986) Afterload reduction. A comparison of captopril and nifedipine in dilated cardiomyopathy. Brit Heart J 55:391–399
5. Packer M, Medina N, Yushak M (1986) Comparative hemodynamic and clinical effects of long-term treatment with prazosin and captopril for severe chronic congestive heart failure secondary to coronary artery disease or idiopathic dilated cardiomyopathy. Am J Cardiol 57:1323–1327
6. Takeda A (1989) Morphological and biochemical abnormalities in new cardiomyopathic Syrian hamsters. Jikeikai Med J 36:129–148
7. Kato M, Takeda A (1990) The experimental animal model. Cardiomyopathic hamster. J Mol Cell Cardiol 22(Suppl II):22
8. Nagano M, Takeda N, Ohkubo YT, Nakamura I, Takeda A (1988) Histopathological myocardial damage and myosin isoenzyme pattern in cardiomyopathic Syrian hamster (in Japanese). Annual report of the research committee of idiopathic cardiomyopathy 1987. The Ministerium of Health and Welfare of Japan, pp 156–157
9. Zusman RM (1988) Eicosanoid: prostaglandins, thromboxane, and prostocyclin. In: The Heart and Cardiovascular System. Raven Press NY, pp 1613–1629

Authors' address:

Prof. Dr. M. Nagano
Department of Internal Medicine
Aoto Hospital
Jikei University School of Medicine
Katsushika-ku, Aoto 6-41
125 Tokyo, Japan

Effects of long-term medication for essential hypertension on cardiac hypertrophy and function

N. Takeda, I. Nakamura, T. Hatanaka, T. Iwai, A. Tanamura,
Y. Obara, and M. Nagano

Department of Internal Medicine, Aoto Hospital,
Jikei University School of Medicine, Tokyo, Japan

Summary: The effects of long-term treatment of hypertensive patients with alacepril (angiotensin-converting enzyme inhibitor) on cardiac mass and function were investigated. A total of 12 patients was examined. Both systolic and diastolic blood pressure were significantly reduced by treatment with alacepril for 1 year. Left ventricular mass, as estimated by echocardiography, was significantly decreased by alacepril treatment, although electrocardiographic and chest x-ray findings were not significantly altered. Cardiac pump function, which was also assessed by echocardiography, was not changed. These results indicate that long-term treatment of hypertension with alacepril induces regression of cardiac hypertrophy without any change in cardiac contractile function.

Key words: Alacepril; angiotensin-converting enzyme (ACE) inhibitor; hypertension; cardiac hypertrophy; cardiac function

Introduction

The treatment of hypertensive patients should be considered in relation to other associated pathophysiological conditions or complications, e.g., renal damage, diabetes, and cerebrovascular or cardiovascular disorders. In the latter condition, except for coronary sclerosis, cardiomegaly occurs at high incidence. This can be regarded as an adaptation to pressure overload in order to maintain cardiac pump function, whereas on the other hand, cardiomegaly itself may induce alteration of coronary circulation. In this study, we investigated the effects of a newly developed angiotensin-converting enzyme inhibitor, alacepril (4, 7, 14, 15), on both left ventricular mass and function as estimated by echocardiography in patients with essential hypertension.

Methods

Twelve hypertensive out-patients at our hospital, who had no diabetes or ischemic change in electrocardiogram (ECG) were investigated. All had been hypertensive for 2–7 years and had remained untreated for at least 2 years. Blood pressure was measured in a sitting position using a manometer (Riva-Rocci type). ECG, chest x-ray film, and echocardiogram were checked at the beginning and after 1 year of alacepril treatment. Alacepril was administered orally at a daily dose of 50 mg for 1 year. Left ventricular mass (LVM) was calculated according to the equation of Hammond et al. (3).

Statistical analysis of data was performed using paired *t*-test.

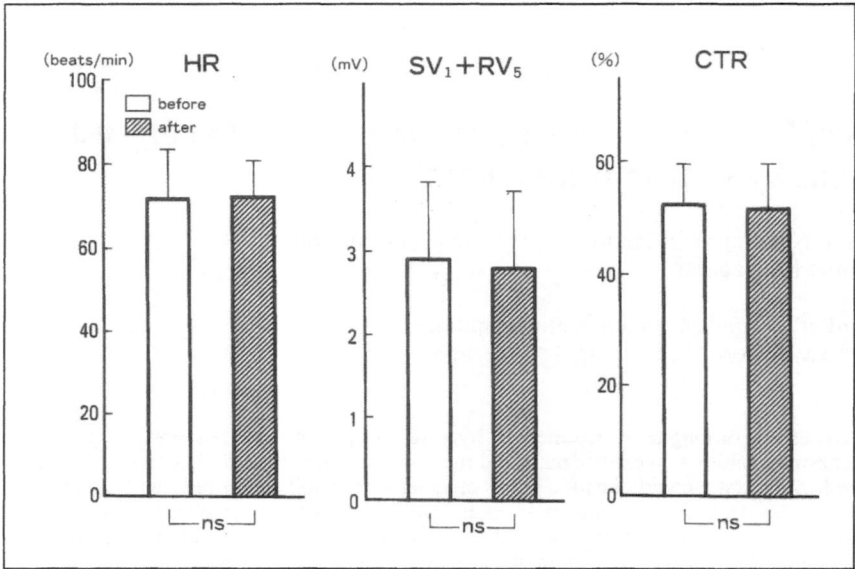

Fig. 1. Electrocardiographic and chest x-ray findings. HR: heart rates, $SV_1 + RV_5$:ECG index CTR: cardiothoracic ratio, ns: not significant; vertical lines indicate SD

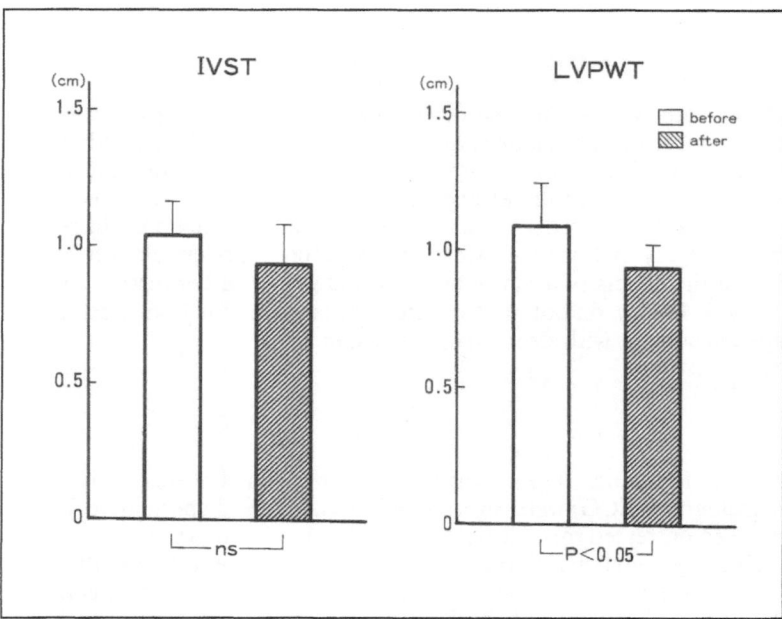

Fig. 2. Echocardiographic findings. IVST: interventricular septal thickness, LVPWT: left-ventricular posterior wall thickness, ns: not significant; vertical lines indicate SD

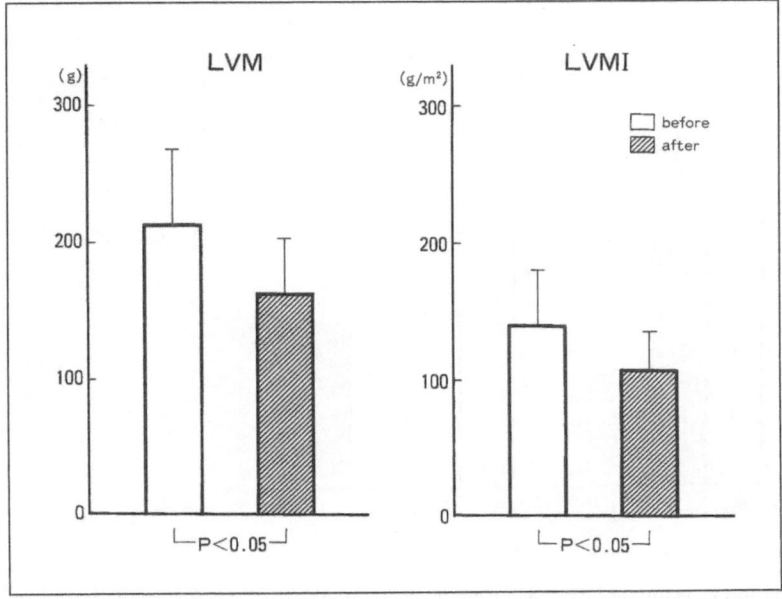

Fig. 3. Left-ventricular mass (LVM) and LVM index (LVMI); vertical lines indicate SD

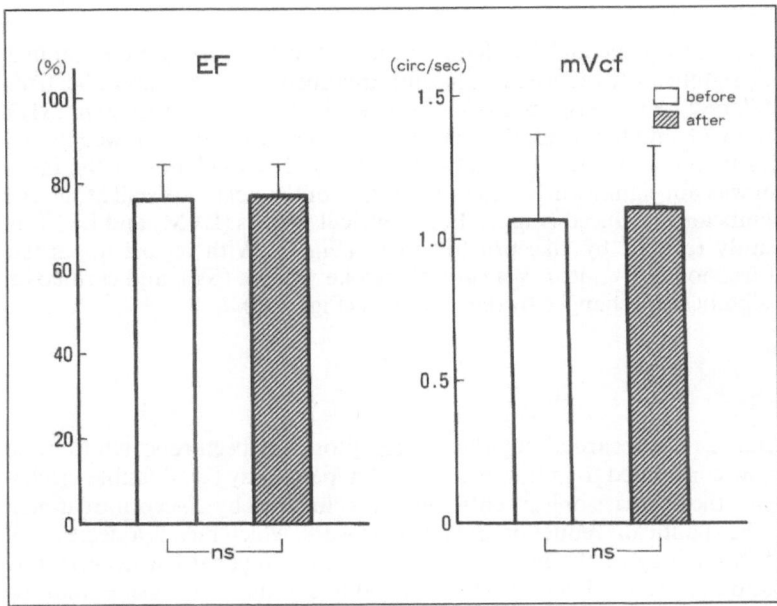

Fig. 4. Cardiac function as estimated by echocardiography (I). EF: ejection fraction, mVcf: mean circumferential shortening velocity, ns: not significant; vertical lines indicate SD

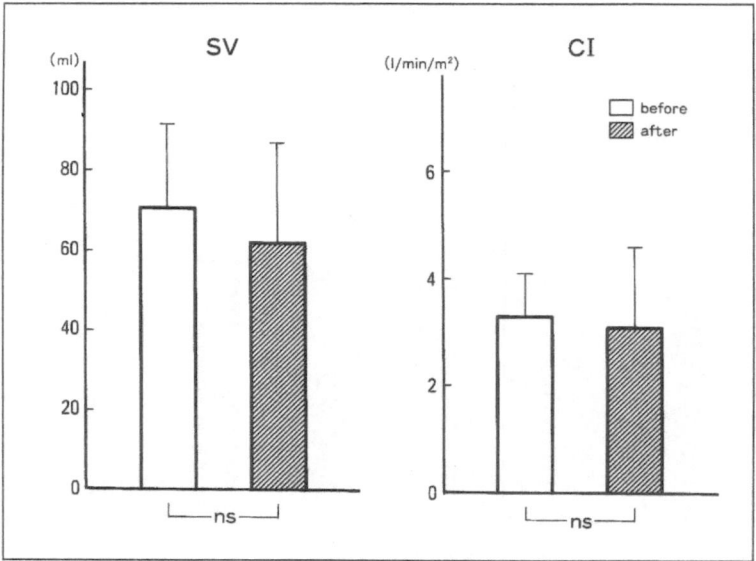

Fig. 5. Cardiac function as estimated by echocardiography (II). SV: stroke volume, CI: cardiac index, ns: not significant; vertical lines indicate SD

Results

In total, 12 patients (seven male and five female, aged 30 to 69 years) were examined. Blood pressure was significantly reduced by alacepril treatment for 1 year (systolic: from 156.7 ± 10.8 to 137.5 ± 12.3 mm Hg, diastolic: from 94.6 ± 10.2 to 83.4 ± 6.2 mm Hg). Both $SV_1 + RV_5$ in ECG, and the cardiothoracic ratio on chest x-ray film showed no significant differences before and after the treatment (Fig. 1). The thickness of the interventricular septum was not significantly reduced, but that of the posterior wall at the end of diastole was significantly reduced (Fig. 2). Left ventricular mass (LVM) and LVM index were significantly reduced by alacepril treatment (Fig. 3). With regard to cardiac function, ejection fraction (EF), mean Vcf (mVcf), stroke volume (SV), and cardiac index (CI) were not significantly changed by the treatment (Figs. 4, 5).

Discussion

Recently, the existence of myocardial angiotensin receptors has been reported (8), and angiotensin II is now considered to induce myocardial hypertrophy (2). Possible mechanisms responsible for the decrease of left ventricular mass induced by alacepril treatment are as follows. 1) The significant reduction of blood pressure, which means a decrease of pressure overload. Stretching of the heart muscle can induce myocardial hypertrophy through the activation of protein kinase C (1, 5, 6), and it is natural to consider that the reduction of blood pressure overload, which is related to muscle stretching, can induce regression of myocardial hypertrophy. 2) ACE inhibitory action itself influences cardiac mass, as mentioned above. 3) The inhibitory action of alacepril on the peripheral adrenergic system (15), which is thought to be related to cardiac hypertrophy (9, 17). 4) Vascular dilatative effects of the kallikrein-kinin and prostaglandin systems, which are activated by alacepril. Cardiac function, on the other hand, was not significantly influenced by long-term treatment with alacepril.

In our former studies with spontaneously hypertensive rats (SHR), myocardial contractility as estimated by the isometric tension development in isolated left ventricular papillary muscles, showed no significant differences between SHR and control Wistar-Kyoto rats (WKY). Long-term treatment of SHR with antihypertensive drugs did not influence the developed isometric tension, despite the regression of cardiac hypertrophy (10–13). This means that the myocardial contractile system was not significantly altered by treatment with the antihypertensive drugs. Cardiac diastolic dysfunction, which is induced by collagen remodeling (16), must also be investigated. The inhibitory effects of ACE inhibitors on cardiac diastolic dysfunction can also be expected for alacepril, although this aspect was not examined in the present study.

References

1. Cooper G, Kent RL, Uboh CE, Thompson EW, Marino TA (1985) Hemodynamic versus adrenergic control of cat right ventricular hypertrophy. J Clin Invest 75:1403–1414
2. Dzau VJ (1988) Cardiac renin-angiotensin system: molecular and functional aspects. Am J Med 84(Suppl 3A):22–27
3. Hammond IW, Devereux RB, Alderman MH, Lutas EM, Spitzer MC, Crowley JS, Laragh JH (1986) The prevalence and correlates of echocardiographic left ventricular hypertrophy among employed patients with uncomplicated hypertension. J Am Coll Cardiol 7:639–650
4. Hosoki K, Takeyama K, Minato H, Fukuya F, Kawahara S, Kadokawa T (1986) Effect of alacepril on renin-angiotensin-aldosterone system and kallikrein-kinin-prostaglandin system in experimental animals. Arzneim-Forsch 36:77–83
5. Izumo S, Nadal-Ginard B, Mahdavi V (1988) Protooncogene induction and reprogramming of cardiac gene expression produced by pressure overload. Proc Natl Acad Sci USA 85:339–343
6. Komuro I, Kurabayashi N, Takaku F, Yazaki Y (1988) Expression of cellular oncogenes in the myocardium during the developmental stage and pressure-overloaded hypertrophy of the rat heart. Circ Res 62:1075–1079
7. Matsuno Y, Taira N, Fujitani B, Ito T, Kadokawa T (1986) General pharmacology of the novel angiotensin converting enzyme inhibitor alacepril. Arzneim-Forsch 36:55–62
8. Re RN (1987) Cellular mechanisms of growth in cardiovascular tissue. Am J Cardiol 60:1041
9. Simpson P (1983) Norepinephrine-stimualted hypertrophy of cultured rat myocardial cells in an alpha 1 adrenergic response. J Clin Invest 72:732–738
10. Takeda N, Kanemura M, Noma K, Ohkubo T, Nagano M (1987) Influences of long-term treatment with antihypertensive drugs on left ventricular myosin isoenzyme pattern in spontaneously hypertensive rats. In: Beamish RE, Panagia V, Dhalla NS (eds) Pharmacological aspects of heart disease. Nijhoff, Boston, pp 119–124
11. Takeda N, Nakamura I, Hatanaka T, Ohkubo T, Nagano M (1988) Effects of bunitrolol on myocardial contractility and left ventricular myosin isoenzyme pattern. Arzneim-Forsch 38:1280–1282
12. Takeda N, Nakamura I, Ohkubo T, Iwai T, Tanamura A, Nagano M (1989) Effects of long-term treatment with the α_1-blocker bunazosin on cardiac hypertrophy and myocardial contractile energetics in SHR. J Mol Cell Cardiol 21(Suppl II):S65
13. Takeda N, Ohkubo T, Iwai T, Tanamura A, Nagano M (1990) Influence of long-term arotinolol treatment on myocardial mechanics and ventricular myosin isoenzymes in spontaneously hypertensive rats. Arch int Pharmacodyn 305:63–68
14. Takeyama K, Minato H, Fukuya F, Kawahara S, Hosoki K, Kadokawa T (1985) Antihypertensive activity of alacepril, an orally active angiotensin converting enzyme inhibitor, in renal hypertensive rats and dogs. Arzneim-Forsch 35:1502–1507

15. Takeyama K, Minato H, Ikeno A, Hosoki K, Kadoma T (1986) Antihypertensive mechanism of alacepril: effect on norepinephrine-induced vasoconstrictive response in vitro and in vivo. Arzneim-Forsch 36:74–77
16. Weber KT, Janicki JS, Shroff SG, Pick R, Chen RM, Bashey RI (1988) Collagen remodeling of the pressure-overloaded, hypertrophied nonhuman primate myocardium. Circ Res 62:757–765
17. Yamori Y, Ooshima A, Tarazi RC (1980) Prevention of cardiovascular structural changes in norepinephrine-induced hypertension by alpha and beta blockers. Clin Exp Hypertension 2:347–357

Authors' address:

Dr. Nobuakira Takeda
Department of Internal Medicine
Aoto Hospital
Jikei University School of Medicine
Aoto 6-41-2, Katsushika-ku
Tokyo 125, Japan

Part V: Cardioprotection: Dietetic and Pharmacological Treatments

Phenomenon of the adaptive stabilization of sarcoplasmic and nuclear structures in myocardium

F. Z. Meerson, I. Yu. Malyshev, and A. B. Shneider

Institute of General Pathology and Pathological Physiology of the USSR AMS, Moscow, USSR

Summary: In adaptation of rats to repeated stress exposure, a mechanism gradually forms at the level of heart to provide a considerable increase in the organ resistance to reperfusion paradox and toxic concentrations of catecholamines and Ca^{2+}. Sarcoplasmic reticulum and mitochondria isolated from the hearts of adapted animals are highly resistant to autolysis, and nuclei to the damaging action of one-chain DNA. These changes are named phenomenon of the adaptive stabilization of structures (PhASS). An important role of myocardial heat shock protein (HSP) accumulation in the mechanism of PhASS is shown. The development of PhASS is accompanied by an increased resistance of myocardium to ischemic necrosis.

Key words: Adaptation; stress; autolysis; DNA; stress-limiting systems

Introduction

In the past decade, it was shown that repeated action of nondamaging short-term stressful situations results in adaptation of the organism. This adaptation does not only increase the resistance to severe stress, but also exerts a broad protective cross-effect, protecting the organism against direct ischemic, chemical toxicity, cold, and even radiation damages [for review, see (7)]. With respect to the heart it was established that animals adapted to repeated immobilization or emotional painful stress exposure gain a high resistance to ischemic and reperfusion arrhythmias and cardiac fibrillation. Adaptation to repeated stress also prevents disturbances of the heart electric stability in experimental myocardial infarction and eliminates seemingly stable disturbances of the electric stability in post-infarction cardiosclerosis (7).

In recent years is appeared that adaptation to repeated stress is accompanied by an activation of central mechanisms which limit stress reaction, namely, GABAergic, opioidergic, and serotonergic systems (10). Simultaneously, an activation of such local stress-limiting systems as prostaglandin, antioxidant, and the up-regulation of adenosinergic receptors (6) is observed in executive organs. These data have led us to a hypothesis which is illustrated by the scheme in Fig. 1. The hypothesis is based on the fact that just the coordinated activation of central and local stress-limiting systems is the cause of the cardioprotective effect of adaptation.

However, the most important question has remained open, i.e., to what extent the adaptive protection of the heart against various injuries depends on central mechanisms, and to what extent it is determined by mechanisms formed at the level of heart itself under the action of repeated stress exposure.

The simplest approach to this problem was to determine to what extent the cardioprotective effect of adaptation observed in vivo was preserved in isolated hearts and in cellular organelles isolated from myocardium of adapted animals.

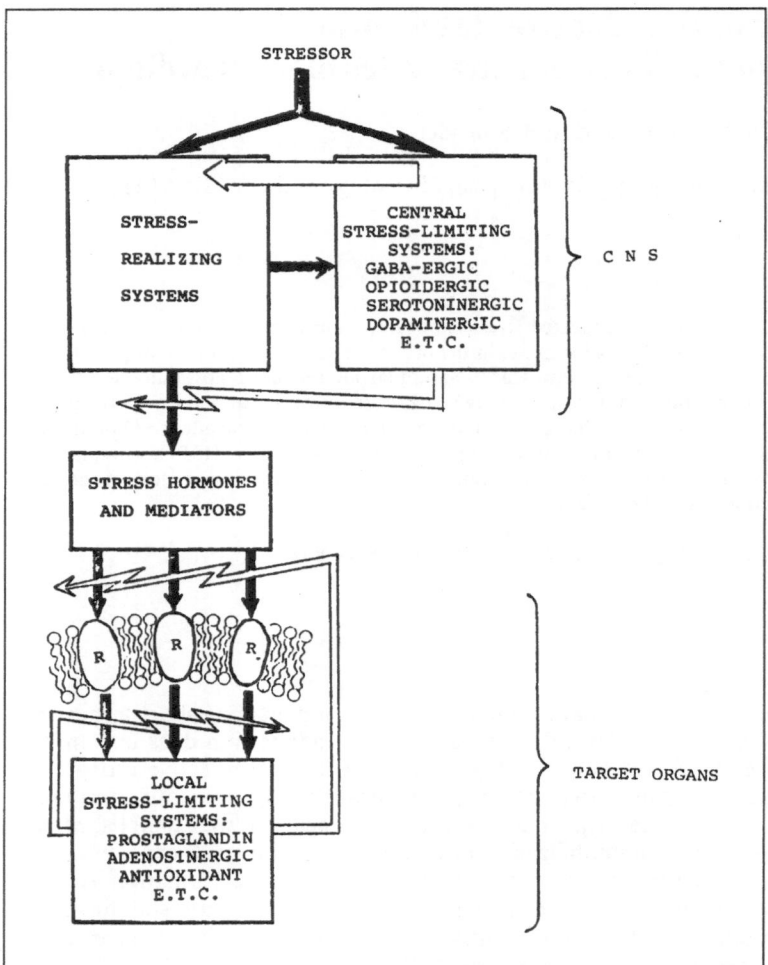

Fig. 1. Central and local stress-limiting systems

Method of adaptation

Wistar male rats were adapted to stress exposure by short-term fixation on their backs for 1 h during 18 days every second day, as described earlier (9). At the end of the immobilization course, none of the animals had any stress damage.

Results and Discussion

It was shown that such course of preliminary adaptation considerably enhanced the resistance of isolated hearts to the Hearse's reperfusion paradox (4), toxic concentrations of catecholamines, and toxic concentrations of Ca^{2+}.

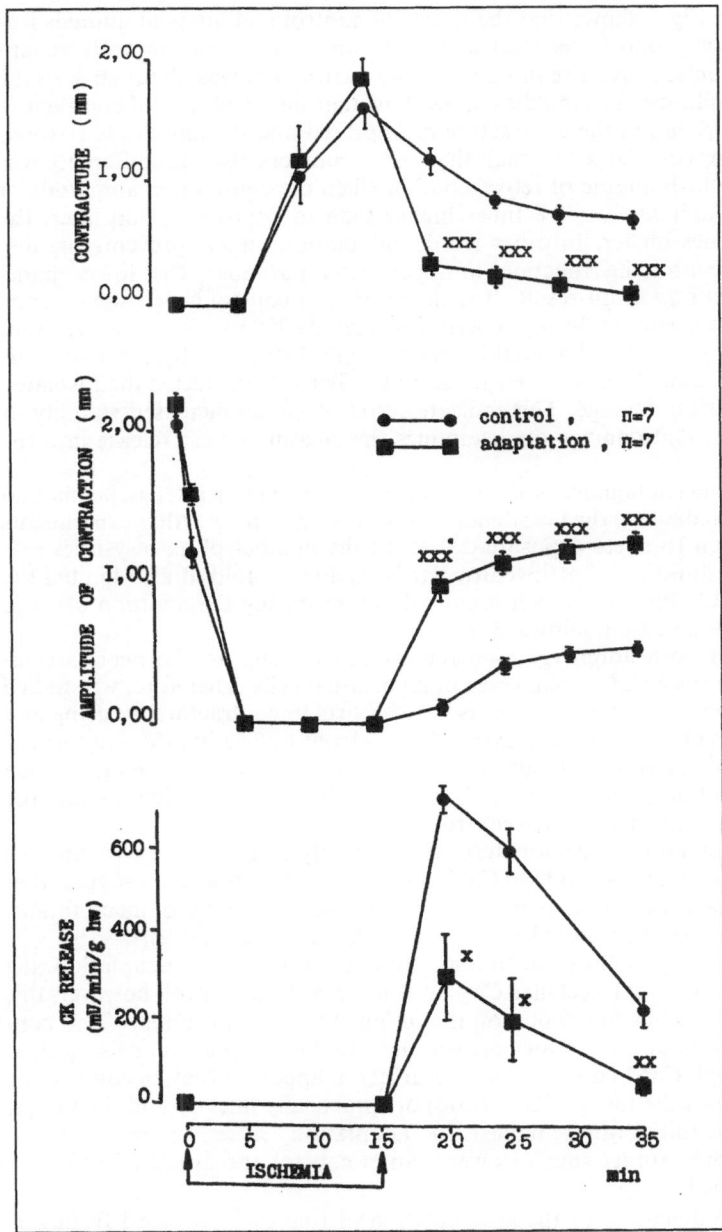

Fig. 2. Effect of adaptation to stress exposure on the contracture, contraction amplitude, and CK release from rat isolated heart in ischemia and reperfusion. Abscissa = time, min. Results are expressed as means ± SE. Significance of difference from the control – (*)p < 0.05; (**)p < 0.01; (***)p < 0.001

The upper curve in Fig. 2 shows that the hearts of control and adapted animals isolated according to Langendorff responded to a 15-min total ischemia with an approximately similar contracture. The intensity of the contracture was about 80% of the initial contraction amplitude. The middle curves show that the amplitude of contracture is depressed. In reoxygenation the contracture disappeared and the amplitude restored much faster in the hearts of adapted animals than in the control ones. This difference was especially large in the fifth minute of reoxygenation when the contraction amplitude of hearts from adapted animals was 8.8 times higher than in control. 20 min later, the amplitude was 2.5 times higher. In other words, adaptation largely prevents the disturbances of heart contractile function in reperfusion paradox. The lower panel demonstrates the most important result. It is shown that in control hearts the creatine kinase release into the perfusate during reperfusion exceeds 700 mU per min per gram heart weight, while in the adapted animal hearts it is only 250 mU. Thus, it is obvious that the adaptation of animals to repeated stress quite efficiently protected their isolated hearts against reperfusion damage. This indicates, first of all, an increased stability of sarcolemma and, thus, that damage predetermines the creatine kinase release into the perfusate.

An abundance of catecholamines is the second important factor after ischemia and reperfusion which both damage the heart under natural conditions. Further experiments showed that adaptation to stress exposure decreased the number of extrasystoles 6.5-fold, and reduced the duration of atrioventricular blockade 2.5-fold; it also limited the depression of contractile function which usually develops during the addition of toxic adrenalin doses into the perfusing solution (5).

It is important that both adrenergic and reperfusion damage to the heart are induced by the appearance of Ca^{2+} abundance in myocardial cells. Therefore, we studied the effect of adaptation on the resistance of isolated hearts to contracture-inducing and arrhythmogenic effects of the increase in external Ca^{2+} from 1.36 to 10 mM. It appeared that, in the hearts of adapted animals, the maximum value of contracture which developed under the action of increased Ca^{2+} was three times less, and that the number of extrasystoles was five times less than in control.

Thus, preliminary adaptation to short-term stress greatly increases the resistance of isolated hearts of adapted animals to high Ca^{2+} concentrations. These data suggest that adaptation somehow increased the activity and the resistance to damage of membranous mechanisms responsible for the removal of Ca^{2+} excess from myocardial cells.

Our recent experiments (11) have shown that, both in control and in adaptation, the rate of Ca^{2+} uptake grew as extracellular Ca^{2+} was increased. In control, however, this value reached a plateau, while in adaptation it continued to grow at similar Ca^{2+} concentrations. Then the rate of Ca^{2+} transport was increased in adapted animals, both at physiological and at high Ca^{2+} concentrations. Further, it appeared that, in control, the storage at 4° C decreased the rate of Ca^{2+} transport practically linearly and, in 4 days, only about 20% of the initial rate remained. In "adaptation" series, the rate of Ca^{2+} transport reduced during storage much slower than in control and appeared to be 2.5 times as high as in control.

In homogenates the dynamics of the accumulation of free Ca^{2+} released from sarcoplasmic reticulum and mitochondria can serve as another criterion of the state of membranous structures of the myocardium. In 4 days of storage of control preparations, the Ca^{2+} content increased by 62% of the initial level. Adaptation to stress exposure decelerated by 2.5 times the growth of Ca^{2+} level and, in 4 days of storage, the Ca^{2+} content did not significantly differ from the initial level. This striking fact of a practically complete absence of Ca^{2+} leakage from intracellular Ca^{2+} stores following preliminary adaptation indicates a significant increase in the stability of membranous structures in the process of adaptation.

In order to evaluate the revealed stabilization of sarcoplasmic reticulum membranes, we had to decide whether it is a particular phenomenon characteristic only of these organelles, or if it is a general regularity which all cellular structures conform to.

To solve this question, the dynamics of inactivation of respiration and phosphorylation were studied in isolated mitochondria during storage of mitochondrial suspension at 4° C. It was shown (8) that, in conditions of a complete oxidation-phosphorylation uncoupling, the oxygen consumption during succinate oxidation by preparations from adapted animals was initially similar to that in control. During storage of mitochondria from adapted animals, however, the oxygen consumption fell much slower than in control, and in 2 days it appeared to be higher by 50% than in control. Adaptation to stress exerted a similar effect on the dynamics of phosphorylation. As a result, in 2 days of storage, the rate of phosphorylation was twice as high as in control.

Thus the obtained results evidence that, in adaptation to stress exposure, a mechanism is realized at the level of heart (which provides the stabilization of structures of sarcolemma, sarcoplasmic reticulum, and mitochondria) that is essentially the main structures of the myocardial cell. We named this "a phenomenon" of the adaptive stabilization of structures – PhASS.

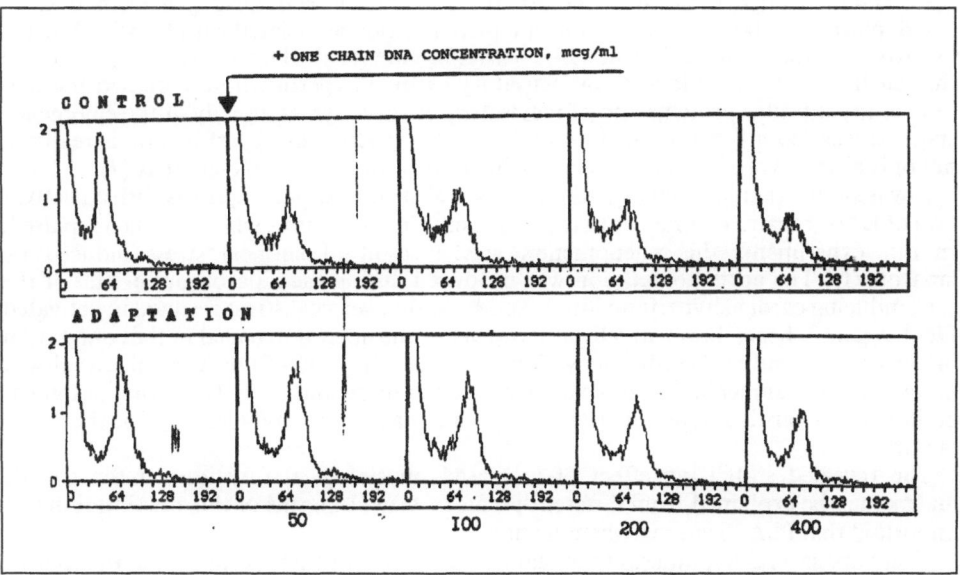

Fig. 3. Effect of adaptation to stress exposure on the resistance of nuclear DNA from myocardial cells to the damaging action of one-chain exogenous DNA. Upper part of figure: histograms of the nuclear DNA distribution in control; lower part: the same after adaptation. Histograms: ordinate – number of nuclei, thousands; abscissa: fluorescence intensity of DNA-bound dye in relative units, analyzer channels. The nuclei containing normal diploid DNA are within the range of 48 to 112 channels. To the left of the arrow: histograms of nuclear suspensions in control and adaptation without addition of one-chain DNA. To the right of the arrow: histograms of the nuclei following the addition of one-chain DNA in concentration of 50, 100, 200, 400 µg/ml (as indicated under the histograms)

Further, a question arose whether the PhASS occurs only in cytoplasmic structures or if it also develops at the level of DNA genetic matrix. In order to solve this problem, we estimated the effect of adaptation on the resistance of isolated myocardial nuclei to the damaging effect of one-chain exogenous DNA, according to Watson's method (13). One-chain DNA is known to activate nuclear proteases and, in effect, can trigger the process of DNA destruction in cellular nuclei.

Histograms in Fig. 3 demonstrate the effect of adaptation on the magnitude of fluorescence peak of myocardial nuclei with normal DNA content. The nuclei were stained with ethidium bromide, a DNA-binding dye. It is also seen that, prior to the administration of one-chain DNA into the nuclei suspension, the magnitude of fluorescence peak in control was similar to that in adaptation and, therefore, the number of nuclei with normal diploid DNA content was also similar. After the administration of one chain DNA, a dramatic decrease in the fluorescence peak was observed and, therefore, the nuclei destruction occurred in control animals. In adaptation, this phenomenon was absent. The magnitude of fluorescence peak decreased only slightly, even at high one-chain DNA concentrations.

Quantitative study of this phenomenon showed that, in control, almost half of the nuclei were already damaged at one-chain DNA concentration of 50 µg/ml. In adaptation, this phenomenon was 5.5 times less pronounced. When the one-chain DNA concentration was increased, this protective effect of adaptation remained. Thus, PhASS is realized not only in cytoplasmic structures but also at the level of DNA genetic matrix.

Adaptation to stress is not a unique adaptive reaction associated with PhASS. Indeed, as early as in the 1970s, Zak et al. (14), Aschenbrenner et al. (1), and later we (7) showed that such adaptive reaction as compensatory cardiac hyperfunction increased the lifetime of myofibrillar proteins and of respiratory chain enzymes already at the emergency stage. It was recently established that this stabilizing effect of hyperfunction is realized, not only at the level of cellular organelles, but also at the level of DNA matrix (7).

It was shown that internal organs respond to a sufficiently strong stress with an activation of DNA repair. This means that stress results in disruptions which are then repaired. In our experiments this phenomenon was a result of surgical stress induced by laparotomy. The aorta coarctation was produced during the laparotomy in half of the rats, inducing cardiac hyperfunction. It appeared that surgical stress resulted in activated DNA repair in heart, brain, and liver. However, if the operation ended in the coarctation of aorta, which induced cardiac hyperfunction, the activation of DNA repair was absent in the myocardium while it completely remained in brain and liver. Therefore, in our experiments, in cardiac hyperfunction the genetic matrix was stabilized by local cellular factors.

The revealed stabilizing effect of increased physiological function on the genetic matrix may be explained from different points of view. In terms of this presentation it is important that PhASS is a real phenomenon.

There are several hypotheses to explain PhASS. One of them results from the following statement. Repeated stressful situations inevitably involve many repeated effects of stress hormones on so-called calcium-mobilizing receptors which activate the inositol triphosphate-diacylglycerol regulatory system via phospholipase C.

Estimating the situation given in Fig. 4, one should keep in mind that inositol triphosphate affects specific receptors in sarcoplasmic reticulum in order to release Ca^{2+} therefrom. Thus, this is an intracellular messenger of urgent adaptive reactions. At the same time, diacylglycerol is a messenger of long-term adaptation; it can activate transcription, growth, and proliferation of cells via protein kinase C and sarcolemmal sodium-hydrogen exchanger. Outstanding works by Hammond et al. (3), Currie and

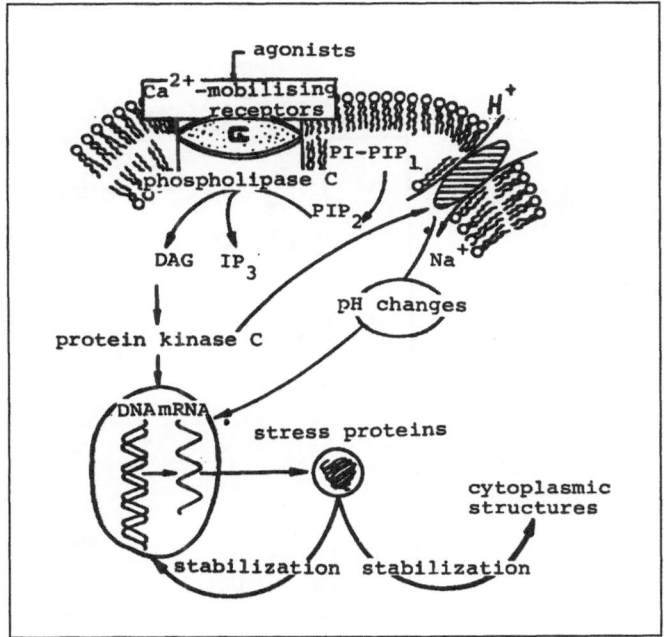

Fig. 4. Hypothetic mechanism of the stabilization of cellular structures in repeated stress exposure. G = G-protein; PIP_1 = phosphoinositol phosphate; PIP_2 = phosphoinositol diphosphate; IP_3 = inositol triphosphate; DAG = diacylglycerol. (For further explanation, see text.)

White (2), Schwartz (12), and others have shown that such activation of genetic apparatus during hyperfunction and hypertrophy, heat shock, and hypoxia, i.e., different, but a priori stressful situations, results in accumulation of heat shock proteins (HSPs). These stress proteins normalize function of the damaged nuclei, eliminate disturbances of mRNA splicing and of ribosome formation in nucleoli. They possess a wonderful capacity to disaggregate anomalous protein-to-protein hydrophobic bonds. Thus, stress proteins eliminate and limit injuries of protein structures.

The scheme reflects a hypothesis that, in repeated stress, the increase in diacylglycerol concentration activates genes which determine the synthesis of stress proteins. These proteins realize PhASS, both at the level of cellular organelles and at the level of the genetic matrix itself.

In order to approach testing of this hypothesis, we had to solve at least two problems: 1) to learn whether PhASS is accompanied by an increase in the heart thermal stability, and 2) it was important to directly measure the content of HSP in myocardium of animals adapted to stress.

The curves in Fig. 5A show that, in control, the heating of perfusion solution from 37° to 42° C results in a depression of the contraction amplitude of isolated hearts by the development of contracture and, what is most important, heating results in a massive release of creatine kinase into the perfusate. In fact, by the 15th min of the hot solution perfusion, the amplitude reduced sixfold. The creatine kinase activity in perfusate reached 300 mU/min/g wet weight. In adaptation the amplitude was 2.5 times as high as in control and the enzyme release into the perfusate was practically absent. Thus, we can

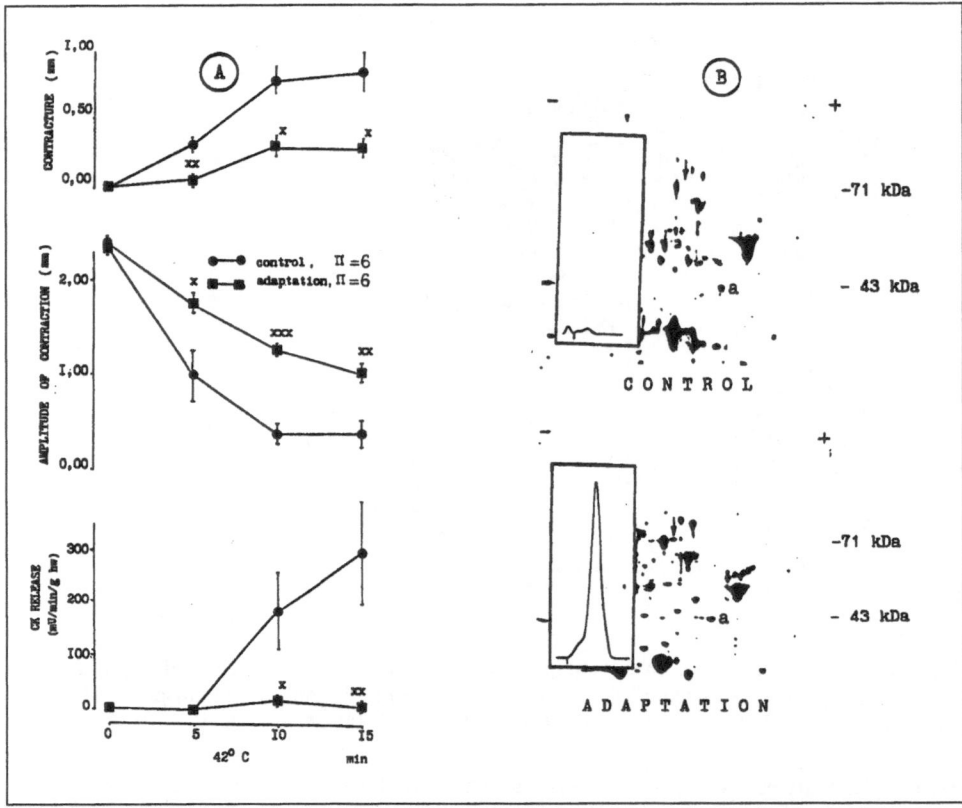

Fig. 5. Effect of adaptation to stress exposure on the contracture, amplitude of contractions, and CK release from isolated heart at high temperature (42°) (A) and on myocardial protein profiles (B). (x)p < 0.05; (xx)p < 0.01; (xxx)p < 0.001.

say that the considerable increase in the heart thermal stability is one of the PhASS components, as well as the increased resistance of the heart to the reperfusion paradox and to toxic catecholamine concentrations.

It is quite important that, in our experiments, the PhASS components never developed as a result of a single stress exposure, but always followed a series of such exposures (i.e., formed as a result of adaptation). This fact allows to suggest that PhASS is connected with the accumulation of stress proteins, HSPs in particular.

Figure 5 B allows to compare protein profiles obtained from the control hearts and the hearts after adaptation. We can see that in the gels obtained from the control hearts, the large inducible HSP 71 is practically indetectable. The site of its localization is seen as a small "mist". However, in the hearts of adapted animals, an intense staining with sharp contours appears in the same region. To the left of the pictures there are corresponding densitograms of this protein. Laser densitometry is known to provide the determination of both the protein concentration in gel and of the width of zone which this protein occupies. This fact allows to compare the amounts of HSP 71 in control and in adaptation

Table 1. Effect of adaptation to stress exposure on stereometric indices of the ischemic heart damage (mean ± SEM)

Experimental series	Volume of ischemic zone, % of the left-ventricular myocardium volume	Volume of necrotic zone, % of the ischemic zone volume	Volume of ischemic myo-cardium not subjected to necrosis, % of the ischemic zone volume (restoration zone)	Volume of necrosis, % of the left-ventricular myocardium volume
Control (n = 14)	36.8 ± 3.6	73.5 ± 3.8	26.5 ± 1.7	27.0 ± 1.4
Adaptation (n = 11)	34.3 ± 4.1	44.7 ± 4.1*	55.3 ± 2.0*	15.3 ± 1.4*

Significance of differences: *$p > 0.05$; n = number of animals.

in relative values. It is seen that the adaptation increased the content of this protein at least by 37 times.

A single stress does not result in such an accumulation of HSP 71. Thus, the matter is one of the adaptive accumulation of this stress protein simultaneously with the PhASS development. This coincidence can be regarded as evidence in favor of the role of HSP in the PhASS genetic mechansim. Of course, HSPs form only one of the links of the complex PhASS mechanism. On the whole, this mechanism is still waiting to be investigated.

At the same time, the existence of PhASS itself is beyond doubt and, what is more, PhASS works: it protects the myocardium against ischemic necroses.

While carrying out our recent morphological investigation, we used a well-known statement that there are three zones to be determined in the myocardium following the coronary artery ligation: a) a large zone of primary ischemia; 2) a relatively small zone of restoration, and 3) a zone of necrosis which is distinctly seen in 2 days.

It follows from Table 1 that, in our experiments, the course of adaptation to short-term stress does not affect the volume of ischemic zone 5 min after the left coronary artery ligation in rat. However, the volume of necrotic tissue which was measured 2 days after the artery ligation was reduced by more than 40% in the hearts of adapted animals. This protective action became possible because a considerably lesser part of the primarily ischemic tissue was subjected to necrosis than in control.

Therefore, adaptation to stress has no anti-ischemic effect, but it possesses a strong cytoprotective effect. We believe that this effect is an expression of PhASS.

Conclusion

In conclusion, it should be noted that the PhASS is a generalized phenomenon: in adaptation it develops, not only in the heart, but in other organs as well. Further analysis of PhASS mechanisms has a basic significance. Practical significance of the PhASS is determined by the fact that the PhASS is inducible without any stress, by a course of special physiotherapeutic procedures which can be efficiently used in clinic.

References

1. Aschenbrenner V, Druyan R, Albin R, Rabinovitz M (1970) Haem a, cytochrome c and total protein turnover in mitochondria from rat heart and liver. Biochem J 119:157–168
2. Currie RW, White FP (1981) Trauma-induced protein in rat tissues: a physiological role for a "heat shock protein"? Science 214:72–73
3. Hammond DL, Lai JK, Markert CL (1982) Diverse forms of stress lead to a new pattern of gene expression through a common and essential metabolic pathway. Proc Natl Acad Sci USA 79:3485
4. Hearse DJ, Humphrey SM, Chain EB (1973) Abrupt reoxygenation of the anoxic potassium arrested perfused rat heart. J Mol Cell Cardiol 5:395–401
5. Malyshev IYu (1989) Adaptation of the organism to stress exposure increases the heart resistance to adrenotoxic damage (in Russian). Bull Exper Biol Med 4:411–413
6. Meerson FZ (1988) The role of lipid peroxidation in the myocardium in stress and the antioxidant protection of the heart. In: Singal PK (ed) Oxygen radicals in the pathophysiology of heart disease. Kluwer Academic Publishers, Boston, pp 285–301
7. Meerson FZ (1991) Adaptive protection of the heart: protecting against stress and ischemic damage. CRC Press, Boca Raton
8. Meerson FZ (1990) Phenomenon of the adaptive stabilization of structures and protection of the heart (in Russian). Kardiologiya 3:6–12
9. Meerson FZ, Malyshev IYu, Sazontova TG (1990) Adaptation to stress exposure prevents arrhythmogenic and contractural effects of the excess of Ca^{2+} on the heart by increased activity of sarcoplasmic reticulum. Basic Res Cardiol 85:96–103
10. Meerson FZ, Pshennikova MG, Belkina LM, Abdikaliev NA, Malyshev IYu (1989) Prevention of ischemic arrhythmias by activation of stress-limiting systems of the organism. CV World Report 2:205–212
11. Meerson FZ, Sazontova TG, Arkhipenko YuV (1990) Increased resistance of cardiac sarcoplasmic reticulum Ca^{2+} pump to autolysis after adaptation of rats to stress. Biomed Sci 1:373–378
12. Schwartz K, Boheler KR, Chassagne C, Bastie D, Mercadier JJ (1990) The mechanogenic transduction of the hypertrophied mammalian myocardium. J Mol Cell Cardiol 22(Suppl II):8
13. Watson JV, Nakeff A, Chambers SH, Smith PS (1985) Flow cytometric fluorescence emission spectrum analysis of Hoechst 33343 strained DNA in chicken thymocytes. Cytometry 6:310–315
14. Zak R, Aschenbrenner V, Rabinowitz M (1971) Synthesis and degradation of myosin in cardiac hypertrophy. J Clin Invest 50:1020

Author's address:

Prof. F. Z. Meerson
Institute of General Pathology
and Pathological Physiology
USSR Academy of Medical Sciences
Baltiyskaya str. 8
Moscow-315, USSR

Cardioprotection: endogenous protective mechanisms promoted by prostacyclin

L. Szekeres, J. Pataricza, Z. Szilvássy, É. Udvary, and Á. Végh

Institute of Pharmacology, Albert Szent-Györgyi Medical University, Szeged, Hungary

Summary: Evidence is accumulating that acute stress situations such as ischemia, adrenergic dominance, and ouabain intoxication enhance production of endogenous substances (PgI_2, adenosine, NO) which may protect the myocardium from harmful consequences of these stress situations. PgI_2 and its stable analogue 7-oxo-PgI_2 exert an early direct- and induce a delayed indirect antiischemic, antiarrhythmic, and cytoprotective effect. The direct action is shortlasting; it protects from myocardial ischemia and arrhythmias, at least partly, by its vasodilating, antiaggregatory, and "membrane-stabilizing" effects. The delayed, long-lasting PgI_2-induced protection from postocclusion, reperfusion- and ouabain-arrhythmias is dose- (optimal 50 µg/kg) and time- (optimal 48 h after treatment) dependent. Its mechanism is probably based on a 7-oxo-PgI_2 induced increase in the activity of Na/K-ATP-ase, and further, on a reduced sensitivity to β-adrenergic agonists and to changes at the cardiac membrane level, resulting in a prolongation of the action potential duration and the effective refractory period.

Key words: Endogenous cardioprotective mechanisms; prostacyclin; early and delayed effect; antiischemic effect; antiarrhythmic effect; ouabain toxicity

Introduction

Life-threatening situations such as heart attack and alarm reactions associated with increased sympathetic drive or arrhythmias due to digitalis overdose are survived by a substantial number of patients. Survival is partly, but not only genetically determined. Observations show that repeated or persistent mild stresses such as physical exercise or moderate hypoxia may increase resistance against consequences of such alarm situations. Evidence is accumulating that endogenous substances such as prostacyclin (PgI_2), adenosine, and nitric oxide (NO) released during mild stresses may protect the heart from deleterious effects of the above-mentioned life-threatening situations.

The present paper is devoted to our observations concerning the cardioprotective actions of prostacyclin and its analogue, which is stable in solution: 7-oxo-PgI_2 [synthetized by Kovács et al. (4)].

Prostacyclin, a metabolite of the arachidonate cascade promotes endogenous cardioprotective mechanisms: 1) directly, by ischemic release of PgI_2 during preconditioning; and 2) indirectly, by a late appearing cardioprotective action induced by endogenous or exogenous PgI_2 (or its stable analogues, e.g., 7-oxo-PgI_2).

Ischemic release of PgI_2 during preconditioning

Preconditioning is a brief ischemic stress (e.g., a brief coronary artery occlusion) which may protect the heart from consequences of sustained periods of ischemia, such as irreversible cell injury (6, 8, 9), as well as from fatal arrhythmias (3, 23, 24).

In anesthetized thoracotomized dogs Végh et al. (24) have shown that the protection of two short (5 min) preconditioning occlusions from elevation of the ST-segment in the epicardial ECG, as well as from arrhythmias appearing during sustained occlusion (25 min) and the following reperfusion period could be greatly reduced by inhibition of the cyclooxygenase by means of meclophenamate. Thus, ischemic release of PgI_2 could at least partly account for the otherwise shortlasting [no more than 1 h (23)] cardioprotection. The protection could be at least partly attributed to the vasodilating antiaggregatory and "membrane-stabilizing" effects of PgI_2. Reduced sensitivity to β-adrenergic stimuli may also play a role, as shown by Szilvássy and Szekeres (unpublished results) in conscious rabbits, in which ventricular pacing at 500/min rate for 5 min significantly moderated the isoproterenol-induced tachycardia and shortening of the ventricular effective refractory period up to 2 h.

Late appearing cardioprotective action of PgI_2

In addition to the above described short-lasting "direct" protective effect of prostacyclin, a later appearing and long-lasting cardioprotective action after administration of PgI_2 and its stable analogue 7-oxo-PgI_2 was described by us in 1983 (12).

We have shown that 7-oxo-PgI_2 induces a dose- and time-dependent (optimal: 48 h after 50 µg/kg dose of 7-oxo-PgI_2 = in the following: "pretreatment") protection from:
– coronary-occlusion-induced ischemic ST-segment elevation (11, 12, 21);
– early postocclusion and reperfusion arrhythmias in anesthetized dogs (12, 13, 21), and late arrhythmias appearing in conscious dogs 24 h after recovery from two-stage coronary occlusion (25);
– ischemic loss of intracellular K_i^+, gain in Na_i^+ and reperfusion-induced accumulation of Ca_i^{2+} in myocardial cells of isolated guinea pig hearts exposed to 25 min global ischemia followed by 15 min reperfusion (14, 10).
– In isolated guinea pig hearts subjected to the same procedure, pretreatment prevented ischemia-induced early structural changes, such as shortening of sarcomeres, swelling of mitochondria, and – in the reperfusion phase – accumulation of Ca deposits in the mitochondria (10).
– In isolated guinea pig hearts subjected to the same procedure, pretreatment moderated postischemic and reperfusion-induced elevation of the left-ventricular end-diastolic pressure and diminution of coronary blood flow (21, 22).
– Pretreatment also moderated ischemic breakdown of ATP and CP and accumulation of lactate in excised rat hearts incubated in Ringer solution for 1 min (20, 14).

All these protective actions appeared already in the isolated heart in the absence of extracardiac factors such as nervous and hormonal influences or blood constituents such as platelets, white and red blood cells.

Pretreatment did not affect the above parameters under normal conditions, but protected against harmful consequences of myocardial ischemia and reperfusion (26).

There was but one exception, namely:
– Pretreatment distinctly prolonged the effective refractory period and repolarization time (QT) in normal conscious rabbits and guinea pigs, and in anesthetized dogs (17). In isolated papillary muscle preparation of rabbits incubated for 20 min with 10^{-8} mol/l 7-oxo-PgI_2, prolongation of ERP and APD_{90} appeared only 2 h after washout of the substance (15).
– Pretreatment doubled the ouabain dose necessary to evoke extrasystoles, VT, VF, and cardiac arrest in anesthetized guinea pigs (18). It also increased the doses needed to

produce toxic ouabain effects in anesthetized dogs; at the same time, it reduced the positive inotropic ED_{25} dose and, thus, nearly doubled the therapeutic range of ouabain (16, 18).

In addition to these *cardiac* protective effects, some *extracardiac* effects contributing to the protective action could be observed:

- a prolongation of the bleeding time (antithrombotic effect) (14) (probably via increased capillary permeability) as well as
- an antiadrenergic effect (diminution of the isoproterenol induced increase in heart rate and blood pressure in conscious rabbits, as well as that of the positive chrono- and inotropic action of the same drug in the isolated rabbit atrial muscle, but increased vasoconstrictory action phenylephrine) was observed (14).

Possible mode of the PgI_2-induced late protective actions

The first question to be answered is whether a direct effect of PgI_2 could contribute to the late protection induced by PgI_2 and 7-oxo-PgI_2? On the basis of the following evidence it is unlikely that the action is a direct effect of PgI_2 or 7-oxo-PgI_2. Their biological half-life is short (4–5 min), but protective effects appeared later (even at large 250 μg dose not earlier then 2 h after drug administration) when platelet activation inhibitory effect and vasodilatory actions characteristic for PgI_2 were already over. Maximal cardioprotection appeared 24–48 h after drug administration, suggesting that a longer time is needed for the full development of the cardioprotective action. Since this time is required for the "de novo" protein synthesis via transcription, this may suggest involvement of protein synthesis in the protective mechanism.

The acute effect of this dose of PgI_2 and of 7-oxo-PgI_2 is an increase of the degree of ischemia (due to the fall in BP and to that of coronary perfusion pressure) and this dose is also arrhythmogenic (19): a) indirectly, by aggravating ischemia; and b) by increasing transmembrane influx of Ca^{2+} (7) and inhibiting K^+, Na^+ ATPase (2), like digitalis and ischemia (the latter due to accumulation of FFAs and of long-chain acyl-carnitines and acyl CoA). This is in contrast to the PgI_2-induced delayed protective action against ischemia and arrhythmias.

This is true even if PgI_2 in low doses does not affect electrophysiological parameters in dogs, however, in the presence of ischemia (occlusion) even low doses (50 μg/kg) are highly arrhythmogenic (19).

On the basis of the following evidence a trigger effect of PgI_2 (and 7-oxo-PgI_2) initiating the development of cardioprotective (metabolic and membrane) changes is more probable. Evidence for this is our finding that, in the isolated papillary muscle preparation, no substantial change in VFRP and APD was seen during short (20 min) incubation with 7-oxo-PgI_2, however, marked prolongation of both parameters appeared 2 h after washout, i.e., in the absence of 7-oxo-PgI_2.

Accordingly, the following factors might be involved in 7-oxo-PgI_2 induced protection from harmful effects of ischemia or ouabain. Both ischemia (NA release) and PgI_2 activate adenylate-cyclase, enhancing cAMP level. Since available phosphodiesterase (PDE) is not sufficient to split all excess cAMP, this latter will accumulate and produce harmful effects (Fig. 1) such as:

- accumulation of free fatty acids (FFA) by activation of triglyceride (TG) lipase. FFA will block Na^+/K^+-ATPase responsible for restoring equilibrium of these cations on both sides of the cardiac membrane after each cycle, and the consequence is cellular potassium loss and sodium gain.

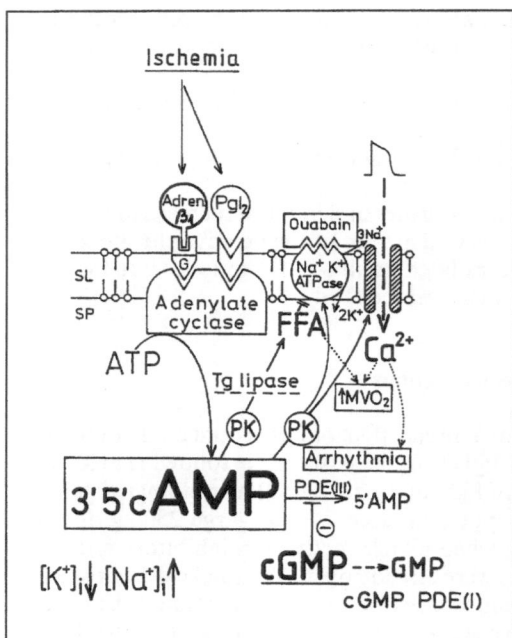

Fig. 1. Some myocardial ischemia-induced metabolic changes responsible for ischemic damage. Abbreviations: SL = sarcolemma; SP = sarcoplasma;   PK = protein-kinase; MVO_2 = myocardial   oxygen   uptake; G = G-protein;   cGMP = cyclic guanyl-monophosphate; cGMP PDE = cGMP splitting PDE (I)

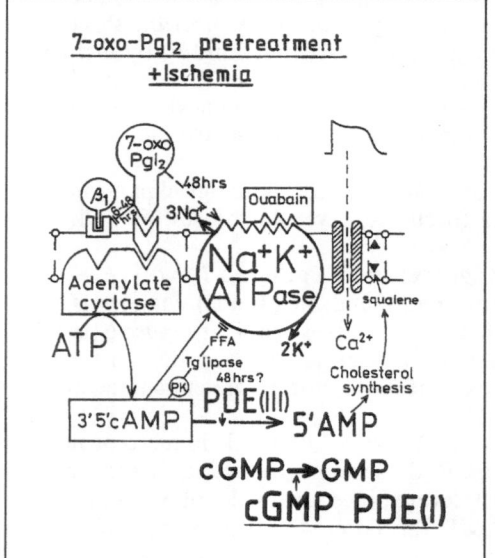

Fig. 2. Effect of 7-oxo-PgI$_2$ pretreatment on metabolic changes produced by myocardial ischaemia. Abbreviations as in Fig. 1

– FFAs also increase myocardial O_2 uptake and aggravate ischemia.
– cAMP activates Ca^{2+}-channels; free cellular Ca^{2+} level rises, promoting the appearance of arrhythmias.

There is now evidence that 7-oxo-PgI_2 initiated induction of enzymes counteracting the harmful effects of ischemia and ouabain.

Dzurba et al. (1) have shown that activity and amount of Na^+/K^+- ATPase in isolated rat heart sarcolemma is nearly doubled by 7-oxo-PgI_2 pretreatment of the animal. This change accounts for: a) prevention of ischemic cellular K^+ loss and Na^+ gain, and b) reduction of ouabain toxicity (Fig. 2).

Krause et al. (5) have found that in rat Langendorff heart preparations from 7-oxo-PgI_2 pretreated animals the isoproterenol-induced increase in contractile force, cAMP content, and phosphorylase A was markedly reduced as compared with the untreated controls. They have also observed an increased activity (amount?) of cGMP hydrolyzing PDE in the particulate fraction of the myocardium of 7-oxo-PgI_2 pretreated rats. The rise in cGMP hydrolysis after 7-oxo-PgI_2 treatment may explain, at least partly, the antiadrenergic effect of pretreatment at the level of cAMP-breakdown.

At lower cytosolic cGMP level the rate of cAMP hydrolysis may accelerate as a consequence of a weakening of the cGMP-induced inhibition of cAMP-PDE III-subtype.

This finding may account for sufficient breakdown of excess cAMP formed in ischemia (Fig. 2).

Conclusions

In sum, the delayed cardioprotective effect induced by 7-oxo-PgI_2 appears as a protection from:
– myocardial ischemia;
– early and late postinfarction arrhythmias;
– reperfusion arrhythmias;
– toxic effects of cardiac glycosides;
– ischemic loss of K^+ and accumulation of Na^+ (and after reperfusion of Ca^{2+}) in myocardial cells;
– early morphologic changes due to ischemia and reperfusion.

The possible mechanism of 7-oxo-PgI_2-induced late cardioprotective effects can be summarized as follows:
– reduced sensitivity to β-adrenergic stimuli;
– increased activity and amount of sarcolemmal Na^+/K^+-ATPase coping with ischemia, and reperfusion-induced loss of K^+ and gain of Na^+ and Ca^{2+} in myocardial cells, as well as with the toxic effects of digitalis;
– increased activity of available myocardial PDE capable of splitting excess cAMP;
– antiarrhythmic electrophysiological changes such as prolongation of ERP and APD (Endogenous Class III antiarrhythmic action);
– hemodynamic changes (bradycardia, moderation of the ischemic rise of the left-ventricular end-diastolic pressure).

References

1. Dzurba A, Ziegelhöffer A, Breier A, Vrbjar N, Szekeres L (1991) Increased activity of sarcolemmal (Na,K)-ATPase is involved in the late cardioprotective action of 7-oxo-prostacyclin. Cardioscience 2:105–108

2. Karmazyn M, Dhalla NS (1983) Physiological and pathophysiological aspects of cardiac prostaglandins. Can J Physiol Pharmacol 61:1207–1225
3. Komori S, Parratt JR, Szekeres L, Végh Á (1990) Preconditioning reduces the severity of ischaemia and reperfusion-induced arrhythmias in both anesthetized rats and dogs. J Physiol Lond 423:16P
4. Kovács G, Simonidesz V, Tömösközi I, Körmöczy P, Székely I, Papp Behr Á, Stadler I, Szekeres L, Papp G (1982) A new stable prostacyclin mimic, 7-oxo-prostaglandin I_2. J Med Chem 25:105–107
5. Krause EG, Bartel S, Luthardt G, Szilvássy Z, Szekeres L (1990) The cytoprotective effect of 7-oxo-prostacyclin (7-oxo) is related to a rise in particulate cGMP hydrolysing PDE activity in the myocardium. J Mol Cell Cardiol 22(Suppl 3):S33
6. Li GC, Vasquez JA, Gallagher KP, Lucchesi BR (1989) Preconditioning with simple or multiple brief coronary artery occlusions limits infarct size. J Mol Cell Cardiol 21(Suppl 1):481
7. Moffat MP (1987) Concentration-dependent effects of prostacyclin on the response of the isolated guinea pig heart to ischemia and reperfusion: possible involvement of the slow inward current. J Pharm Exp Ther 242:292–299
8. Schott R, Rohmann S, Braun E, Winkler B, Jörgen S, Schaper W (1989) The effect of ischemic preconditioning on myocardial oxygen consumption MVO_2 and infarct size in pigs. J Mol Cell Cardiol 21(Suppl 1):482
9. Schott RJ, Rohmann S, Braun ER, Schaper W (1988) Ischemic preconditioning reduces infarct size in swine myocardium. Circ Res 66:1133–1142
10. Szekeres L, Bálint Zs, Karcsú S, Tósaki Á, Udvary É (1989) On the 7-oxo-PgI$_2$ induced late appearing long-lasting cytoprotective effect. Prostaglandins in Clinical Research: Cardiovascular System. Liss Inc, pp 143–147
11. Szekeres L, Koltai M, Pataricza J, Takáts I, Udvary É (1984) On the late antiischaemic action of the stable PgI$_2$ analogue: 7-oxo-PgI$_2$-Na and its possible mode of action. Biomed Biochim Acta 43:S135–S142
12. Szekeres L, Krassói I, Udvary É (1983) Delayed antiischaemic effect of PgI$_2$ and of a new stable PgI$_2$ analogue 7-oxo-Prostacyclin-Na in experimental model angina in dogs. J Mol Cell Cardiol 15(Suppl):394
13. Szekeres L, Krassói I, Pataricza J, Udvary É (1985) Delayed antiischaemic effect of Prostaglandin I$_2$ and of new stable Prostaglandin I$_2$ analogue, 7-oxo-Prostacyclin-Na, in experimental model angina in dogs. In: Dhalla NS, Hearse DJ (eds) Advances in Myocardiology, Vol. 6. New York, Plenum Press, pp 607–618
14. Szekeres L, Németh M, Szilvássy Z, Tósaki Á, Udvary É, Végh Á (1988) On the nature and molecular basis of prostacyclin induced late cardiac changes. Biomed Biochim Acta 47:S6–S11
15. Szekeres L, Németh M, Papp JGy, Udvary É (1990) Short incubation with 7-oxo-Prostacyclin induces long-lasting prolongation of repolarization time and effective refractory period in rabbit papillary muscle preparation. Cardiovasc Res 24:37–41
16. Szekeres L, Szilvássy Z, Udvary É, Végh Á (1989) 7-oxo-PgI$_2$ induced late appearing protection against ouabain induced cardiac arrhythmias in anaesthetized guinea pigs. Pharmacol Res Comm Vol 20(Suppl 1):77–78
17. Szekeres L, Szilvássy Z, Udvary É, Végh Á (1989) 7-oxo-PgI$_2$ induced late appearing and long-lasting electrophysiological changes in the heart in situ of the rabbit, guinea-pig, dog and cat. J Mol Cell Cardiol 21:545–554
18. Szilvássy Z, Szekeres L, Udvary É, Végh Á (1988) On the 7-oxo-PgI$_2$ induced lasting protection against ouabain arrhythmias in anaesthetized guinea pigs. Biomed Biochim Acta 47:S35–S38
19. Taniguchi M, Szekeres L, Udvary É (1989) On the acute cardiac effects of 7-oxo-PgI$_2$ during coronary occlusion and reperfusion. J Mol Cell Cardiol 21(Suppl IV):S48
20. Takáts I, Szekeres L (1985) Effect of 7-oxo-prostacyclin (7-oxo-PgI$_2$). Acta Physiol Hung 66:390
21. Udvary É, Szekeres L (1985) Prostacyclin: antiischaemic or cardioprotective? Proc 4th Cong Hung Pharmacol Soc Budapest, Vol 3. Sect. 7 Prostanoids (eds. V. Kecskeméti, K. Gyires, G. Kovács) 333–338
22. Udvary É, Végh Á, Szekeres L (1988) 7-oxo-PgI$_2$-induced late appearing and long lasting antiischaemic action in dogs. Pharmacol Res Comm Vol 20(Suppl 1):171–172

23. Végh Á, Parratt JR, Szekeres L (1990) Role of time in the protective effect of preconditioning. J Mol Cell Cardiol 22(Suppl 3):S77
24. Végh Á, Szekeres L, Parratt JR (1990) Protective effects of preconditioning of the ischemic myocardium involve cyclo-products. Cardiovasc 24:1020–1023
25. Végh Á (1990) 7-oxo-PgI$_2$ induced delayed protective action from late postocclusion arrhythmias in conscious dogs. In: Slezak J (ed) Ischemia and Reperfusion Injury of the Heart East European Subsection Meeting, International Society for Heart Research, May 13–18, 1990, Smolenice, Czechoslovakia, p 93
26. Végh Á, Udvary É, Szekeres L, Szilvássy Z (1988) 7-oxo-PgI$_2$ induced late appearing and long lasting antiischaemic and antiarrhythmic action in dogs. Biomed Biochim Acta 47:S31–S34

Authors' address:

Prof. Dr. L. Szekeres
University Medical School of Szeged
Institute of Pharmacology
Dóm tér 12
H-6701 Szeged, Hungary

Long-term treatment in arterial hypertension for protecting hypertrophic myocardium

M. Vogt, W. Motz, and B. E. Strauer

Medizinische Klinik und Poliklinik B der Heinrich-Heine-Universität Düsseldorf, Abteilung für Kardiologie, Pneumologie und Angiologie, FRG

Summary: The cardiac organ manifestation of arterial hypertension comprises the myocardium itself with left-ventricular hypertrophy, the interstitium with perivascular and interstitial fibrosis, and the coronary circulation with disease of large and small coronary arteries. The consequences of the sum and interactions of these cardiac organ manifestations have an impact on left-ventricular systolic and diastolic function, the ischemic risk, and the occurrence of arrhythmias in hypertensive patients. As the prognosis of arterial hypertension is determined, to a considerable extent, by these cardiac complications, the aim of treatment of hypertensive heart disease is reversal of the myocardial hypertrophy in order to prevent later progression to hypertensive failure. A further goal of therapy is reversal of hypertensive coronary microangiopathy in order to improve the coronary reserve and to reduce the ischemic risk. Regression of hypertrophy can be induced by suitable antihypertensive drugs (calcium channel blockers of the dihydropyridine type, ACE inhibitors, and sympatholytic substances). While normal systolic function was maintained in the compensated stage of hypertensive hypertrophy and was not significantly influenced by antihypertensive therapy, diastolic function was impaired in a very early stage of arterial hypertension. Both the phase of isovolumic relaxation and the phase of early diastolic filling were impaired, while after long-term antihypertensive treatment with Ca-channel blockers of the dihydropyridine type or ACE inhibitors, only the latter one was improved. From preliminary results there is clinical evidence that hypertensive disease of small coronary arteries can be reversed after long-term antihypertensive treatment with a consequently improved coronay reserve and a reduced ischemic risk.

Moreover, to what extent the prognosis of hypertensive heart disease can be improved by reversal of myocardial hypertrophy and disease of small coronary arteries is yet unknown.

Key words: Left-ventricular hypertrophy; arterial hypertension; regression of hypertrophy; coronary reserve; antihypertensive drugs

Introduction

Arterial hypertension is the most common cause of chronic pressure overload of the heart. The great importance of recognition and adaquate therapeutic management of arterial hypertension results from the high incidence in the population and the prognostic significance of arterial hypertension.

The hypertensive damage to the target organ "heart" comprises myocardial hypertrophy, alterations of the interstitium, and disease of large and small coronary arteries, and determines essentially the prognosis of arterial hypertension (Fig. 1). Left ventricular hypertrophy represents the main structural adaptation of the heart to sustained pressure overload. According to the Framingham Study, electrocardiographic signs and echocardiographic assessment of left-ventricular hypertrophy in hypertensive patients are associated with an increased cardiovascular mortality (12, 17) and, particularly, with an increased incidence of sudden death (13). With respect to the coronary circulation arterial hypertension is an important risk factor for the development of coronary artery disease. However, angina pectoris is often a complaint in hypertensive patients, even in the ab-

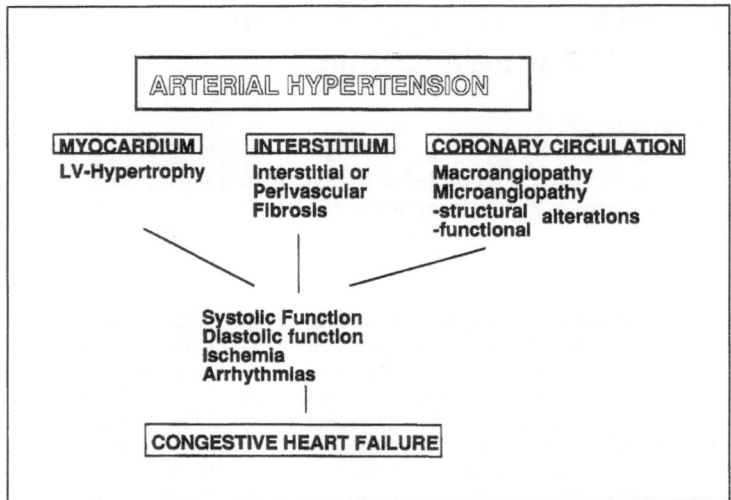

Fig. 1. Cardiac organ manifestations of arterial hypertension. Morphologic and functional consequences

sence of coronary artery disease. The pathophysiologic background of the clinical symptom of chest pain in these patients is often a restricted coronary regulatory capacity on the basis of coronary microangiopathy (26, 32, 33, 36, 38).

Left-ventricular hypertrophy

Left-ventricular hypertrophy seems to be primarily an adaptational process of the heart to cope with increased hemodynamic load. Concentric left-ventricular hypertrophy with an increase in mass-to-volume ratio renormalizes systolic wall stress, i.e., myocardial afterload, in spite of increased left-ventricular pressure, i.e., ventricular afterload. As a consequence of renormalized systolic wall stress, external myocardial shortening and, thus, systolic pump function are maintained in the compensated stage of arterial hypertension. Accordingly, myocardial oxygen consumption per unit weight of myocardium remains normal (32).

However, epidemiologic studies have shown the prognostic significance of left-ventricular hypertrophy for the development of congestive heart failure (12, 13). In this context, it has to be regarded that detection and follow-up of left-ventricular hypertrophy are feasible in the clinical routine by electro- and echocardiographic assessment, and that left-ventricular hypertrophy is, therefore, indeed the most impressive phenomenon of the cardiac manifestation of arterial hypertension, but that alterations on the level of contractile proteins, cardiac cell organelles, and tissue composition are inherent processes of hypertrophic growth which are more difficult to assess, but may be decisive in the further course of arterial hypertension. Long-term treatment of the hypertensive heart has therefore focused on prevention or regression of left-ventricular hypertrophy. Clinical studies have shown that not all forms of antihypertensive therapy lead to regression of myocardial hypertrophy. In a concept of differential antihypertensive therapy, factors which can modify the degree of pressure-induced left-ventricular hyper-

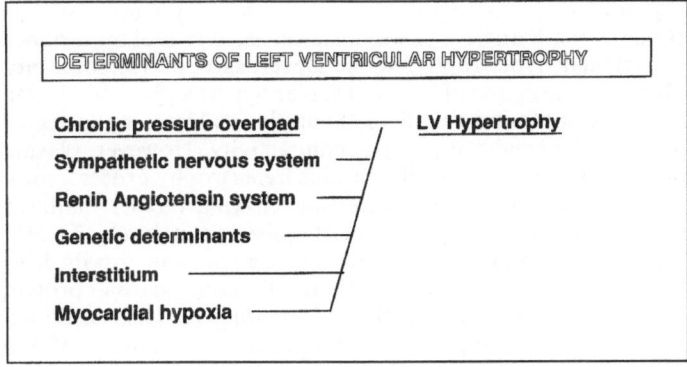

Fig. 2. Determinants of left-ventricular hypertrophy and the factors which can modify the degree of pressure-induced left-ventricular hypertrophy

trophy have to be considered. Apart from arterial blood pressure, the degree of left-ventricular hypertrophy is governed by the sympathoadrenergic system, the renin-angiotensin-aldosterone system, and genetic determination (Fig. 2).

Sen and Tarazi (30) emphasized the trophic role of catecholamines and the sympathetic nervous system in the process of cardiac hypertrophy. Due to reflex-induced stimulation of the sympathetic nervous system, hydralazine, a vasodilating agent with direct relaxing effect on the smooth vascular muscle, failed to induce a regression of left-ventricular hypertrophy in spite of effective lowering of blood pressure (30). On the other hand, a decrease in the level of circulating norepinephrine as a result of additional administration of methyldopa was paralleled by a pressure-unrelated decrease in left-ventricular muscle mass without further reduction in blood pressure (4). Based on the observation that chronic infusion of subhypertensive doses of norepinephrine led to left-ventricular hypertrophy in the dog, Laks described norepinephrine as a myocardial hypertrophy hormone (16). In this context α_1-adrenoceptors seem to be of special relevance. Simpson was able to show that norepinephrine stimulates the growth of isolated cultured myocardial cells through α_1-adrenoceptors (31). In addition, prazosin, an α_1-blocking agent, was found to be effective in lowering blood pressure and in regressing left-ventricular muscle mass without any alteration of the plasma catecholamine levels (34). A further indication of the trophic role of the sympathetic nervous system is provided by the finding that treatment with clonidine, a sympatholytic agent, was followed by a marked decrease in left-ventricular muscle mass in relation to the reduction in blood pressure (34).

The role of β-adrenergic antagonists in the clinical therapeutic reversal of cardiac hypertrophy is discussed controversially. Wikstrand et al. (39) could demonstrate only a very protracted regression of hypertrophy after 12 months of therapy with metoprolol, whereas other investigators using metoprolol or atenolol described a significant regression of cardiac hypertrophy (1, 27). Treatment for 12 months with acebutolol, a β-blocker with intrinsic sympathomimetic activity, did not produce any regression of cardiac hypertrophy, but when therapy in the same patients was switched to atenolol, a β-blocker without intrinsic sympathomimetic activity, there was regression of cardiac hypertrophy while blood pressure remained at comparable levels (27). This suggests that the intrinsic activity plays an important role in the reversal of cardiac hypertrophy during treatment with β-adrenergic antagonists. Also, the influence of the antihypertensive treatment on the renin-angiotensin-aldosterone system is of importance for the regression of left-ventricular hypertrophy. While Devereux et al. (2) could not demonstrate a correlation between the extent of left-ventricular hypertrophy and plasma renin levels in hypertensives, Gross (8) found a significant correlation between the degree of hypertensive hypertrophy and the height of plasma renin activity. However, plasma renin per se seems not to play the decisive role for the cardiac hypertrophy process, since antihypertensive treatment with an angiotensin-converting enzyme (ACE) inhibitor leads to regression of cardiac hypertrophy, despite regularly raised renin levels (23, 29). The trophic action of the renin-angiotensin aldosterone system was ascribed to angiotensin II. Sen et al. (29) reported that angiotensin II stimulates myocardial protein biosynthesis. Presumably, the observed trophic action of angiotensin II is mediated secondarily by catecholamines, because angiotensin II enhances the effects of the sympathetic tone due to its peripheral and central action on the autonomic nervous system, and it stimulates catecholamine secretion by the adrenal medulla.

After chronic treatment with diuretics, no reversal of cardiac hypertrophy was demonstrated, even though arterial blood pressure was reduced to normotensive levels (22, 40). Diuretics stimulate the sympathetic nervous system and, as a rule, elevated levels of angiotensin II were found during diuretic treatment (40). Both factors may be responsible for the failure of diuretic therapy to produce reversal of hypertrophy.

When left-ventricular hypertrophy is diagnosed echocardiographically or in the ventriculogram, an additional pathologic, genetically determined form of hypertrophy, such as hypertrophic obstructive or nonobstructive cardiomyopathy can never principally be ruled out. Marked asymmetric spetal hypertrophy is, however, also seen in about 14% of hypertensives, so that asymmetric left-ventricular hypertrophy is not specific for hypertrophic cardiomyopathy (33). Because essential hypertension is genetically determined, the capacity of the heart to respond with hypertrophy might also be, at least in part, genetically determined. Every case of hypertensive cardiac hypertrophy could contain an individually varying genetic component which might help to explain the varying responses of the myocardium to antihypertensive treatment in different patients. In the course of cardiac hypertrophy, marked structural changes take place in the myocardium which might no longer be amenable to the molecular processes involved in regression of hypertrophy. The progressive increase in myocardial connective tissue might be a particular hindrance to potential regression processes (10, 24). Investigations in patients with valvular aortic stenosis after aortic valve replacement showed that on account of collagen persistence, regression of myocardial hypertrophy can be accompanied by a relative increase in the amount of connective tissue, and, thus, myocardial fibrosis may be responsible for the failure to achieve reversal of hypertrophy (10). However, experimental studies in spontaneously hypertensive rats have shown that antihypertensive treatment with nifedipine can regress myocardial collagen in parallel with cardiac muscle mass, when treatment started in the stage of hemodynamic compensation (24).

Systolic function

Apart from the contractile state, systolic wall stress, i.e., myocardial afterload is the decisive determinant of external myocardial shortening and, thus, of ejection fraction. In the concentric type of hypertrophy with normal intracavitary dimensions and an increment in left-ventricular wall thickness due to myocardial hypertrophy, systolic wall stress is kept normal inspite of elevated intraventricular pressure. Accordingly, invasive studies in patients with chronic left-ventricular pressure-overload have clearly demonstrated that systolic pump function is not impaired as long as left-ventricular systolic wall stress is not increased (32). Thus, in this compensated stage the aim of antihypertensive treatment is a regression of left-ventricular hypertrophy with respect to prevention of later myocardial insufficiency, rather than an improvement in systolic function. Most studies could show that systolic function is not altered significantly when regression of hypertrophy is in proportion to blood-pressure reduction (23, 37). A possibly negative inotropic effect of the antihypertensive drug is generally exceeded by the favorable effect of reduction in afterload (21, 25).

In the further course of arterial hypertension with ongoing pressure-overload, as a rule, the concentric hypertrophy changes to eccentric hypertrophy with progressive tendency in the development of chronic dilatation and heart failure. Chronic dilatation is a structural dilatation which arises from fiber slippage and rearrangement of the heart muscle cells in the myocardium, and it is characterized by insufficient increase in wall thickness relative to ventricular radius (18). According to La Place's relation, the unfavorable geometric conditions necessitate a corresponding increase in systolic wall stress development. Based on the force-shortening relation, diminution in external myocardial shortening must occur with increasing wall stress, while oxygen consumption increases and cardiac efficiency decreases (11, 32). If clinical symptoms and signs of congestive heart failure occur, the therapeutic principles of the medical management of heart failure apply. In contrast to concentric hypertrophy, at this stage of hypertensive heart disease reversal of hypertrophy is no longer attempted. Although digitalis glycosides, diuretics, positive inotropic drugs, and reduction of left-ventricular afterload are regularly accompanied by a partial reduction in left-ventricular diastolic volume with improvement of global left-ventricular function, a reduction in wall thickness might have detrimental effects.

Diastolic function

Adequate diastolic filling of the left ventricle is a prerequisite for systolic pump function. Diastolic filling is determined by active processes of relaxation, by loading conditions (pre- and afterload) of the left ventricle, by heart rate and sympathetic drive to the heart, by passive elastic properties of the left ventricle, and by coronary blood flow and myocardial perfusion (5). In the past few years echocardiographic studies have shown abnormalities in left-ventricular diastolic function in patients with arterial hypertension (5, 9, 37). These abnormalities with a prolongation of left-ventricular relaxation and an impaired early diastolic filling occur early in the evolution of arterial hypertension, when ejection fraction and cardiac output are still normal.

In a former study, we analyzed left-ventricular diastolic function in hypertensive patients by means of digitized M-mode echocardiography. The peak rate of left-ventricular internal dimension change (MLVD), as an index of early diastolic filling, and the relaxation time index (RTI), as an index of isovolumic relaxation were determined. In comparison to healthy normotensives, RTI was significantly increased and MLVD significantly reduced in the hypertensive patients (Fig. 3). Long-term therapy with nitrendipine, a Ca-channel blocker of the dihydropyridine type, induced a regression of left-ventricular hypertrophy by about 14% in parallel to the decrease in systolic blood pressure. While RTI remained nearly unchanged, MLVD was significantly increased after therapy. The increase in MLVD is synonymous with an improvement of early diastolic filling, which is in accordance to the findings of Giles et al. (7). Since a decrease

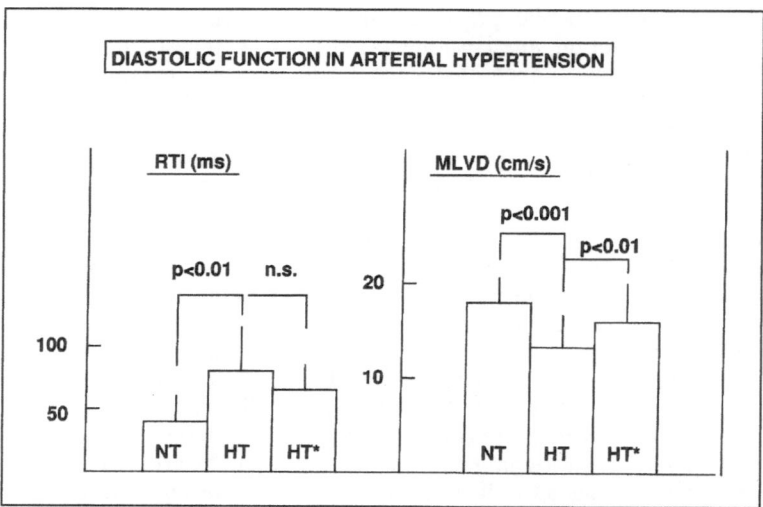

Fig. 3. Echocardiographic parameters of left-ventricular diastolic function. Relaxation-time-index (RTI) as an index of isovolumic relaxation and peak rate of left-ventricular diastolic internal dimension change (MLVD) as an index of early diastolic filling were determined by digitized M-mode echocardiography. Note the increase of RTI and the decrease of MLVD in untreated hypertensive patients (HT) in comparison to healthy normotensives (NT): after long-term antihypertensive treatment MLVD was significantly increased (HT*)

of left-ventricular peak systolic pressure per se would lead to a shortening of the relaxation time without any change of the relaxation velocity, the lack of significant reduction of RTI suggested that no change of the relaxation velocity had occurred during therapy with nitrendipine. Thus, the enhanced early diastolic filling seems to be the consequence of an increased left-ventricular distensibility, rather than being the consequence of functional alterations on the subcellular level. The increased left-ventricular distensibility was primarily due to an altered ventricular geometry with a reduction in the degree of left-ventricular hypertrophy. The improvement of diastolic function with enhanced early diastolic filling is of clinical significance in hypertensive patients. Isovolumic relaxation and early or rapid diastolic filling are essential determinants of an adequate left-ventricular diastolic filling and, hence, are a prerequisite of systolic function. Hanrath et al. (9) could demonstrate that, in healthy normotensives, 62% of ventricular dimension change occurs during the rapid filling phase and 16% during atrial contraction, while in hypertensives only 51% of ventricular dimension change occurs during the rapid filling phase, and 23% occurs during atrial contraction. Ventricular dimension change during the slow-filling phase did not differ significantly between normotensives and hypertensives. Accordingly, when early diastolic filling is diminished, an adequate ventricular filling can only be achieved by recruitment of compensatory mechanisms, which include an increase in left atrial pressure and a more vigorous contribution of atrial contraction. These alterations on the level of the left atrium implicate a higher incidence of atrial flutter or atrial fibrillation in hypertensive patients, with consecutive depression of the cardiocirculatory power capacity (20). Long-term antihypertensive treatment with prevention or regression of left-ventricular hypertrophy can be expected to have a favorable effect on these alterations.

Coronary circulation

Angina pectoris is a frequent symptom in hypertensive patients. The ischemic risk of the hypertensive patient results from the different cardiac manifestations of arterial hypertension. Since arterial hypertension is an important risk factor for the development of coronary heart disease, the occurrence of angina pectoris in hypertensive patients often reflects coronary atherosclerotic artery disease (12). However, even hypertensive patients with smooth coronary arteries frequently have chest pain. The pathophysiologic background of the clinical symptom angina pectoris in these patients is a restricted coronary regulatory capacity, i.e., a limitation in coronary vasodilator reserve (26, 32, 38). Left-ventricular hypertrophy was emphasized as the essential cause of limitation of coronary vasodilator reserve (19, 26).

In a former study, we analyzed the underlying mechanisms of an impaired coronary vasodilator reserve in hypertensive patients with a normal coronary angiogram (38). The role of left-ventricular hypertrophy and extravascular compressive forces, the impact of metabolic influences, as well as the role of the coronary factors were addressed. In this study coronary blood flow was measured quantitatively by the gaschromatographic argon method, as described in detail elsewhere (35), and maximal coronary vasodilation was achieved by application of dipyridamole intravenously. In comparison with healthy normotensives, coronary reserve, which is defined as the ratio of coronary resistance under baseline conditions to minimal coronary resistance after maximal coronary dilation, was significantly reduced by about 38% in the hypertensive patients. No significant correlation was found between minimal coronary resistance or coronary reserve and left-ventricular muscle mass. Thus, the reduction in coronary regulation capacity in hypertensives does not parallel the degree of left-ventricular hypertrophy. In hypertensive dogs with left-ventricular hypertrophy Tomanek et al. (36) found a rarefiaction of coronary arterioles rather than an increase in wall/lumen ratio in coronary resistance vessels. They postulated that rarefiaction of arterioles was a specific feature of hypertensive hypertrophy. However, our data, showing reduced coronary reserve even in the absence of left-ventricular hypertrophy, suggest that the impaired coronary reserve is not due to a reduced capillary density which might result from myocardial hypertrophy without concomitant neovascularization. Furthermore, in these patients with hemodynamically compensated hypertensive heart disease, no significant difference in myocardial oxygen consumption per unit weight myocardium could be detected in comparison to the normotensives, and diastolic wall stress has not shown a significant impact on minimal coronary vascular resistance.

Since extravascular compressive forces, i.e., systolic and diastolic wall stress seem to play a minor role, and since no increase in myocardial oxygen consumption under basic conditions was evident, the impaired coronary reserve in hypertensive patients seems to be the consequence of primary vascular alterations. Recently, quantitative morphometric studies in spontaneously hypertensive rats revealed a significant media hypertrophy of the small coronary resistance vessels along with severely increased minimal coronary resistance (15). Structural abnormalities of the small coronary resistance vessels in hypertensive patients were described 20–30 years ago by Furuyama (6) and Kathke (14). In our hypertensive patients with microvascular angina pectoris both significant media hypertrophy and perivascular fibrosis were detectable by morphologic studies (28). Media hypertrophy leads to an increment in the wall/lumen ratio which causes progressive luminal encroachment during smooth muscle contraction and, therefore, can support the process of flow autoregulation and contribute to the protection of the tissue against overperfusion. However, a reduction in luminal diameter even when

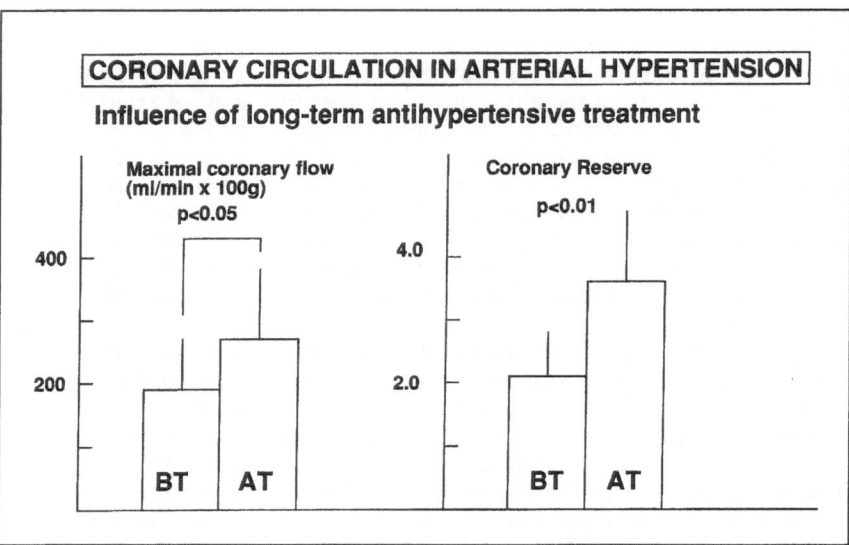

Fig. 4. Maximal coronary flow per unit weight myocardium and coronary reserve in hypertensive patients with microvascular angina pectoris are depicted before (BT) and after (AT) long-term antihypertensive treatment

vascular smooth muscle is fully relaxed might also be the pathologic anatomic background of an impaired coronary regulatory capacity in hypertensive patients.

In experimental studies in spontaneously hypertensive rats a long-term treatment with Ca-channel blocking agents of the dihydropyridine type have shown a regression of the media hypertrophy, along with significant reduction of minimal coronary resistance (3, 15).

In a preliminary study, we could show, for the first time, an improvement of coronary regulatory capacity after long-term antihypertensive treatment in hypertensive patients with microvascular angina pectoris. In 16 hypertensive patients (age: 54 ± 5 years) with microvascular angina, coronary reserve was determined before and after a 12-month antihypertensive treatment with Ca-channel blockers, ACE-inhibitors, and β-blocking agents, as a monotherapy or in combination. To exclude a direct pharmacologic effect, antihypertensive treatment was interrupted 1 week before control measurement. While coronary flow (87 ± 16 vs 93 ± 32 ml/min $\times$ 100 g; n.s.) under basic conditions remained nearly unchanged, maximal coronary flow after dipyridamole was significantly increased (270 ± 111 vs 189 ± 77 ml/min $\times$ 100 g; $p < 0.05$). Minimal coronary resistance (0.45 ± 0.18 vs 0.64 ± 0.24 mm Hg $\times$ min $\times$ 100 g/ml; $p < 0.05$) was markedly reduced after antihypertensive treatment, and coronary reserve (3.26 ± 1.09 vs 2.13 ± 0.69; $p < 0.01$) increased accordingly (Fig. 4). Since the flow measurements by the gas-chromatographic argon-method are weight-related, it could be argued that, due to a regression of left-ventricular hypertrophy, total coronary flow was the same as before therapy. However, while the maximal coronary flow per unit weight myocardium increased by about 43%, left-ventricular hypertrophy decreased only by 9%. Thus, the total maximal coronary flow is really increased. The improvement of coronary reserve is, therefore, not linked to a regression of myocardial hypertrophy. The increase in coronary reserve is mainly due to a decrease in minimal coronary vascular resistance and therefore seems to be the consequence of a regression of structural alterations of the coronary microvasculature such as media hypertrophy or perivascular fibrosis.

In conclusion, hypertensive heart disease is characterized by the sum and interactions of the hypertensive damage to the target organ "heart" with myocardial hypertrophy, interstitial fibrosis, and disease of large and small coronary arteries. Depending on the degree and type of the hypertensive cardiac manifestations, an appropriate differential form of antihypertensive therapy is required. In the absence of atherosclerotic coronary heart disease the aim of the therapeutic measures is to reverse myocardial hypertrophy, fibrosis and disease of the coronary resistance vessels. Both regression of left-ventricular hypertrophy and reversal of the hypertensive disease of small coronary arteries can be induced by suitable antihypertensive drugs (Ca-channel blockers of the dihydropyridine type, angiotensin-converting enzyme inhibitors, and sympatholytic substances). However, the two processes are not necessarily related. While normal systolic function is maintained for a long time in hypertensive heart disease, diastolic function is impaired in a very early stage; however, it can be partially improved by long-term antihypertensive treatment. Moreover, to what extent the prognosis of hypertensive heart disease can be influenced by reversal of cardiac hypertrophy and coronary microangiopathy has still to be evaluated.

References

1. Corea L, Bentivoglio M, Verdecchia P, Providenca M, Motolese M (1984) Left ventricular hypertrophy regression in hypertensive patients treated with metoprolol. J Clin Pharmacol 22:363–370
2. Devereux RB, Savage DD, Drayer JIM, Laragh JH (1982) Left ventricular hypertrophy and function in high, normal and low-renin forms of essential hypertension. Hypertension 4:524–531
3. Eisenlohr H, Schmiebusch H, Strauer BE (1988) Regression of media hypertrophy in hypertensive coronary resistance vessels by antihypertensive therapy. Circulation 78(Suppl II):II 169
4. Fouad FM, Nakashima Y, Tarazi RC, Salcedo EE (1982) Reversal of left ventricular hypertrophy in hypertensive patients treated with methyldopa. Am J Cardiol 49:795–801
5. Fouad FT (1987) Left ventricular diastolic function in hypertensive patients. Circulation 75(Suppl I):I48–II55
6. Furuyama M (1962) Histometrical investigations of arteries in reference to arterial hypertension. Tokoku J Exp Med 76:388
7. Giles TD, Sander GE, Roffidal LC, Thomas MG, Given MB, Quiros AC (1987) Comparison of nitrendipine and hydrochlorothiazide for systemic hypertension. Am J Cardiol 60:103–110
8. Gross F (1971) The renin angiotensin system and hypertension. Ann Intern Med 75:777
9. Hanrath P, Mathey D, Kremer P, Bleifeld W (1981) Left ventricular relaxation and filling pattern in different forms of left ventricular hypertrophy. In: Strauer BE (ed) The Heart in Hypertension. Springer, Berlin Heidelberg New York, pp 377–386
10. Hess OM, Ritter M, Schneider J, Grimm K, Turina M, Krayenbühl HP (1984) Diastolic stiffness and myocardial structure in aortic valve disease before and after valve replacement. Circulation 69:865–885
11. Jacob R, Vogt M, Rupp H (1986) Pathophysiological mechanisms in cardiac insufficiency induced by chronic pressure-overload – an attempt to analyze specific factors in animal experiment. Basic Res Cardiol 81(Suppl 1):203–216
12. Kannell WB, Gordon T, Offutt D (1969) Left ventricular hypertrophy by electrocardiogram: prevalence, incidence and mortality in the Framingham Study. Ann Intern Med 71:89–105
13. Kannel WB, Doyle JT, McNamara PM, Quickenton P, Gordon T (1975) Precursors of sudden coronary death: factors related to the incidence of sudden death. Circulation 51:606–613

14. Kathke N (1955) Die Veränderungen der Coronararterienzweige des Myokards bei Hypertonie. Beitr Path Anat 155:405
15. Klepzig M, Eisenlohr H, Steindl S, Schmiebusch H, Strauer BE (1986) Mediahypertrophie bei Koronargefäßen spontan hypertoner Ratten. Z Kardiol 75(Suppl 1):32
16. Laks NM (1979) Norepinephrine – the myocardial hypertrophy hormone? Am Heart J 91:674–675
17. Levy D, Garrison RJ, Savage DD, Kannel WB, Castelli WP (1990) Prognostic implications of echocardiographically determined left ventricular mass in the Framingham Heart Study. N Engl J Med 322:1561–1566
18. Linzbach AJ (1960) Heart failure from the point of view of quantitative anatomy. Am J Cardiol 5:370–382
19. Marcus ML, Doty DB, Hiratzka LF, Wright CB, Eastham CL (1983) Decreased coronary reserve: a mechanism for angina pectoris in patients with aortic stenosis and normal coronary arteries. N Engl J Med 307:1362–1367
20. Marriott HJL, Myerburg RJ (1978) Recognition and treatment of cardiac arrhythmias and conduction disturbances. In: Hurst JW (ed) The Heart. McGraw Hill, New York, p 637
21. Motz W, Ippisch R, Strauer BE (1983) Nifedipin hat keine negativ inotrope Wirkung in hohen, antihypertensiv wirksamen Dosen. Z Kardiol 73(Suppl I):102
22. Motz W, Klepzig M, Stellwaag M, Strauer BE (1987) Regression der Herzhypertrophie unter Saluretika? Klin Wochenschr 65 (Suppl):165
23. Motz W, Strauer BE (1988) Rückbildung der hypertensiven Herzhypertrophie durch chronische Angiotensin-Konversionsenzymhemmung. Z Kardiol 77:53–60
24. Motz W, Strauer BE (1989) Left ventricular function and collagen content after regression of hypertensive hypertrophy. Hypertension 13:43–50
25. Muiesan G, Agabiti-Rosei E, Romanelli G, Muisan ML, Castellano M, Beschi M (1986) Adrenergic activity and left ventricular function during treatment of essential hypertension with calcium antagonists. Am J Cardiol 57:44D
26. Pickard AD, Gorlin R, Smith H, Abrose J, Meller J (1981) Coronary flow studies in patients with left ventricular hypertrophy of the hypertensive type: evidence for an impaired coronary vascular reserve. Am J Cardiol 47:547–554
27. Sau F, Seguro C, Merano G, Cherchi A (1986) Atenolol but not acebutolo reverses left ventricular hypertrophy secondary to arterial hypertension. J Am Coll Cardiol 7(Suppl A):A186
28. Schwartzkopff B, Frenzel H, Vogt M, Motz W, Strauer BE (1989) Myocardial structure in patients with reduced coronary reserve in hypertensive heart disease. Circulation 80(Suppl II): II-539
29. Sen S, Tarazi RC, Bumpus FM (1979) Cardiac effects of angiotensin-antagonists in normotensive rats. Clin Sci 56:439–444
30. Sen S, Tarazi RC (1983) Regression of myocardial hypertrophy and influence of adrenergic system. Am J Physiol 244:H97
31. Simpson P (1983) Norepinephrine-stimulated hypertrophy of cultured rat myocardial cell is an alpha-1-adrenergic response. J Clin Invest 72:732–738
32. Strauer BE (1979) Ventricular function and coronary hemodynamics in hypertensive heart disease. Am J Cardiol 44:999–1006
33. Strauer BE (1983) Hypertensive heart disease. Springer, Berlin Heidelberg New York
34. Strauer BE, Bayer F, Brecht HM, Motz W (1985) The influence of sympathetic nervous activity on regression of cardiac hypertrophy. J Hypertension 3(Suppl 4):S39–S44
35. Tauchert M, Kochsiek K, Heiss HW, Rau G, Bretschneider HJ (1971) Technik der Organdurchblutungsmessung mit der Argon-Methode. Z Kreislaufforsch 60:871–880
36. Tomanek RJ, Palmer PJ, Pfeiffer GL, Schreiber KL, Eastham CL, Marcus ML (1986) Morphometry of canine coronary arteries, arterioles and capillaries during hypertension and left ventricular hypertrophy. Circ Res 58:38–46
37. Vogt M, Kreutz KU, Motz W, Strauer BE (1989) Hypertrophieregression nach Nitrendipin: Einfluß auf systolische und diastolische Funktion. Z Kardiol 78:469–477
38. Vogt M, Motz W, Schwartzkopff B, Strauer BE (1990) Coronary microangiopathy and cardiac hypertrophy. Eur Heart J 11(Suppl B):133–138

39. Wikstrand J, Trimarco B, Ricciardelli B, DeLuca N, Volope M (1984) Reversal of cardiovascular changes during antihypertensive treatment: functional consequences and time course of reversal as judged from clinical studies. Hypertension 6:III348–III367
40. Wollam GL, Hall DW, Porter VD, Douglas MB, Unger DJ, Blumenstein BA, Cotsonis GA, Knudtson ML, Felner JM, Schlant RC (1983) Time course of regression of left ventricular hypertrophy in treated hypertensive patients. Am J Med 75(Suppl):100A–110A

Authors' address:

Dr. Martin Vogt
Medizinische Klinik und Poliklinik B
der Heinrich-Heine-Universität Düsseldorf
Abteilung für Kardiologie, Pneumologie und Angiologie
Moorenstraße 5
W-4000 Düsseldorf 1, FRG

Subject Index

A

activity, sympathetic 125, 127, 130, 133, 138, 139, 155
adaptation 3, 205
adrenaline, concentration of 149, 152
adrenergic system 57, 58, 61, 133, 149
adrenoceptor, α- 13, 20, 225
–, β- 13, 20
afterload, ventricular 167, 169, 171, 224
aldolase 191
aldosterone 25, 26, 27, 28, 29, 125, 127, 128, 146
angiotensin converting enzyme 28, 149
– II 27, 28, 29, 129, 149, 226
antibody, anticardiac 102
–, antiendothelial 103
–, antimembrane 112
–, antimyolemmal 101, 102, 103, 104
–, antisarcolemmal 101, 102, 104
–, natural 101, 102, 104, 108
arrhythmia 215, 216
arteriography, coronary 176
ATPase, activity, Ca^{2+} 73
–, –, myofibrillar 5, 85, 86
–, –, Na^+-K^+ 13, 146, 217, 219
atrial natriuretic factor 16, 125, 127
atropine 137
autoantibody 101, 102
autoantigenes, cardiac 105
autolysis 205

B

baroreceptor 133, 138, 141
baroreflex 133, 134, 137, 138, 141
biopsy, endomyocardial 103, 175, 176
blockade, vagal 129, 137

C

Ca^{2+} excess 208
Ca^{2+} concentration, myoplasmic 99 ff
–, toxic 206
Ca^{2+} pump 20
Ca^{2+} sensitizer 91

cAMP 57, 58, 62, 218, 219
captopril 188, 192
cardiomyopathy 187
–, dilative 4, 7, 101, 102, 105
–, hypertrophic 226
cardioprotection 205, 215, 216
carnitine 68, 70, 71, 74
catecholamines 127, 149, 152, 205, 215
–, toxic concentrations of 206
cation transporter 13
cell, endothelial 25
–, myocyte 25, 39, 58, 93, 104
–, non-myocyte 25
–, smooth muscle 25
channel, Ca^{2+} 13, 19, 20
chemiluminescence 115
cineangiography 175, 176
collagen, fibrillar 25, 26
–, myocardial 26, 28, 39
cross-bridge, configuration of, strong-binding 83
–, –, weak-binding 83
–, force-generating 85
–, nonforce-generating 85
–, turnover 83
consumption, oxygen 5, 169
contracture 208
coronary circulation 167, 172, 229
coronary reserve 6, 223, 229, 230
corticosterone 152
creatinphosphokinase 162, 191, 208

D

depression, postexcitatory 144
desipramine 152
diabetes mellitus 67
diacylglycerol 210, 211
dilatation, left ventricular 15, 49, 52, 159, 160, 161, 162, 163
–, structural 7
disease, aortic valve 175, 176
–, coronary artery 14, 223
–, inflammatory heart 102

distensibility, left ventricular   5, 228
DNA content   210

E

efficiency of the heart   167, 172
ejection fraction   49, 51, 162, 175, 176, 177, 200, 226
electrocardiogram   193, 197, 200, 226
electron probe microanalysis   93, 94
enalapril   188, 193
energetics, cardiac   5, 6
etomoxir   72, 73
exchange, Na^+-Ca^{2+} 13, 20, 21

F

fibroblast, cardiac   25
fibrosis, cardiac   7, 25, 26, 27, 28, 29, 33, 35, 37, 41, 226
finite element method   46
fistula, aorto-caval   4, 5, 8
flow, coronary   169, 172, 230
–, lymph, cardiac   30
–, renal plasma   129, 130
force, isometric   85, 86
force-velocity relation   84
Frank-Starling mechanism   5, 7, 8
free fatty acid   8, 66, 67, 71, 73

G

gene expression, cardiac   58, 65
–, –, MHC-α 57, 72, 73, 74, 75
–, –, MHC-β 57, 73
glomerular filtration rate   130
glucose utilization   65, 69, 70, 71

H

hamster, cardiomyopathic   188
heart failure, congestive   13, 14, 16, 17, 18, 125, 129, 133, 134, 159, 163, 167, 169, 173, 175, 187, 224, 227
–, high-output   8
–, model   45
–, size   45, 159
–, thermal stability   212
–, weight   35, 36
heat shock protein   211
hyperaldosteronism   28
hypercontraction   159
hyperinsulinemia   65, 66
hyperplasia   4, 6
hypertension   25, 26, 27, 28, 29, 33, 66, 67, 197, 223
–, renovascular   6, 26
–, secondary   66
hyperthyroidism   4

hypertrophy, cardiac   3, 4, 5, 6, 8, 9, 15, 17, 25, 26, 39, 40, 61, 70, 161, 167, 169, 175, 197, 223, 224
–, cellular   33, 175
–, concentric   161, 227
–, eccentric   8, 161, 227
–, media   33, 39, 41, 229, 230
–, regression of   223
hypothyroidism   4

I

index, cardiac   175, 176, 177, 200
–, left ventricular muscle mass   177
–, relaxation time   227
infarction, myocardial   13, 15, 116, 159, 161
inhibitor, angiotensin converting enzyme   149, 150, 155, 187, 197, 230
–, kininase   187
inositol triphosphate   210
insulin   66
–, resistance   65, 66
ischemia, myocardial   115, 116, 205, 206, 207, 215

L

length-tension diagram, myocardial   49
lymph flow, cardiac   30

M

metabolic syndrome   65, 71
metabolism, fatty acid   66, 67
–, glucose   66, 68
metoprolol   138
microangiopathy, coronary   224
microarteriopathy   35, 41
microfluospectroscopy   93
mitochondria   96, 209
moxonidine   34
mRNA   57, 58
myocarditis   101, 102, 103, 105, 107, 108
myocyte, cardiac   25, 58, 93
–, human   104
–, isolated   94
–, ultrastructure of   39
myofibril, volume   37, 38, 176, 178
myosin heavy chain, cardiac gene expression of   57, 71
–, mRNA   60, 61
–, isoenzyme pattern, ventricular   5, 6, 57, 58, 188, 191

N

nifedipine   34
nitric oxide   215
nitroglycerin   138

noradrenaline (norepinephrine), plasma 127, 149, 152
nuclei, isolated myocardial 210

O

obesity 66
occlusion, coronary 14, 116, 216
one-chain DNA 210
outflow, sympathetic 149, 152, 155
overflow, noradrenaline 151
oxygen, radical 115

P

pacing, cardiac 126, 134
patch-clamp technique 94
peptide, atrial natriuretic 125, 127, 128, 129, 130
pericarditis 103, 107
perimyocarditis 102, 103, 105, 107
phenylephrine 138
pressure, blood 35, 36, 128, 133, 137, 138, 149, 150, 152, 153, 197, 200
–, atrial 134
–, coronary perfusion 167
–, end-diastolic 175, 176, 177
–, mean aortic 169
–, mean arterial 126, 133, 134
–, overload 4, 223
–, ventricular 25, 133
pressure-volume diagram 4, 46
prostacyclin 215

R

radionuclide ventriculography, tomographic 159, 162
ramipril 149, 150
rat, diabetic 69, 72
–, Goldblatt II 4, 6, 8
–, hyperthyreotic 6
–, spontaneous hypertensive (SHR) 4, 7, 33, 34, 70, 149, 167
–, swim-trained 6

renin-angiotensin-aldosterone system 25, 125, 127, 129, 130
reperfusion paradox 205, 206, 208, 212
resistance, coronary 167, 169, 172, 229, 230
–, peripheral vascular 126, 130, 133, 169

S

sarcolemma, receptor of 13
sarcoplasmic reticulum (SR) 20, 96, 205, 209
–, Ca^{2+}-pump 65, 73, 74
saturation, venous oxygen 126
shortening velocity, unloaded 6, 84
sodium diet 27
staircase, positive 96
stenosis, aortic 4, 6, 7, 175, 176
stiffness, fiber 85, 86
–, myocardial 25, 26, 163
stroke volume 45, 46, 49, 51, 160, 162, 167, 169, 200
sympathetic nervous system 129, 133, 225

T

treatment, antihypertensive 74, 197, 224, 228, 230
triglyceride 66, 67, 73

U

uncoupling, oxidation-phosphorylation 209
utilization, fatty acid 67
–, glucose 65, 69, 70, 71

V

vagotomy 140
vasopressin 125, 129
ventricular function, diastolic 6, 159, 227
ventricular geometry 45, 159
voltage clamp 93, 94
volume overload 4

W

wall stress 5, 8, 45, 46, 161, 171, 224, 226
work, pressure-volume 167, 171
working capacity, ventricular 4, 8

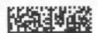